Neurobiology Research on Neurodegenerative Disorders

Guest Editor
Grazyna Lietzau

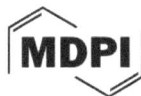

Basel • Beijing • Wuhan • Barcelona • Belgrade • Novi Sad • Cluj • Manchester

Guest Editor
Grazyna Lietzau
Division of Anatomy and
Neurobiology
Medical University of Gdańsk
Gdańsk
Poland

Editorial Office
MDPI AG
Grosspeteranlage 5
4052 Basel, Switzerland

This is a reprint of the Special Issue, published open access by the journal *Brain Sciences* (ISSN 2076-3425), freely accessible at: https://www.mdpi.com/journal/brainsci/special_issues/J79G12EC24.

For citation purposes, cite each article independently as indicated on the article page online and as indicated below:

Lastname, A.A.; Lastname, B.B. Article Title. *Journal Name* **Year**, *Volume Number*, Page Range.

ISBN 978-3-7258-4239-1 (Hbk)
ISBN 978-3-7258-4240-7 (PDF)
https://doi.org/10.3390/books978-3-7258-4240-7

Cover image courtesy of Grazyna Lietzau
Microscopic image of dopaminergic neurons in the substantia nigra pars compacta of the mouse brain.

© 2025 by the authors. Articles in this book are Open Access and distributed under the Creative Commons Attribution (CC BY) license. The book as a whole is distributed by MDPI under the terms and conditions of the Creative Commons Attribution-NonCommercial-NoDerivs (CC BY-NC-ND) license (https://creativecommons.org/licenses/by-nc-nd/4.0/).

Contents

About the Editor vii

Grażyna Lietzau
Neurobiology Research on Neurodegenerative Disorders
Reprinted from: *Brain Sci.* **2024**, *14*, 1121, https://doi.org/10.3390/brainsci14111121 1

Yeong Jin Kim, Bo-Ram Mun, Kyu Yeong Choi and Won-Seok Choi
Oral Administration of Probiotic Bacteria Alleviates Tau Phosphorylation, Aβ Accumulation, Microglia Activation, and Memory Loss in 5xFAD Mice
Reprinted from: *Brain Sci.* **2024**, *14*, 208, https://doi.org/10.3390/brainsci14030208 7

Hai Lu, Ming Chen and Cuiqing Zhu
Intranasal Administration of Apelin-13 Ameliorates Cognitive Deficit in Streptozotocin-Induced Alzheimer's Disease Model via Enhancement of Nrf2-HO1 Pathways
Reprinted from: *Brain Sci.* **2024**, *14*, 488, https://doi.org/10.3390/brainsci14050488 21

Nijee S. Luthra, Angela Clow and Daniel M. Corcos
The Interrelated Multifactorial Actions of Cortisol and Klotho: Potential Implications in the Pathogenesis of Parkinson's Disease
Reprinted from: *Brain Sci.* **2022**, *12*, 1695, https://doi.org/10.3390/brainsci12121695 36

Paolo Solla, Qian Wang, Claudia Frau, Valentina Floris, Francesco Loy, Leonardo Antonio Sechi and Carla Masala
Olfactory Impairment Is the Main Predictor of Higher Scores at REM Sleep Behavior Disorder (RBD) Screening Questionnaire in Parkinson's Disease Patients
Reprinted from: *Brain Sci.* **2024**, *13*, 599, https://doi.org/10.3390/brainsci13040599 55

Nicolaas I. Bohnen, Jaimie Barr, Robert Vangel, Stiven Roytman, Rebecca Paalanen, Kirk A. Frey, et al.
GABA$_A$ Receptor Benzodiazepine Binding Sites and Motor Impairments in Parkinson's Disease
Reprinted from: *Brain Sci.* **2023**, *13*, 1711, https://doi.org/10.3390/brainsci13121711 66

Giuseppe Schirò, Vincenzo Di Stefano, Salvatore Iacono, Antonino Lupica, Filippo Brighina, Roberto Monastero and Carmela Rita Balistreri
Advances on Cellular Clonotypic Immunity in Amyotrophic Lateral Sclerosis
Reprinted from: *Brain Sci.* **2022**, *12*, 1412, https://doi.org/10.3390/brainsci12101412 75

Sharad Kumar Suthar and Sang-Yoon Lee
The Role of Superoxide Dismutase 1 in Amyotrophic Lateral Sclerosis: Identification of Signaling Pathways, Regulators, Molecular Interaction Networks, and Biological Functions through Bioinformatics
Reprinted from: *Brain Sci.* **2023**, *13*, 151, https://doi.org/10.3390/brainsci13010151 86

Ching-Yi Lin, Veronica Vanoverbeke, David Trent, Kathryn Willey and Yu-Shang Lee
The Spatiotemporal Expression of SOCS3 in the Brainstem and Spinal Cord of Amyotrophic Lateral Sclerosis Mice
Reprinted from: *Brain Sci.* **2024**, *14*, 564, https://doi.org/10.3390/brainsci14060564 98

Emanuele Porru, Erik Edström, Lisa Arvidsson, Adrian Elmi-Terander, Alexander Fletcher-Sandersjöö, Anita Lövgren Sandblom, et al.
Ventriculoperitoneal Shunt Treatment Increases 7 Alpha Hy-Droxy-3-Oxo-4-Cholestenoic Acid and 24-Hydroxycholesterol Concentrations in Idiopathic Normal Pressure Hydrocephalus
Reprinted from: *Brain Sci.* **2022**, *12*, 1450, https://doi.org/10.3390/brainsci12111450 112

Chiara Abbatantuono, Federica Alfeo, Livio Clemente, Giulio Lancioni, Maria Fara De Caro, Paolo Livrea and Paolo Taurisano
Current Challenges in the Diagnosis of Progressive Neurocognitive Disorders: A Critical Review of the Literature and Recommendations for Primary and Secondary Care
Reprinted from: *Brain Sci.* **2023**, *13*, 1443, https://doi.org/10.3390/brainsci13101443 . . . . **121**

Klaus Thanke Aspli, Jan O. Aaseth, Trygve Holmøy, Kaj Blennow, Henrik Zetterberg, Bjørn-Eivind Kirsebom, et al.
CSF, Blood, and MRI Biomarkers in Skogholt's Disease—A Rare Neurodegenerative Disease in a Norwegian Kindred
Reprinted from: *Brain Sci.* **2023**, *13*, 1511, https://doi.org/10.3390/brainsci13111511 . . . . **133**

About the Editor

Grazyna Lietzau

Grazyna Lietzau, PhD, DSc, is a researcher and lecturer at the Medical University of Gdańsk, Poland. She serves as the head of the Molecular Biology Laboratory in the Division of Anatomy and Neurobiology and coordinates Research Team X, which focuses on the molecular and biochemical mechanisms underlying civilization diseases.

Dr. Lietzau earned her PhD in Neurobiology from the Medical University of Gdańsk in 2013. Her doctoral thesis explored the NF-κB-mediated regulation of stroke-induced neuroprotective and neurodegenerative processes in the brain. She completed her postdoctoral training at the Department of Clinical Science and Education, Karolinska Institutet, Sweden. As a member of the NeuroCardioMetabol group, she studied the impact of metabolic diseases such as obesity and type 2 diabetes (T2D) on neuroplasticity and neurogenesis during aging and the effects of T2D on stroke recovery. Her research also examined the mechanisms of action and therapeutic potential of various anti-diabetic drugs, including GLP-1 receptor agonists and dipeptidyl peptidase-4 inhibitors, in reversing T2D-induced functional and structural changes in the central nervous system.

Currently, Dr. Lietzau's research interests include investigating the processes underlying neurodegeneration in patients with metabolic diseases, such as hypercholesterolemia and T2D, as well as exploring the effects of lipid-lowering drugs on memory and cognition.

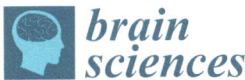

Editorial

Neurobiology Research on Neurodegenerative Disorders

Grażyna Lietzau

Division of Anatomy and Neurobiology, Faculty of Medicine, Medical University of Gdańsk, Dębinki 1, 80-211 Gdańsk, Poland; grazyna.lietzau@gumed.edu.pl

The aim of the following Special Issue was to call for research in the field of neurodegenerative disorders (NDDs). Despite the growing interest in this field over the past few decades, the unquestionable progress in understanding the mechanisms underlying NDDs and numerous attempts to find effective therapies, many questions remain unanswered. Moreover, since it is not possible to reverse the progressive degeneration of neurons in various regions of the central nervous system (CNS), NDDs are still considered incurable. As such, further research is warranted. The scope of this Special Issue covers articles on diagnostics, mechanisms underlying NDDs, and new or modified therapeutic strategies.

Despite the decreasing trend in dementia observed recently in North America and Europe [1], given population growth and ageing trends, the number of people affected by dementia is expected to increase worldwide [1]. This makes dementia a rapidly growing global public health problem. To meet this challenge, new studies are being designed and attempts are being made to develop new treatments. Numerous studies have been conducted to test the effectiveness of various substances in treating dementia, including Alzheimer's disease (AD), using animal models of the disease. Various doses and routes of administration have been tested in different studies. The results of two such studies are presented in this Special Issue. Lu et al. investigated mechanisms at the base of the neuroprotective action of Apelin-13 (Contribution 1), the endogenous ligand of the apelin receptor (APJ) involved in processes in the CNS such as inflammation, oxidative stress, apoptosis, and autophagy. The researchers used a streptozotocin (STZ)-induced model of AD, in which STZ (3 mg/kg) was injected into the lateral ventricles of C57BL/6J mice. The above model is a widely used model of sporadic AD. The results showed that the intranasal administration of Apelin-13 (1 mg/kg) improved cognitive function in AD mice. The functional outcome correlated with the enhancement of synaptic plasticity and the attenuation of oxidative stress. The authors conclude that intranasal administration of Apelin-13 may prove to be a promising therapeutic strategy for neurodegenerative diseases such as AD.

Kim et al. studied the effect of gut microbiome composition on the pathology and progression of AD (Contribution 2). They report that orally administered probiotics, *Bifidobacterium lactis*, *Levilactobacillus brevis*, and *Limosilactobacillus fermentum*, improve spatial and recognition memory and have neuroprotective effects in 5XFAD mice. These transgenic mice are a commonly used model of AD-like amyloid pathology with a relatively early onset and aggressive age-dependent progression. Based on the improvement of cognitive function and the observed reduction in amyloid-β accumulation, decreased microglial activation, and ameliorated increased tau phosphorylation in 5xFAD mice, the authors suggest that probiotics may prove to be an effective neuroprotective intervention in AD. Although animal models of NDDs have certain limitations, they represent a useful tool for studying disease mechanisms and exploring the neuroprotective potential of new or modified therapeutic strategies. The endogenous substances used in the two aforementioned studies affected well-known mechanisms involved in AD: oxidative stress and inflammation. Importantly, they improved cognitive function. However, there is a long way to go to determine their effectiveness in patients with AD.

Parkinson's disease (PD) is the second most common progressive NDD [2]. In addition to the characteristic motor symptoms (tremor, bradykinesia, rigidity, and postural instability), patients with PD also experience non-motor symptoms such as psychological dysfunctions (depression, anxiety, and apathy) and cognitive impairment/dementia [3]. Most patients also develop olfactory dysfunction and sleep disorders, including REM sleep behavior disorder (RBD). Although in recent years more attention has been paid to the non-motor symptoms of PD, many issues related to the role of olfaction in the development and progression of NDDs, as well as the interrelationships between different non-motor symptoms, still await explanation. In their study, Solla et al. investigated the association between olfactory impairment and RBD in PD (Contribution 3). The aim of the study was to determine the role of olfactory dysfunction and other factors (i.e., age at onset, sex, cognitive abilities, and motor symptoms) as potential predictors of higher scores on the RBD screening questionnaire. The authors opined that because new disease-modifying drugs will have the greatest chance of being effective in the early stages of NDDs, identifying olfactory dysfunction and RBD as early as possible may be useful both in clinical practice and in clinical trials of potentially neuroprotective treatments. The main finding of the study was the demonstration of a strong association between olfactory impairment and the studied sleeping disorder. The authors reported that the presence of more severe olfactory impairment strongly correlated with a more symptomatic expression of RBD.

PD is a complex disorder affecting many processes in the CNS. The risk of this NDD increases with age, with the peak incidence occurring in the eighth decade of life. Stress hormones, such as cortisol, may contribute to neurodegeneration. Stress-induced mitochondrial dysfunction, neuroinflammation, and oxidative stress can directly damage dopaminergic neurons in the substantia nigra or increase the vulnerability of these cells to other damaging factors. Consequently, stress exacerbates the symptoms of PD [4]. In their review, Luthra et al. summarize the current knowledge on the role of two hormones, cortisol and Klotho, in PD (Contribution 4). While cortisol is a well-known stress hormone, Klotho is an aging-suppressor protein that has been shown to protect against stress-induced damage, particularly oxidative stress and inflammation, which are often exacerbated by chronic high levels of cortisol. The authors conclude that aging and stress are associated with increased cortisol and decreased Klotho levels, whereas exercise and certain genetic variants lead to decreased cortisol response and increased Klotho levels in PD individuals. Together, they influence the clinical presentation of PD. Elucidating the interacting pathways and the role of antagonistic factors may allow for a better understanding of the complexity of PD and potentially enable the development of more effective therapies.

Another interesting topic included in this Special Issue is addressed by Bohnen and colleagues (Contribution 5). In their study, they investigated the relationship between the CNS regional availability of $GABA_AR$ benzodiazepine binding sites and motor impairments in PD. A total of 11 male patients with PD underwent [^{11}C]flumazenil $GABA_AR$ benzodiazepine binding site and [^{11}C]dihydrotetrabenazine vesicular monoamine transporter type-2 (VMAT2) PET imaging and clinical assessment. The results indicated that decreased availability of $GABA_AR$ benzodiazepine binding sites in the thalamus, reflecting increased GABAergic activity, correlated with increased axial motor impairments in PD, independently of the degree of nigrostriatal neurodegeneration. The findings suggest that $GABA_AR$ benzodiazepine binding site allosteric modulator drugs could be effective in managing axial motor impairments in PD. Since there is still no cure for PD and available therapies such as levodopa/carbidopa, deep brain stimulation, and rehabilitation only alleviate symptoms, it is crucial to search for new treatment options.

Although amyotrophic lateral sclerosis (ALS) is a rare disease (prevalence in Europe: ~10–15/100,000; worldwide annual incidence: ~1.9/100,000), it represents the most aggressive NDD [5]. Selective and progressive degeneration of motor neurons both in the spinal cord and brain usually leads to death within 2–5 years of diagnosis. The projected increase in the number of individuals with ALS between 2015 and 2040 is 69% (prognoses for 10 geographical regions) [6]. Such alarming statistics necessitate taking action to better understand this NDD and design effective treatments or at least limit the effects of ALS in order to prolong patients' lives and improve their quality of life. In their study, Lin et al. investigated the spatiotemporal expression of suppressor of cytokine signaling-3 (SOCS3) in the brainstem and spinal cord of ALS mice (Contribution 6). SOCS3 is a regulator of neuroinflammation that acts primarily by inhibiting the JAK-STAT signaling pathway and controlling the activity of microglia and the production of pro-inflammatory cytokines. The results of in vivo and in vitro studies showed a negative regulatory effect of SOCS3 on neuronal survival and axon regeneration [7], and the authors hypothesized that it participates in ALS progression. As a model of ALS, the B6.Cg-Tg (SOD1*G93A)1Gur/J mouse has been used in a number of studies. The SOD1-G93A transgenic mouse is one of the commonly used ALS models in preclinical studies, involving neurodegeneration of both upper and lower motor neurons. The results of a study showed upregulation of SOCS3 in the pre-Bötzinger complex of the brainstem and in the ventral horn of cervical and lumbar segments of the spinal cord, accompanied by increased astrogliosis and microglia activation as well as neuronal loss in these areas. These results correlated with the progression of ALS from the pre-symptomatic to early symptomatic stage. The authors conclude that SOCS3 is involved in the neuroinflammation-associated non-cell-autonomous pathway in the course of ALS and that it may be a potential therapeutic target for balancing the neuroinflammatory response to regulate ALS progression. Despite recent criticism that the use of transgenic mice has not yielded rapid advances in the prevention and treatment of ALS, they remain a useful tool in studying the pathogenic processes in ALS and tracking disease progression.

In the next article included in this Special Issue, Suthar et al. explore the relationship between superoxide dismutase 1 (SOD1) and ALS (Contribution 7). SOD1 is an antioxidant enzyme that protects cells from free radical-mediated damage. Mutations in the SOD1 gene result in cellular stress and the development of ALS. Furthermore, the number of SOD1 variants that cause ALS is increasing (Contribution 7). Suthar et al. used a bioinformatics approach (including ingenuity pathway analysis) to analyze the signaling pathways, regulatory functions, and network molecules of SOD1. They reported that SOD1-mediated toxicity is related to swelling and oxidative stress and the key signaling pathways involving this enzyme are degradation of superoxide radicals, apelin adipocyte, NRF2-mediated oxidative stress response, ALS, and sirtuin signaling (Contribution 7). Further analysis facilitated the identification of specific molecules in the SOD1-ALS pathway. Modern bioinformatics tools enable the analysis of large data sets, and the obtained results may indicate further directions for in vivo research on ALS.

The third ALS-related article included in this Special Issue is a review by Schirò et al., in which the authors discuss cellular clonotypic immunity in ALS (Contribution 8). This NDD is primarily known for the progressive degeneration of motor neurons; however, increasing evidence suggests that immune mechanisms, including adaptive immunity, might play a role in its development or progression. The role of clonotypic T cells in ALS is complex. From one perspective, regulatory T cells (Tregs), specific T cell clones that are responsible for maintaining immune tolerance and controlling excessive immune responses, may play a protective role by reducing inflammation and potentially slowing disease progression. Conversely, the clonal expansion of cytotoxic T cells (CD8+ T cells) contributes to motor neuron damage by promoting inflammation and attacking neurons or glial cells in the CNS, exacerbating neurodegeneration. A high percentage of CD8+ cells in ALS patients correlates with a higher risk of death [8]. These and other aspects of immune cell function in ALS are summarized in the review. The authors conclude that the prognosis of ALS may be influenced by the balance between CD4+ and CD8+ cells and between Treg and Teff cells (effector T lymphocytes) (Contribution 8). Attempts have been made to treat ALS with immunomodulatory agents. Studies involving larger cohorts and a better understanding of the immune mechanisms at the onset and progression of ALS may enable the development of more effective treatment strategies.

Skogholt's disease (SD) is a disease characterized by white matter lesions in the brain and myelin damage in the peripheral nerves, with high concentrations of copper and iron in the CSF, first described in the 1980s in southeastern Norway by a local physician, Jon Skogholt [9]. This rare disorder is only present in a familial line in Hedmark County, Norway. Aspli et al. performed a neurochemical analysis of plasma and cerebrospinal fluid and morphometric segmentation of the brain using MRI (Contribution 9). The results showed increased concentrations of $A\beta_{1-42}$, $A\beta_{1-40}$, $A\beta_{x-38}$, $A\beta_{x-40}$, phosphorylated and total tau protein, GFAP, PDGFRβ, and β-trace protein in the CSF, in addition to decreased white matter volume and choroid plexus volume and increased gray matter volume and cortical thickness in 11 patients with SD compared to the control group. Further research involving larger cohorts is warranted to better characterize this NDD and to find effective treatment methods.

Early diagnosis of cognitive decline provides better prospects for halting its progression. Neurocognitive disorders (NCDs) have many etiologies such as AD, vascular disease, Lewy body disease, frontotemporal disorders, PD, Huntington's disease, multiple sclerosis, traumatic brain injury, prion disease, and others. Current challenges in the diagnosis of progressive NCDs are presented in the review by Abbatantuono et al. (Contribution 10). The authors conducted searches on online databases (PubMed and Scopus) to investigate the neurocognitive stages characterized by signs and clinical manifestations preceding the onset of mild and/or major NCDs. They discuss the diagnostic criteria and stadial models for NCDs in the context of their usefulness in primary and secondary care. The review focuses on the following stages of neurocognitive decline: the preclinical stage, the transitional stage, the prodromal or mild stage, and major NCD. The authors conclude that the identification and monitoring of individuals at all stages from preclinical to overt dementia are essential for optimizing clinical efforts against neurocognitive decline.

Another type of neurocognitive disorder is normal pressure hydrocephalus in which the accumulation of CSF in the brain ventricles leads to a range of symptoms, including cognitive decline. Idiopathic normal pressure hydrocephalus (iNPH) is the most common form of hydrocephalus in the adult population and may accompany NDDs such as AD and PD [10]. Porru et al. analyzed levels of oxysterols before and after ventriculoperitoneal shunt surgery and reported a significantly lower level of these oxygenated derivatives of cholesterol in iNPH patients before surgery and an increase in 24-OH and 7HOCA levels following surgery (Contribution 11). Based on the obtained results, the scientists conclude that oxysterols present in the CSF may find potential use as biomarkers in the diagnosis and management of iNPH.

The projections of an increase in the incidence of NDDs worldwide in the coming years are alarming and the situation requires urgent attention. Multidirectional actions combining prevention, early diagnosis, and therapies that halt disease progression, in addition to the search for neuroregenerative therapies, should prove effective in the fight against NDDs in the long term. Identifying new biomarkers, better understanding the role of the immune system and hormonal regulation in NDDs, and the use of bioinformatics tools to discover connections between different pathways and processes in the course of NDDs are just some of the research approaches presented in this Special Issue. Different approaches and increased efforts focused on various aspects of NDDs should shed more light on their development and course and, consequently, lead to the development of more effective treatments.

Funding: This work was supported by the National Science Centre (NCN, Poland): 2023/07/X/NZ7/01480 and the Ministry of Science and Higher Education (ST-11).

Conflicts of Interest: The author declares no conflicts of interest.

List of Contributions

1. Lu, H.; Chen, M.; Zhu, C. Intranasal Administration of Apelin-13 Ameliorates Cognitive Deficit in Streptozotocin-Induced Alzheimer's Disease Model via Enhancement of Nrf2-HO1 Pathways. *Brain Sci.* **2024**, *14*, 488. https://doi.org/10.3390/brainsci14050488.
2. Kim, Y.J.; Mun, B.-R.; Choi, K.Y.; Choi, W.-S. Oral Administration of Probiotic Bacteria Alleviates Tau Phosphorylation, Aβ Accumulation, Microglia Activation, and Memory Loss in 5xFAD Mice. *Brain Sci.* **2024**, *14*, 208. https://doi.org/10.3390/brainsci14030208.
3. Solla, P.; Wang, Q.; Frau, C.; Floris, V.; Loy, F.; Sechi, L.A.; Masala, C. Olfactory Impairment Is the Main Predictor of Higher Scores at REM Sleep Behavior Disorder (RBD) Screening Questionnaire in Parkinson's Disease Patients. *Brain Sci.* **2023**, *13*, 599. https://doi.org/10.3390/brainsci13040599.
4. Luthra, N.S.; Clow, A.; Corcos, D.M. The Interrelated Multifactorial Actions of Cortisol and Klotho: Potential Implications in the Pathogenesis of Parkinson's Disease. *Brain Sci.* **2022**, *12*, 1695. https://doi.org/10.3390/brainsci12121695.
5. Bohnen, N.I.; Barr, J.; Vangel, R.; Roytman, S.; Paalanen, R.; Frey, K.A.; Scott, P.J.H.; Kanel, P. GABA$_A$ Receptor Benzodiazepine Binding Sites and Motor Impairments in Parkinson's Disease. *Brain Sci.* **2023**, *13*, 1711. https://doi.org/10.3390/brainsci13121711.
6. Lin, C.-Y.; Vanoverbeke, V.; Trent, D.; Willey, K.; Lee, Y.-S. The Spatiotemporal Expression of SOCS3 in the Brainstem and Spinal Cord of Amyotrophic Lateral Sclerosis Mice. *Brain Sci.* **2024**, *14*, 564. https://doi.org/10.3390/brainsci14060564.
7. Suthar, S.K.; Lee, S.-Y. The Role of Superoxide Dismutase 1 in Amyotrophic Lateral Sclerosis: Identification of Signaling Pathways, Regulators, Molecular Interaction Networks, and Biological Functions through Bioinformatics. *Brain Sci.* **2023**, *13*, 151. https://doi.org/10.3390/brainsci13010151.
8. Schirò, G.; Di Stefano, V.; Iacono, S.; Lupica, A.; Brighina, F.; Monastero, R.; Balistreri, C.R. Advances on Cellular Clonotypic Immunity in Amyotrophic Lateral Sclerosis. *Brain Sci.* **2022**, *12*, 1412. https://doi.org/10.3390/brainsci12101412.
9. Aspli, K.T.; Aaseth, J.O.; Holmøy, T.; Blennow, K.; Zetterberg, H.; Kirsebom, B.-E.; Fladby, T.; Selnes, P. CSF, Blood, and MRI Biomarkers in Skogholt's Disease—A Rare Neurodegenerative Disease in a Norwegian Kindred. *Brain Sci.* **2023**, *13*, 1511. https://doi.org/10.3390/brainsci13111511.
10. Abbatantuono, C.; Alfeo, F.; Clemente, L.; Lancioni, G.; De Caro, M.F.; Livrea, P.; Taurisano, P. Current Challenges in the Diagnosis of Progressive Neurocognitive Disorders: A Critical Review of the Literature and Recommendations for Primary and Secondary Care. *Brain Sci.* **2023**, *13*, 1443. https://doi.org/10.3390/brainsci13101443.
11. Porru, E.; Edström, E.; Arvidsson, L.; Elmi-Terander, A.; Fletcher-Sandersjöö, A.; Sandblom, A.L.; Hansson, M.; Duell, F.; Björkhem, I. Ventriculoperitoneal Shunt Treatment Increases 7 Alpha Hy-Droxy-3-Oxo-4-Cholestenoic Acid and 24-Hydroxycholesterol Concentrations in Idiopathic Normal Pressure Hydrocephalus. *Brain Sci.* **2022**, *12*, 1450. https://doi.org/10.3390/brainsci12111450.

References

1. Nichols, E.; Steinmetz, J.D.; Vollset, S.E.; Fukutaki, K.; Chalek, J.; Abd-Allah, F.; Abdoli, A.; Abualhasan, A.; Abu-Gharbieh, E.; Akram, T.T.; et al. Estimation of the Global Prevalence of Dementia in 2019 and Forecasted Prevalence in 2050: An Analysis for the Global Burden of Disease Study 2019. *Lancet Public Health* **2022**, *7*, e105–e125. [CrossRef] [PubMed]
2. Ben-Shlomo, Y.; Darweesh, S.; Llibre-Guerra, J.; Marras, C.; San Luciano, M.; Tanner, C. The Epidemiology of Parkinson's Disease. *Lancet* **2024**, *403*, 283–292. [CrossRef] [PubMed]
3. WHO Parkinson Disease 2023. Available online: https://www.who.int/news-room/fact-sheets/detail/parkinson-disease (accessed on 14 August 2024).
4. Dodiya, H.B.; Forsyth, C.B.; Voigt, R.M.; Engen, P.A.; Patel, J.; Shaikh, M.; Green, S.J.; Naqib, A.; Roy, A.; Kordower, J.H.; et al. Chronic Stress-Induced Gut Dysfunction Exacerbates Parkinson's Disease Phenotype and Pathology in a Rotenone-Induced Mouse Model of Parkinson's Disease. *Neurobiol. Dis.* **2020**, *135*, 104352. [CrossRef] [PubMed]
5. Logroscino, G.; Urso, D.; Tortelli, R. The Challenge of Amyotrophic Lateral Sclerosis Descriptive Epidemiology: To Estimate Low Incidence Rates across Complex Phenotypes in Different Geographic Areas. *Curr. Opin. Neurol.* **2022**, *35*, 678–685. [CrossRef] [PubMed]

6. Arthur, K.C.; Calvo, A.; Price, T.R.; Geiger, J.T.; Chiò, A.; Traynor, B.J. Projected Increase in Amyotrophic Lateral Sclerosis from 2015 to 2040. *Nat. Commun.* **2016**, *7*, 12408. [CrossRef] [PubMed]
7. Sun, F.; Park, K.K.; Belin, S.; Wang, D.; Lu, T.; Chen, G.; Zhang, K.; Yeung, C.; Feng, G.; Yankner, B.A.; et al. Sustained Axon Regeneration Induced by Co-Deletion of PTEN and SOCS3. *Nature* **2011**, *480*, 372–375. [CrossRef] [PubMed]
8. Cui, C.; Ingre, C.; Yin, L.; Li, X.; Andersson, J.; Seitz, C.; Ruffin, N.; Pawitan, Y.; Piehl, F.; Fang, F. Correlation between Leukocyte Phenotypes and Prognosis of Amyotrophic Lateral Sclerosis. *eLife* **2022**, *11*, e74065. [CrossRef] [PubMed]
9. Hagen, K.; Boman, H.; Mellgren, S.I.; Lindal, S.; Bovim, G. Progressive Central and Peripheral Demyelinating Disease of Adult Onset in a Norwegian Family. *Arch. Neurol.* **1998**, *55*, 1467–1472. [CrossRef] [PubMed]
10. Williams, M.A.; Malm, J. Diagnosis and Treatment of Idiopathic Normal Pressure Hydrocephalus. *Continuum* **2016**, *22*, 579–599. [CrossRef] [PubMed]

Disclaimer/Publisher's Note: The statements, opinions and data contained in all publications are solely those of the individual author(s) and contributor(s) and not of MDPI and/or the editor(s). MDPI and/or the editor(s) disclaim responsibility for any injury to people or property resulting from any ideas, methods, instructions or products referred to in the content.

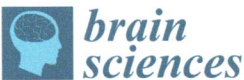

Article

Oral Administration of Probiotic Bacteria Alleviates Tau Phosphorylation, Aβ Accumulation, Microglia Activation, and Memory Loss in 5xFAD Mice

Yeong Jin Kim [1], Bo-Ram Mun [1], Kyu Yeong Choi [2,3] and Won-Seok Choi [1,*]

[1] School of Biological Sciences and Technology, College of Natural Sciences, College of Medicine, Chonnam National University, Gwangju 61186, Republic of Korea; vitalogy1032@gmail.com (Y.J.K.); boram5490@gmail.com (B.-R.M.)
[2] Gwangju Alzheimer's and Related Dementia Cohort Research Center, Chosun University, Gwangju 61452, Republic of Korea; khaser@gmail.com
[3] Kolab, Inc., Gwangju 61436, Republic of Korea
* Correspondence: choiw@chonnam.ac.kr; Tel.: +82-62-530-1912

Abstract: The gut–brain axis (GBA) plays a significant role in various neurodegenerative disorders, such as Alzheimer's disease (AD), and the gut microbiome (GM) can bidirectionally communicate with the brain through the GBA. Thus, recent evidence indicates that the GM may affect the pathological features and the progression of AD in humans. The aim of our study was to elucidate the impact of probiotics on the pathological features of AD in a 5xFAD model. Probiotics (*Bifidobacterium lactis*, *Levilactobacillus brevis*, and *Limosilactobacillus fermentum*) were orally administered in 5xFAD mice to modify the GM composition. Additionally, freeze-dried food containing phosphatidylserine was used as the positive control. Behavioral pathogenesis was assessed through the cross maze and Morris water maze tests. Our findings revealed that probiotic administration resulted in significant improvements in spatial and recognition memories. Furthermore, the neuroprotective effects of probiotics were substantiated by a reduction in amyloid-β accumulation in critical brain regions. Microglial activation in 5xFAD mice was also attenuated by probiotics in the hippocampus and cerebral cortex. Moreover, elevated tau phosphorylation in 5xFAD mice was ameliorated in the probiotics-treated group. The results highlight the potential use of probiotics as a neuroprotective intervention in AD.

Keywords: Alzheimer's disease; tau; amyloid beta; microglia; probiotics

1. Introduction

Alzheimer's disease (AD) is a chronic, progressive neurodegenerative disease that affects brain functions, including memory and cognition. The core pathophysiology of AD has been postulated as the intraneuronal aggregation of hyperphosphorylated tau, a microtubule-associated protein, which leads to the formation of neurofibrillary tangles, and the interstitial aggregation of insoluble forms of the amyloid-β (Aβ) peptide, which results in neuritic plaques [1]. Less than 1% of cases are characterized by the familial type of AD, which is associated with autosomal dominant inheritance, Aβ overexpression, and onset often before the age of 65 years [2]. In the sporadic form of AD, both genetic and environmental risk factors play a role. Plaque formation in the brain has toxic effects on neurons and occurs due to the overproduction or decreased clearance of Aβ [3]. Additionally, substantial evidence suggests that neuroinflammation plays a key role in the pathophysiology of AD. Specifically, the accumulation of activated microglia around damaged areas is a hallmark of neuroinflammation in AD. Moreover, microglia can be activated by pathogens and improperly deposited proteins such as Aβ in AD [4].

The brain interacts with the gut either through the nervous system or through chemical substances that cross the blood–brain barrier (BBB). The gut microbiota (GM) produces amino acids and monoamines that, through the lymphatic and vascular systems, reach the central nervous system (CNS) where they can affect its activity [5]. Additionally, aging causes substantial changes in the content and function of the gut–brain axis (GBA), which can have an impact on health and age-related disorders [6]. Emerging evidence suggests the GBA's role in neurodegenerative disease progression through diverse pathways [7]. Bacterial metabolites contribute to immune and metabolic changes, potentially increasing intestinal and blood–brain barrier permeability, modulating inflammatory responses, and influencing microglial maturation, which is crucial for CNS homeostasis and regulating inflammation. Notably, research has identified a correlation between gut dysbiosis and the aggregation of Aβ, the formation of tau proteins, and the onset of neuroinflammation and oxidative stress, all of which are implicated in AD [8].

Recent studies indicate that the consumption of specific probiotics can ameliorate a range of diseases, including sepsis, cancer, and neurodegeneration, via antioxidant and anti-inflammatory pathways [9]. Clinical studies have provided strong evidence supporting potential interventions of probiotics for neurodegenerative diseases. Of these strains, lactic acid bacteria (LAB), such as *Lactobacillus* and *Bifidobacterium*, are the most widely utilized probiotics [10]. According to a preclinical study, probiotics may improve cognitive function in animal models of cognitive impairment [11]. It has been demonstrated that mixed cultures of LAB and Bifidobacterium strains exert a synergistic effect on host health, leading to the enhanced production of short-chain fatty acids and modulation of the immune response [12]. Thus, it is important to investigate the possible therapeutic advantages of probiotics on brain health in degenerative diseases like AD [13].

In this study, we investigated the effect of probiotics on amyloid-induced pathology in an AD model. The 5xFAD mice, containing APP and presenilin mutants, are commonly used as an AD model, constituting approximately 10% of all AD studies that employ an animal model [14]. These mice develop amyloid pathology, with plaques appearing in the brain between 2 to 4 months of age [15]. In contrast, the 3xTG mouse model, which contains APP, presenilin, and tau mutants, exhibits a much slower disease progression and amyloid deposition starting around 6 months. For our study, we used 4-month-old 5xFAD mice and investigated the effect on tau, Aβ, and microglial activity.

2. Materials and Methods

2.1. Animals

Four-month-old 5XFAD (APP K670N/M671L [Swedish], APP I716V [Florida], APP V717I [London], PSEN1 M146L, and PSEN1 L286V; Jackson Laboratory, Bar Harbor, ME, USA) mice and wild-type (WT) littermates were housed under a regular 12 h light/12 h dark cycle at room temperature (20–25 °C) and supplied with food and water [16]. For the experiment, each mouse (WT: male n = 7, female n = 8; 5xFAD: male n = 16, female n = 16) was placed into an individual cage. All protocols for the animal experiments were approved by the Institutional Animal Care and Use Committee of Chonnam National University (CNU IACUC-YB-2022-154; CNU IACUC-YB-2023-156) [17].

2.2. Probiotics and Phosphatidylserine Supplementation

The mice were divided into four groups: 5xFAD, 5xFAD/Probiotics, 5xFAD/Phosphatidylserine (PS), and WT. Starting from 4 months of age, the probiotics group was supplemented daily with 8×10^7 CFU of probiotics (*Bifidobacterium lactis* KL101, *Limosilactobacillus fermentum* KL271, and *Levilactobacillus brevis* KL251; Kolab, Inc., Gwangju, Republic of Korea) in 8 mL sterilized water for 3 months. The probiotics were prepared as described with minor modifications [9]. The bacterial cultures were stored at 4 °C and used in their live state. PS significantly improved cognitive function when administered to AD patients [18]. Several studies confirmed the efficacy of PS in AD patients and an animal model [19–21]. In the rodent model, the effective dose was 15–30 mg/kg and we used 21mg/kg daily in this study. The PS group, as a positive control, was fed freeze-dried food containing PS for 3 months.

2.3. Open Field Test

After 2 months of probiotics supplementation, the mice were subjected to behavior tests. Locomotor activity was measured in an open-field test as described [22]. Each mouse was placed in the center of the arena (40 × 40 × 40 cm) and allowed to freely explore for 5 min for prehabituation. In the main test, the movement of each mouse was recorded for 20 min and analyzed using ANY-maze software ver. 6.32 (Stoelting, Wood Dale, IL, USA).

2.4. Cross Maze

Each mouse was placed in a cross-shaped maze with four arms and monitored. The duration of the examination period was 10 min. The rate of spontaneous alternation was determined using the following formula: actual alternation/(possible alternation [total number of arm entries] − 3) × 100 (%) [17].

2.5. Morris Water Maze

The Morris water maze (MWM) test utilized a circular, open pool, which was filled with opaque water, with a diameter of 114 cm [23]. The water became opaque using non-toxic paint and the temperature was maintained at ~24 °C. A hidden platform (17 × 10.5 cm) was strategically positioned in the target quadrant below the water surface [24]. The mice were then subjected to the acquisition and probe phases. In the acquisition phase, each mouse underwent training, which involved four trials per day for 4 days [25]. During each trial, the mice were given a 60 s time limit to swim, and the trial concluded as soon as they reached the platform. Following the completion of each trial, the mice were allowed to remain on the platform for 20 s. After finishing the 4-day acquisition phase, a probe test was performed without the platform, lasting for 90 s. The movement of each mouse was then recorded, and time spent in the designated target quadrant and the latency to reach the platform were analyzed using ANY-maze software.

2.6. Immunohistochemistry

The animals were euthanized after a 3-month period of receiving treatments. Subsequently, their brains were extracted, fixed in a 4% paraformaldehyde solution, and then soaked in phosphate-buffered saline (PBS) with 30% sucrose overnight. The brain tissues were then embedded in optimum cutting temperature (OCT) freezing media, sliced (30 μm thickness), and mounted on glass slides. Brain sections were permeabilized using 0.15% Triton X-100 in PBS (PBST) for 30 min and then washed with PBS. The sections were then incubated with 3% bovine serum albumin (BSA) and 3% goat serum in PBS with 0.1% Triton X-100 for 30 min. The primary antibodies, mouse anti-Aβ (6E10, 1:3000; BioLegend, San Diego, CA, USA) and rabbit anti-IBA-1 (1:3000; Wako, Richmond, VA, USA), were applied to the samples for 3 days at 4 °C. The sections were then washed with PBS and incubated with the secondary antibodies, Alexa Fluor 568 anti-mouse IgG or Alexa Fluor 488 goat anti-rabbit IgG (1:2000; Invitrogen, Waltham, MA, USA), overnight at 4 °C.

2.7. Quantification and Image Analysis

Fluorescence images were captured utilizing the EVOS M7000 (Invitrogen, Waltham, MA, USA) microscope. Subsequent quantification and analyses were carried out utilizing ImageJ software ver. 1.53q developed by the National Institutes of Health (NIH, https://imagej.net/ij/). The immunoreactivity of Aβ was calculated as the percent area of immunoreactive cells per slide (%). Regarding the microglia, the relative immunoreactivity was determined based on the stained slides. Images were taken using a Leica Stellaris 5 (Leica, Deerfield, IL, USA) confocal microscope to analyze microglial branches z-stacked at 1.5 μm intervals and compressed to about 15 images.

2.8. Microglia Morphology Analysis

A ramified cell is one that exhibits a complex network of processes originating from the cell body. Changes in microglia ramification indicate a microglial response to altered physiological conditions. ImageJ software (NIH) was consistently employed to process all photomicrographs, converting them into binary and skeletonized images. To analyze the microglial branches, we measured processes from a total of 10–20 microglia for each location in one mouse and summarized the number of branches and the total process length using ImageJ software. In addition to generating skeletonized images, we manually counted the cell bodies in each photomicrograph [26].

2.9. Protein Preparation

The brain cortex was collected in radioimmunoprecipitation assay (RIPA) lysis buffer composed of 25 mM Tris-HCl (pH 7.6), 0.01% Nonidet P-40, 150 mM NaCl, 1% sodium deoxycholate, 0.1% sodium dodecyl sulfate (SDS), 100 mM phenylmethylsulfonyl fluoride (PMSF), and protease inhibitors. These lysates were mechanically homogenized using a 26-gauge needle with 10 repetitions. Subsequently, the samples were centrifuged at 16,100 cfg for 30 min at 4 °C. RIPA lysis buffer was utilized in a volume of 200 µL for small tissue samples and 500 µL for larger tissues, such as the cortex. The protein concentration in the lysates was determined using the bicinchoninic acid (BCA) assay.

2.10. Western Blot

Lysates containing 35 µg of protein were separated on a 10% acrylamide gel through SDS-polyacrylamide gel electrophoresis (PAGE). The separated proteins were subsequently transferred onto polyvinylidene difluoride (PVDF) or nitrocellulose membranes (Amersham, Little Chalfont, UK). To prevent non-specific binding, the membranes were blocked using a blocking buffer composed of 5% skim milk in Tris-buffered saline (TBS) containing 0.1% Tween 20 (TBST) buffer for 30 min at room temperature. Following the blocking step, the membrane was washed four times with TBST for 5 min each time. Afterward, it was incubated with the primary antibody, mouse anti-PHF-1 (1:3000), in TBST overnight at 4 °C. The next day, the membrane was exposed to the goat anti-mouse HRP-conjugated secondary antibody (ENZO, Farmingdale, NY, USA) in TBST at a dilution of 1:10,000 at room temperature for 2 h. Finally, the immunoreactive bands were selectively detected using the enhanced chemiluminescence (ECL) reaction.

2.11. Statistical Analysis

Behavioral data, images, and Western blot data underwent analysis using a two-way analysis of variance (ANOVA) and one-way ANOVA, followed by post hoc analysis utilizing Tukey's post hoc test. All presented data are expressed as the mean ± standard error of the mean (SEM). Statistical significance was determined with a threshold of $p < 0.05$, where values below this threshold were considered statistically significant.

3. Results

3.1. Probiotics Improve Recognition, Memory, and Spatial Memory in 5xFAD Mice

In this study, we investigated the hypothesis that probiotics enhance memory in animal models of AD, as suggested by a preclinical study [11,12]. To test this, we supplied a mixture of probiotic bacteria (*Bifidobacterium lactis*, *Levilactobacillus brevis*, and *Limosilactobacillus fermentum*) and phosphatidylserine (PS) as a positive control or the vehicle for 2 months before the behavior study (Figure 1A). PS improved the pathology and symptoms of AD by inhibiting neuroinflammation, increasing glucose metabolism in the brain, and normalizing N-Methyl-D-aspartate (NMDA) receptor activity [27]. Cognition and memory were evaluated in 5xFAD mice, an AD mouse model, using cross maze, novel object recognition, and MWM tests, while continuing to supply probiotics to the mice. In the cross maze test, the 5xFAD mice treated with probiotics or PS showed a significant improvement in their memory, represented by a higher alternation ratio, compared to that of the untreated 5xFAD mice. However, there was no change in the total arm entry (Figure 1B,C). Similarly, in the novel object recognition test, the 5xFAD mice treated with probiotics or PS exhibited enhanced memory, showing a higher preference index compared to that of the untreated 5xFAD mice, though the difference was not statistically significant (Supplemental Figure S1). Furthermore, in the MWM test to assess hippocampus-dependent spatial learning and memory, a notable increase in the memory (represented by decreased time spent in the target quadrant) was observed in the 5xFAD mice treated with probiotics or PS in the probe test as compared to that of the vehicle-treated 5xFAD mice (Figure 1D–G). These findings strongly suggest that probiotics can have a protective effect on the loss of spatial and recognition memories in the 5xFAD mouse model.

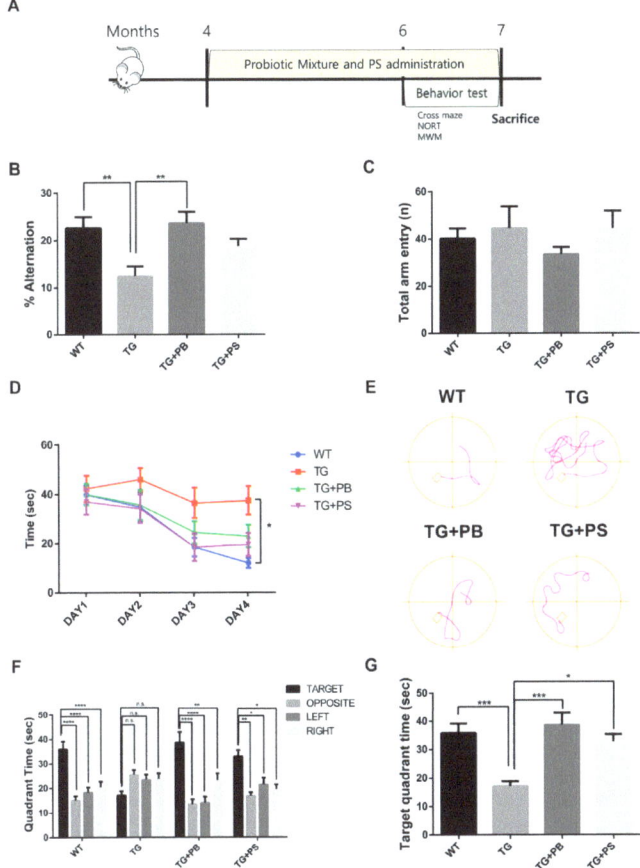

Figure 1. Probiotics alleviated the memory defect in 5xFAD mice. (**A**) The experimental procedure for the mice is displayed. (**B,C**) The cross maze and (**D–G**) Morris water maze were utilized to assess the learning and memory of mice. (**B**) In the cross maze test, the loss of the alternation rate was attenuated by probiotics, (**C**) but no changes in the number of total arm entries of the 5xFAD mice were seen. (**D–G**) Probiotics also diminished the defects in learning and memory in the Morris water maze test. (**D**) Escape latency during the learning phase. (**E**) Representative track plot of Day 4. (**F**) Time spent in each quadrant (seconds) during the probe phase. Treatment, $F_{(3, 35)} = 0.4372$, $p = 0.7278$; Quadrant time, $F_{(3, 105)} = 16.58$, $p < 0.0001$; Interaction Treatment × Quadrant time, $F_{(9,105)} = 5.365$, $p < 0.0001$ was analyzed using two-way ANOVA, post hoc Tukey's test. (**G**) Target quadrant time (seconds) in the probe phase. WT: Wild type, $n = 13$; TG: 5xFAD transgenic mice, $n = 9$; TG + PB: Probiotic-treated 5xFAD transgenic mice, $n = 9$; TG + PS: Phosphatidylserine-treated 5xFAD transgenic mice, $n = 8$. One-way analysis of variance (ANOVA) test; two-way ANOVA test; n.s, not significant; *, $p < 0.05$; **, $p < 0.01$; ***, $p < 0.001$; ****, $p < 0.0001$.

3.2. Probiotics Alleviated Aβ Accumulation in the Hippocampus and Cerebral Cortex of 5xFAD Mice

A recent study found significant variations in the composition of the GM (which regulates the decline in cognitive function) and an increase in Aβ deposition in an AD model [28]. Therefore, we investigated the Aβ-positive area in the hippocampus and cerebral cortex to further evaluate the neuroprotective effects of probiotics. In the tissue staining, a significant decrease in the Aβ (6E10)-positive area was seen in 5xFAD mice that were treated with either probiotics or PS compared to that of the untreated 5xFAD mice (Figure 2). These findings provide compelling evidence of the neuroprotective effects of probiotics, especially in the hippocampus and cerebral cortex, thus highlighting their potential use as a treatment for AD.

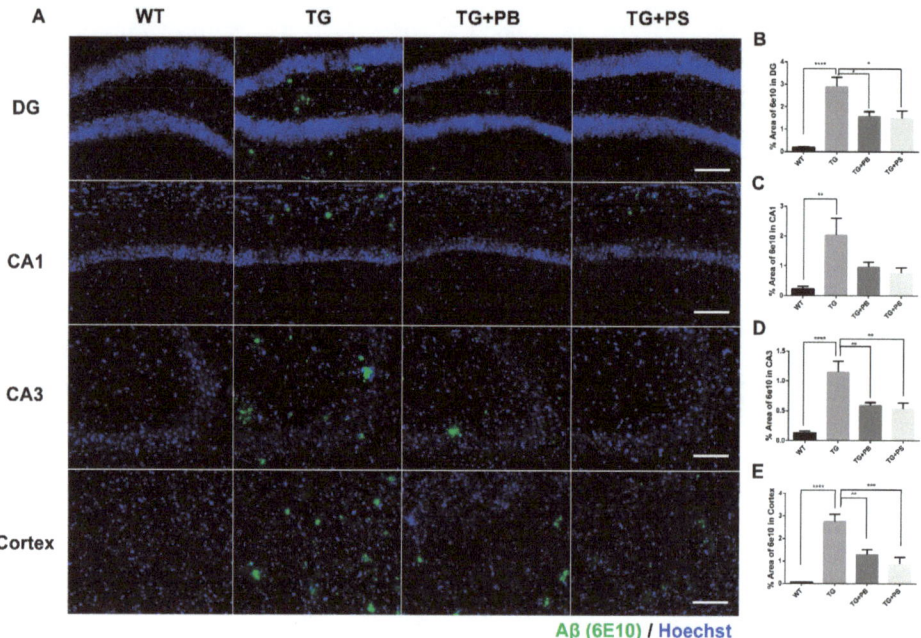

Figure 2. Probiotics decreased amyloid-β (Aβ) accumulation in the hippocampus and cerebral cortex in 5xFAD mice. (**A**) Representative immunohistochemistry images of the hippocampus and cerebral cortex. Scale bar = 100 μm. (**B–E**) Probiotics significantly decreased the Aβ level as quantified as the percent area of Aβ staining (6E10 positive) in the dentate gyrus (DG), Cornu Ammonis (CA) 1, CA3, and cortex in 5xFAD mice. Phosphatidylserine showed a similar protective effect. WT: Wild type, $n = 6$; TG: 5xFAD transgenic mouse, $n = 6$; TG + PB: Probiotics-treated 5xFAD transgenic mice, $n = 6$; TG + PS: Phosphatidylserine-treated 5xFAD transgenic mice, $n = 5$. One-way analysis of variance (ANOVA) test; *, $p < 0.05$; **, $p < 0.01$; ***, $p < 0.001$; ****, $p < 0.0001$.

3.3. Probiotics Reduced Microglial Activation in the Hippocampus and Cerebral Cortex in 5xFAD Mice

Microglial activation is a prominent feature of AD [29] and the impact of the host GM on microglia homeostasis has been suggested [30]. We investigated the effects of probiotics on microglia by evaluating the intensity of the activated microglia in the hippocampus and cerebral cortex in 5xFAD mice. As a result, increased immunoreactivity and activated microglia were observed in the brains of 5xFAD mice (Figure 3). However, 5xFAD mice treated with either probiotics or PS showed a significant reduction in both the number and activity of microglia as compared to that of the vehicle-treated 5xFAD mice (Figure 3). These findings provide compelling evidence for the role probiotics play in alleviating microglial activation in the AD model.

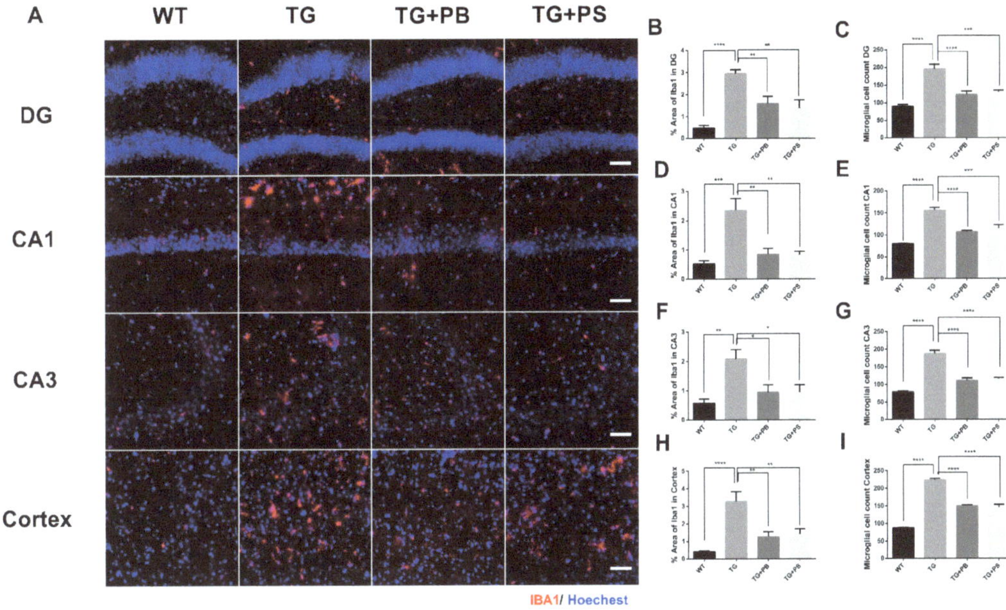

Figure 3. Activation of microglia in 5xFAD mice was reduced by probiotics. (**A**) Representative images of activated microglia (IBA-1) in the hippocampus and cerebral cortex. Scale bar = 100 μm. (**B–I**) Probiotics reduced the stained area of microglia and the number of microglia in the dentate gyrus (DG), Cornu Ammonis (CA) 1, CA3, and cortex in 5xFAD mice treated with either probiotics or phosphatidylserine, as compared to that of the vehicle-treated 5xFAD mice, and as quantified as the percent area of IBA-1 immunoreactivity. WT: Wild type, $n = 6$; TG: 5xFAD transgenic mouse, $n = 6$; TG + PB: Probiotics-treated 5xFAD transgenic mouse, $n = 6$; TG + PS: Phosphatidylserine-treated 5xFAD transgenic mouse, $n = 5$. One-way analysis of variance (ANOVA) test; *, $p < 0.05$; **, $p < 0.01$; ***, $p < 0.001$; ****, $p < 0.0001$.

3.4. Probiotics Suppressed Microglial Activation in 5xFAD Mice

We further analyzed the detailed morphological modification of microglial activation using the microglial skeleton analysis method. Our results indicate that the number of branches and the total process length of the microglia were reduced in the hippocampus and cerebral cortex (Figures 4 and S2) of 5xFAD mice. However, the administration of probiotics and PS attenuated these changes in 5xFAD mice (Figure 4). Taken together, these findings imply that the use of probiotics may efficiently suppress microglial activation in the AD mouse model.

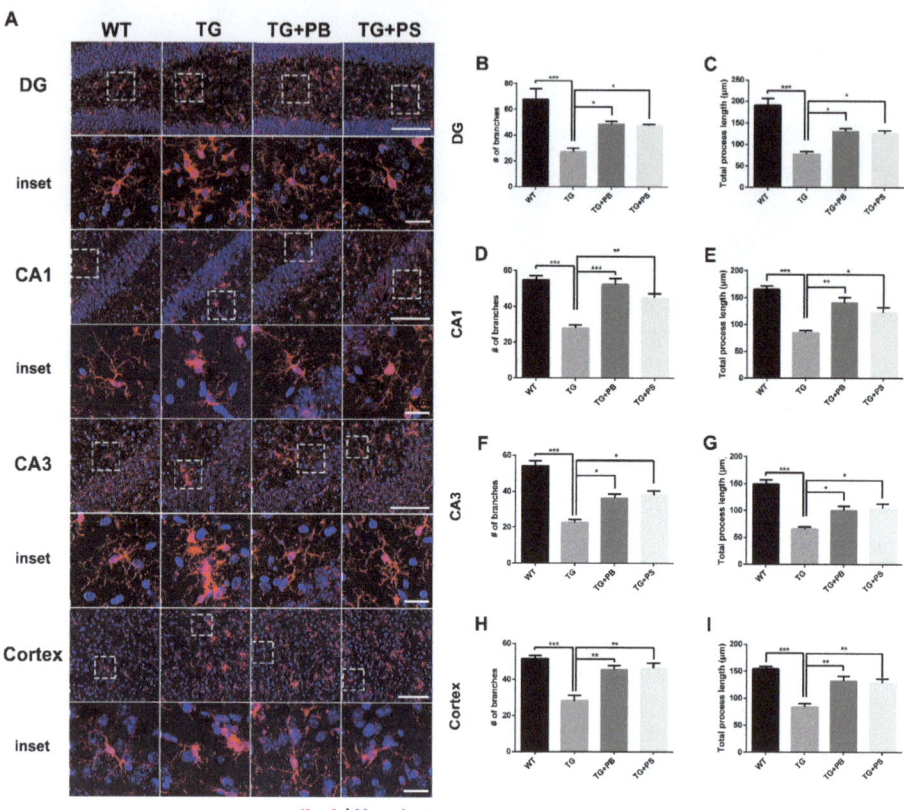

Figure 4. Probiotics suppressed microglial activation in the dentate gyrus (DG), Cornu Ammonis (CA) 1, and CA3 in the hippocampus and cerebral cortex of 5xFAD mice. (**A**) Representative images of microglial processes in the DG, CA1, and CA3 in the hippocampus and cerebral cortex. The inset indicates an enlarged area of the upper white dotted frame. Scale bar = 100 μm, inset scale bar = 20 μm. Our results demonstrate that the administration of probiotics and phosphatidylserine to 5xFAD mice resulted in increased numbers of branches and the total process length of microglia, as compared to that of the 5xFAD mice in the (**B**,**C**) DG, (**D**,**E**) CA1, and (**F**,**G**) CA3 in the (**H**,**I**) hippocampus and cerebral cortex. WT: Wild type, n = 6; TG: 5xFAD transgenic mouse, n = 6; TG + PB: Probiotics-treated 5xFAD transgenic mouse, n = 6; TG + PS: Phosphatidylserine-treated 5xFAD transgenic mouse, n = 5; One-way analysis of variance (ANOVA) test; *, $p < 0.05$; **, $p < 0.01$; ***, $p < 0.001$.

3.5. Probiotics Reduce Phosphorylated Tau in the Cerebral Cortex in 5xFAD Mice

Tau hyperphosphorylation is another distinct pathological feature in the brains of AD patients. Accumulating evidence suggests microglia play a role in the tau level and distribution in AD [31,32]. Recent studies have reported that microglial activation is an important factor that accelerates the aggregation and propagation of tau [32,33]. In this study, we observed the tau phosphorylation level using a phosphorylated tau-specific antibody. In the Western blotting assay, tau phosphorylation was elevated in 5xFAD mice, as compared to that of the WT mice (Figures 5 and S3). However, it was significantly reduced in the 5xFAD group treated with probiotics, which was comparable with the effect of PS treatment (Figure 5). These findings strongly support the idea that probiotics have a beneficial effect in reducing tau phosphorylation in the brain of an AD mouse model.

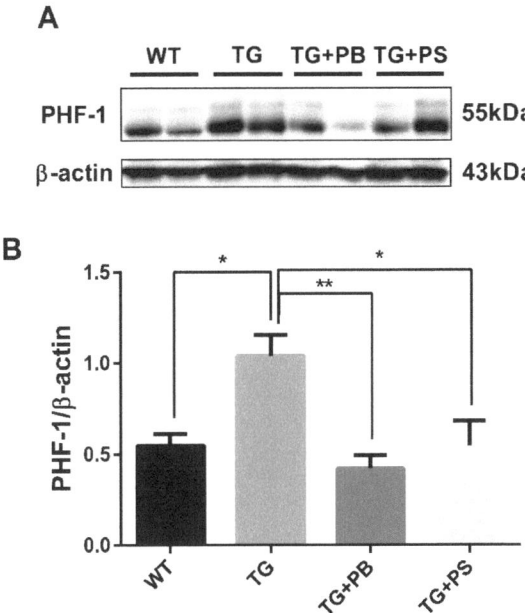

Figure 5. Probiotics reduce p-tau (s396, s404; PHF-1) in the cerebral cortex. (**A**) A representative Western blot of the cerebral cortex revealed that the level of phosphorylated tau (PHF-1) was significantly decreased in the 5xFAD group treated with probiotics when compared to that of the vehicle-treated 5xFAD group. A similar effect was observed in mice subjected to phosphatidylserine. (**B**) Immunoblot quantification of phosphorylated tau. WT: Wild type, n = 4; TG: 5xFAD transgenic mouse, n = 4; TG + PB: Probiotics-treated 5xFAD transgenic mouse, n = 4; TG + PS: Phosphatidylserine-treated 5xFAD transgenic mouse, n = 4. One-way analysis of variance (ANOVA) test; *, $p < 0.05$; **, $p < 0.01$.

Altogether, our data suggest that oral uptake of probiotics alleviated Aβ or tau pathology and memory loss in an AD model, which might be mediated by the attenuation of microglial activation.

4. Discussion

Currently, the existing treatments for AD are primarily focused on symptom management rather than halting or preventing the progression of the disorder. However, therapeutic approaches directly targeting Aβ or tau have had limited application up until now. Recently, significant research efforts have been focused on GM and GBA as alternative mechanisms to regulate AD. This approach showed a potential for the development of novel therapeutic interventions for AD [34]. Specifically, oral bacteriotherapy, which involves orally administering beneficial bacteria, is gaining recognition as a viable strategy for preventing and treating various disorders, including those related to the CNS [11,35,36], given that probiotics may enhance recognition and spatial memories in animal models of cognitive impairment. Therefore, we hypothesized that probiotics may have a therapeutic effect on 5xFAD mice. In our various behavioral tests, we found that probiotics improved recognition and spatial memories in 5xFAD mice.

In the previous report, oral supplementation with *Bifidobacterium breve* had a protective effect against memory impairment in an AD model [37]. The probiotics (*Bifidobacterium lactis*, *Levilactobacillus brevis*, and *Limosilactobacillus fermentum*) also improved LPS-induced cognitive impairment and memory loss in mice [9]. In this study, we used the same combination of live probiotic bacteria strains to investigate their therapeutic effects on AD. The probiotics improved the cognitive defects and memory loss and attenuated Aβ accumulation in 5xFAD mice. Additionally, the protective effect of the combined strains on Aβ and memory in this study was more pronounced than that of the single strain used previously. This suggests a beneficial effect of the combined use of probiotics. However, direct comparisons were not possible because the two studies used different AD models. Hence, further investigation comparing a single strain and multiple strains in a model would give direct evidence of the beneficial effect of combining multiple strains.

A recent study utilized WT and APP$^{swe/PS1\Delta E9}$ transgenic mice to investigate the role of dysbiosis in AD using several methods. The investigation results revealed that dysbiosis induced heightened Aβ accumulation, significantly altered GM composition, and caused a decline in cognitive function, suggesting the importance of the GM in preventing Aβ burden in an AD model [38]. Consequently, our findings show that probiotics notably reduced Aβ accumulation and prevented cognitive/memory dysfunction in the AD model. Although Aβ has long been believed as the main pathological cause of AD, it has been consistently demonstrated that the accumulation and deposition of amyloid-β (Aβ) plaques do not exhibit a direct correlation with neuronal loss or cognitive decline [39–41]. Moreover, many individuals exhibit a substantial burden of amyloid plaques, as assessed through positron emission tomography (PET) scans, yet remain asymptomatic in terms of memory impairment [42]. On the other hand, the mean prevalence of amyloid positivity was 88% among the patients diagnosed with AD, meaning that significant cases of AD are not Aβ-dependent [43]. These brought up questions about the role of Aβ in AD. Nevertheless, the observed efficacy of recently approved anti-Aβ therapies, such as Lecanemab and Donanemab, in mitigating cognitive decline provides further evidence supporting the pathological involvement of amyloid-β (Aβ) in neurodegenerative processes [44].

Furthermore, inflammation-mediated pathways may trigger neurodegenerative diseases via the GBA. Chronic low-grade inflammation observed in older individuals may influence neuroinflammation by affecting glial cells, which may result in cognitive impairment [45]. In AD, neuroinflammation is driven by microglia [46], which can be modified to several morphological types. The hyperramified microglia are one type of activated microglia, which have an enlarged soma and thickened processes. The hyperramified microglia have been described in post-mortem AD, aged, and stressed human brains [47,48], which is possibly involved in stress-related synaptic modifications. On the other hand, dystrophic microglia are described with beading and fragmentation of the branches of the microglia [49]. Dystrophic microglia, which are observed in close proximity to Aβ deposits in the brains of postmortem AD patients, are hypothesized to represent a senescent phenotype of microglia [49,50]. In this condition, microglia lose their capacity to respond to chronic inflammatory stimuli and to perform their neuroprotective functions [47]. In a previous study, the microglia of 5xFAD mice had shorter processes and fewer branches compared to the microglia of WT mice and we observed similar microglial modifications [51]. In our data, probiotics suppressed the modifications of microglia, which can promote toxic activity and suppress the beneficial effects of microglia, leading to neuroinflammation in 5xFAD mice.

One defining pathological characteristic of the brains of patients with AD is the hyperphosphorylation of tau. In AD, patients' brains have been shown to exhibit excessive tau phosphorylation. This impedes the normal attachment of tau to microtubules, leading to AD pathology. Recently, it was proposed that probiotic intake may affect tau phosphorylation [52]. In our findings, probiotics inhibited tau hyperphosphorylation. Specifically, probiotics may suppress lipopolysaccharide (LPS)-generating bacteria and LPS-induced inflammation, which stimulates tau phosphorylation [53].

In summary, the current findings support the potential use of probiotics as an innovative therapeutic strategy for treating AD. We demonstrated the protective effect of probiotics in 5xFAD mice through several memory tests. In the cross maze, novel object recognition, and MWM tests, the probiotic treatment attenuated memory impairment in 5xFAD mice. Moreover, the neuroprotective effects of probiotics in AD were supported by a decreased accumulation of Aβ in the hippocampus and cerebral cortex. Microglial activation was also attenuated in these regions and the group that received probiotics showed a reduction in tau phosphorylation. These findings suggest a protective effect of probiotics to reduce Aβ burden, tau pathology, and microglia-mediated inflammation in the AD model. Future studies will comprehensively identify and elucidate the mechanisms of probiotics in the context of AD.

Supplementary Materials: The following supporting information can be downloaded at: https://www.mdpi.com/article/10.3390/brainsci14030208/s1, Figure S1: Recognition memory defect was alleviated by probiotics in 5xFAD mice; Figure S2: Skeletonized images of microglia; Figure S3: Additional Western blot used for the quantification of phosphorylated tau (PHF-1) in Figure 5B.

Author Contributions: W.-S.C. conceived and designed the experiments. Y.J.K. and B.-R.M. performed the experiments. Y.J.K. and B.-R.M. analyzed the data. K.Y.C. contributed reagents/materials. Y.J.K., B.-R.M. and W.-S.C. wrote the paper. All authors have read and agreed to the published version of the manuscript.

Funding: This research was funded by the R&BD program of the Korea Innovation Foundation funded by the Ministry of Science and ICT (development of the probiotics for dementia prevention based on oral metagenome, Project Number: 2022-DD-RD-0010, KYC); the KBRI Basic Research Program through the Korea Brain Research Institute, funded by the Ministry of Science and ICT (24-BR-03-05, KYC); a grant from the Korea Health Technology R&D Project through the Korea Health Industry Development Institute (KHIDI), funded by the Ministry of Health and Welfare, Republic of Korea (HR22C141105, KYC); the Basic Science Research Program through the National Research Foundation of Korea (NRF), funded by the Ministry of Education (2019R1A2C1004575, WSC); the National Research Foundation of Korea (NRF) grant funded by the Korea government (MSIT) (No. 2022R1H1A092601, WSC); and a grant of the Korea Dementia Research Project through the Korea Dementia Research Center (KDRC), funded by the Ministry of Health and Welfare and Ministry of Science and ICT, Republic of Korea (grant number: HU23C0199, WSC).

Institutional Review Board Statement: The animal study protocol was approved by the Institutional Animal Care and Use Committee of Chonnam National University (CNU IACUC-YB-2022-154, 19 December 2022; CNU IACUC-YB-2023-156, 30 November 2023).

Informed Consent Statement: Not applicable.

Data Availability Statement: The data are not not publicly available due to the confidentiality issues but are available from the corresponding author on reasonable request.

Conflicts of Interest: The author K.Y.C. is a registered director of Kolab. W.-S.C. was an advisory committee member of Kolab. The probiotics (*Bifidobacterium lactis* KL101, *Limosilactobacillus fermentum* KL271, and *Levilactobacillus brevis* KL251) were produced by Kolab, Inc. The remaining authors declare that the research was conducted in the absence of any commercial or financial relationships that could be construed as a potential conflict of interest.

References

1. Reitz, C.; Brayne, C.; Mayeux, R. Epidemiology of Alzheimer disease. *Nat. Rev. Neurol.* **2011**, *7*, 137–152. [CrossRef] [PubMed]
2. Doifode, T.; Giridharan, V.V.; Generoso, J.S.; Bhatti, G.; Collodel, A.; Schulz, P.E.; Forlenza, O.V.; Barichello, T. The impact of the microbiota-gut-brain axis on Alzheimer's disease pathophysiology. *Pharmacol. Res.* **2021**, *164*, 105314. [CrossRef] [PubMed]
3. de Rijke, T.J.; Doting, M.H.E.; van Hemert, S.; De Deyn, P.P.; van Munster, B.C.; Harmsen, H.J.M.; Sommer, I.E.C. A Systematic Review on the Effects of Different Types of Probiotics in Animal Alzheimer's Disease Studies. *Front. Psychiatry* **2022**, *13*, 879491. [CrossRef]
4. Cai, Y.; Liu, J.; Wang, B.; Sun, M.; Yang, H. Microglia in the Neuroinflammatory Pathogenesis of Alzheimer's Disease and Related Therapeutic Targets. *Front. Immunol.* **2022**, *13*, 856376. [CrossRef] [PubMed]
5. Angelucci, F.; Cechova, K.; Amlerova, J.; Hort, J. Antibiotics, gut microbiota, and Alzheimer's disease. *J. Neuroinflamm.* **2019**, *16*, 108. [CrossRef] [PubMed]
6. Xiang, S.; Ji, J.L.; Li, S.; Cao, X.P.; Xu, W.; Tan, L.; Tan, C.C. Efficacy and Safety of Probiotics for the Treatment of Alzheimer's Disease, Mild Cognitive Impairment, and Parkinson's Disease: A Systematic Review and Meta-Analysis. *Front. Aging Neurosci.* **2022**, *14*, 730036. [CrossRef]

7. Czarnik, W.; Fularski, P.; Gajewska, A.; Jakubowska, P.; Uszok, Z.; Mlynarska, E.; Rysz, J.; Franczyk, B. The Role of Intestinal Microbiota and Diet as Modulating Factors in the Course of Alzheimer's and Parkinson's Diseases. *Nutrients* **2024**, *16*, 308. [CrossRef] [PubMed]
8. Dissanayaka, D.M.S.; Jayasena, V.; Rainey-Smith, S.R.; Martins, R.N.; Fernando, W. The Role of Diet and Gut Microbiota in Alzheimer's Disease. *Nutrients* **2024**, *16*, 412. [CrossRef]
9. Lee, S.; Eom, S.; Lee, J.; Pyeon, M.; Kim, K.; Choi, K.Y.; Lee, J.H.; Shin, D.J.; Lee, K.H.; Oh, S.; et al. Probiotics that Ameliorate Cognitive Impairment through Anti-Inflammation and Anti-Oxidation in Mice. *Food Sci. Anim. Resour.* **2023**, *43*, 612–624. [CrossRef]
10. Davari, S.; Talaei, S.A.; Alaei, H.; Salami, M. Probiotics treatment improves diabetes-induced impairment of synaptic activity and cognitive function: Behavioral and electrophysiological proofs for microbiome-gut-brain axis. *Neuroscience* **2013**, *240*, 287–296. [CrossRef]
11. Agahi, A.; Hamidi, G.A.; Daneshvar, R.; Hamdieh, M.; Soheili, M.; Alinaghipour, A.; Esmaeili Taba, S.M.; Salami, M. Does Severity of Alzheimer's Disease Contribute to Its Responsiveness to Modifying Gut Microbiota? A Double Blind Clinical Trial. *Front. Neurol.* **2018**, *9*, 662. [CrossRef]
12. Webberley, T.S.; Masetti, G.; Bevan, R.J.; Kerry-Smith, J.; Jack, A.A.; Michael, D.R.; Thomas, S.; Glymenaki, M.; Li, J.; McDonald, J.A.K.; et al. The Impact of Probiotic Supplementation on Cognitive, Pathological and Metabolic Markers in a Transgenic Mouse Model of Alzheimer's Disease. *Front. Neurosci.* **2022**, *16*, 843105. [CrossRef]
13. Kim, C.S.; Cha, L.; Sim, M.; Jung, S.; Chun, W.Y.; Baik, H.W.; Shin, D.M. Probiotic Supplementation Improves Cognitive Function and Mood with Changes in Gut Microbiota in Community-Dwelling Older Adults: A Randomized, Double-Blind, Placebo-Controlled, Multicenter Trial. *J. Gerontol. A Biol. Sci. Med. Sci.* **2021**, *76*, 32–40. [CrossRef]
14. Forner, S.; Kawauchi, S.; Balderrama-Gutierrez, G.; Kramar, E.A.; Matheos, D.P.; Phan, J.; Javonillo, D.I.; Tran, K.M.; Hingco, E.; da Cunha, C.; et al. Systematic phenotyping and characterization of the 5xFAD mouse model of Alzheimer's disease. *Sci. Data* **2021**, *8*, 270. [CrossRef] [PubMed]
15. Jawhar, S.; Trawicka, A.; Jenneckens, C.; Bayer, T.A.; Wirths, O. Motor deficits, neuron loss, and reduced anxiety coinciding with axonal degeneration and intraneuronal Abeta aggregation in the 5XFAD mouse model of Alzheimer's disease. *Neurobiol. Aging* **2012**, *33*, 196.e29–196.e40. [CrossRef] [PubMed]
16. Ramasamy, V.S.; Samidurai, M.; Park, H.J.; Wang, M.; Park, R.Y.; Yu, S.Y.; Kang, H.K.; Hong, S.; Choi, W.S.; Lee, Y.Y.; et al. Avenanthramide-C Restores Impaired Plasticity and Cognition in Alzheimer's Disease Model Mice. *Mol. Neurobiol.* **2020**, *57*, 315–330. [CrossRef] [PubMed]
17. Jeong, J.; Park, H.J.; Mun, B.R.; Jang, J.K.; Choi, Y.M.; Choi, W.S. JBPOS0101 regulates amyloid beta, tau, and glial cells in an Alzheimer's disease model. *PLoS ONE* **2020**, *15*, e0237153. [CrossRef] [PubMed]
18. Delwaide, P.J.; Gyselynck-Mambourg, A.M.; Hurlet, A.; Ylieff, M. Double-blind randomized controlled study of phosphatidylserine in senile demented patients. *Acta Neurol. Scand.* **1986**, *73*, 136–140. [CrossRef] [PubMed]
19. Nair, S.; Traini, M.; Dawes, I.W.; Perrone, G.G. Genome-wide analysis of *Saccharomyces cerevisiae* identifies cellular processes affecting intracellular aggregation of Alzheimer's amyloid-beta42: Importance of lipid homeostasis. *Mol. Biol. Cell* **2014**, *25*, 2235–2249. [CrossRef] [PubMed]
20. Meng, X.; Wang, M.; Sun, G.; Ye, J.; Zhou, Y.; Dong, X.; Wang, T.; Lu, S.; Sun, X. Attenuation of Aβ25-35-induced parallel autophagic and apoptotic cell death by gypenoside XVII through the estrogen receptor-dependent activation of Nrf2/ARE pathways. *Toxicol. Appl. Pharmacol.* **2014**, *279*, 63–75. [CrossRef] [PubMed]
21. Zhang, Y.Y.; Yang, L.Q.; Guo, L.M. Effect of phosphatidylserine on memory in patients and rats with Alzheimer's disease. *Genet. Mol. Res.* **2015**, *14*, 9325–9333. [CrossRef]
22. Choi, W.S.; Kim, H.W.; Tronche, F.; Palmiter, R.D.; Storm, D.R.; Xia, Z. Conditional deletion of Ndufs4 in dopaminergic neurons promotes Parkinson's disease-like non-motor symptoms without loss of dopamine neurons. *Sci. Rep.* **2017**, *7*, 44989. [CrossRef] [PubMed]
23. Griñán-Ferré, C.; Sarroca, S.; Ivanova, A.; Puigoriol-Illamola, D.; Aguado, F.; Camins, A.; Sanfeliu, C.; Pallàs, M. Epigenetic mechanisms underlying cognitive impairment and Alzheimer disease hallmarks in 5XFAD mice. *Aging* **2016**, *8*, 664–684. [CrossRef]
24. Ennaceur, A.; Delacour, J. A new one-trial test for neurobiological studies of memory in rats. 1: Behavioral data. *Behav. Brain Res.* **1988**, *31*, 47–59. [CrossRef] [PubMed]
25. Ardestani, P.M.; Evans, A.K.; Yi, B.; Nguyen, T.; Coutellier, L.; Shamloo, M. Modulation of neuroinflammation and pathology in the 5XFAD mouse model of Alzheimer's disease using a biased and selective beta-1 adrenergic receptor partial agonist. *Neuropharmacology* **2017**, *116*, 371–386. [CrossRef] [PubMed]
26. Morrison, H.; Young, K.; Qureshi, M.; Rowe, R.K.; Lifshitz, J. Quantitative microglia analyses reveal diverse morphologic responses in the rat cortex after diffuse brain injury. *Sci. Rep.* **2017**, *7*, 13211. [CrossRef]
27. Ma, X.; Li, X.; Wang, W.; Zhang, M.; Yang, B.; Miao, Z. Phosphatidylserine, inflammation, and central nervous system diseases. *Front. Aging Neurosci.* **2022**, *14*, 975176. [CrossRef]
28. Li, Z.; Zhu, H.; Guo, Y.; Du, X.; Qin, C. Gut microbiota regulate cognitive deficits and amyloid deposition in a model of Alzheimer's disease. *J. Neurochem.* **2020**, *155*, 448–461. [CrossRef]
29. Hansen, D.V.; Hanson, J.E.; Sheng, M. Microglia in Alzheimer's disease. *J. Cell Biol.* **2018**, *217*, 459–472. [CrossRef]

30. Erny, D.; Hrabě de Angelis, A.L.; Jaitin, D.; Wieghofer, P.; Staszewski, O.; David, E.; Keren-Shaul, H.; Mahlakoiv, T.; Jakobshagen, K.; Buch, T.; et al. Host microbiota constantly control maturation and function of microglia in the CNS. *Nat. Neurosci.* **2015**, *18*, 965–977. [CrossRef]
31. Ayyubova, G. Dysfunctional microglia and tau pathology in Alzheimer's disease. *Rev. Neurosci.* **2023**, *34*, 443–458. [CrossRef]
32. Wang, C.; Fan, L.; Khawaja, R.R.; Liu, B.; Zhan, L.; Kodama, L.; Chin, M.; Li, Y.; Le, D.; Zhou, Y.; et al. Microglial NF-κB drives tau spreading and toxicity in a mouse model of tauopathy. *Nat. Commun.* **2022**, *13*, 1969. [CrossRef]
33. Stancu, I.C.; Cremers, N.; Vanrusselt, H.; Couturier, J.; Vanoosthuyse, A.; Kessels, S.; Lodder, C.; Brône, B.; Huaux, F.; Octave, J.N.; et al. Aggregated Tau activates NLRP3-ASC inflammasome exacerbating exogenously seeded and non-exogenously seeded Tau pathology in vivo. *Acta Neuropathol.* **2019**, *137*, 599–617. [CrossRef] [PubMed]
34. Bhattacharjee, S.; Lukiw, W.J. Alzheimer's disease and the microbiome. *Front. Cell. Neurosci.* **2013**, *7*, 153. [CrossRef]
35. Hsiao, E.Y.; McBride, S.W.; Hsien, S.; Sharon, G.; Hyde, E.R.; McCue, T.; Codelli, J.A.; Chow, J.; Reisman, S.E.; Petrosino, J.F.; et al. Microbiota modulate behavioral and physiological abnormalities associated with neurodevelopmental disorders. *Cell* **2013**, *155*, 1451–1463. [CrossRef] [PubMed]
36. Wang, T.; Hu, X.; Liang, S.; Li, W.; Wu, X.; Wang, L.; Jin, F. *Lactobacillus fermentum* NS9 restores the antibiotic induced physiological and psychological abnormalities in rats. *Benef. Microbes* **2015**, *6*, 707–717. [CrossRef] [PubMed]
37. Abdelhamid, M.; Zhou, C.; Ohno, K.; Kuhara, T.; Taslima, F.; Abdullah, M.; Jung, C.G.; Michikawa, M. Probiotic *Bifidobacterium breve* Prevents Memory Impairment through the Reduction of Both Amyloid-β Production and Microglia Activation in APP Knock-In Mouse. *J. Alzheimer's Dis.* **2022**, *85*, 1555–1571. [CrossRef]
38. Wang, M.; Cao, J.; Gong, C.; Amakye, W.K.; Yao, M.; Ren, J. Exploring the microbiota-Alzheimer's disease linkage using short-term antibiotic treatment followed by fecal microbiota transplantation. *Brain Behav. Immun.* **2021**, *96*, 227–238. [CrossRef]
39. Katzman, R.; Terry, R.; DeTeresa, R.; Brown, T.; Davies, P.; Fuld, P.; Renbing, X.; Peck, A. Clinical, pathological, and neurochemical changes in dementia: A subgroup with preserved mental status and numerous neocortical plaques. *Ann. Neurol.* **1988**, *23*, 138–144. [CrossRef]
40. Dickson, D.W.; Crystal, H.A.; Mattiace, L.A.; Masur, D.M.; Blau, A.D.; Davies, P.; Yen, S.H.; Aronson, M.K. Identification of normal and pathological aging in prospectively studied nondemented elderly humans. *Neurobiol. Aging* **1992**, *13*, 179–189. [CrossRef]
41. Aizenstein, H.J.; Nebes, R.D.; Saxton, J.A.; Price, J.C.; Mathis, C.A.; Tsopelas, N.D.; Ziolko, S.K.; James, J.A.; Snitz, B.E.; Houck, P.R.; et al. Frequent amyloid deposition without significant cognitive impairment among the elderly. *Arch. Neurol.* **2008**, *65*, 1509–1517. [CrossRef] [PubMed]
42. Chetelat, G.; La Joie, R.; Villain, N.; Perrotin, A.; de La Sayette, V.; Eustache, F.; Vandenberghe, R. Amyloid imaging in cognitively normal individuals, at-risk populations and preclinical Alzheimer's disease. *Neuroimage Clin.* **2013**, *2*, 356–365. [CrossRef] [PubMed]
43. Ossenkoppele, R.; Jansen, W.J.; Rabinovici, G.D.; Knol, D.L.; van der Flier, W.M.; van Berckel, B.N.; Scheltens, P.; Visser, P.J.; Amyloid, P.E.T.S.G.; Verfaillie, S.C.; et al. Prevalence of amyloid PET positivity in dementia syndromes: A meta-analysis. *JAMA* **2015**, *313*, 1939–1949. [CrossRef] [PubMed]
44. Cummings, J.; Osse, A.M.L.; Cammann, D.; Powell, J.; Chen, J. Anti-Amyloid Monoclonal Antibodies for the Treatment of Alzheimer's Disease. *BioDrugs* **2024**, *38*, 5–22. [CrossRef] [PubMed]
45. Di Benedetto, S.; Müller, L.; Wenger, E.; Düzel, S.; Pawelec, G. Contribution of neuroinflammation and immunity to brain aging and the mitigating effects of physical and cognitive interventions. *Neurosci. Biobehav. Rev.* **2017**, *75*, 114–128. [CrossRef] [PubMed]
46. Heppner, F.L.; Ransohoff, R.M.; Becher, B. Immune attack: The role of inflammation in Alzheimer disease. *Nat. Rev. Neurosci.* **2015**, *16*, 358–372. [CrossRef]
47. Bachstetter, A.D.; Van Eldik, L.J.; Schmitt, F.A.; Neltner, J.H.; Ighodaro, E.T.; Webster, S.J.; Patel, E.; Abner, E.L.; Kryscio, R.J.; Nelson, P.T. Disease-related microglia heterogeneity in the hippocampus of Alzheimer's disease, dementia with Lewy bodies, and hippocampal sclerosis of aging. *Acta Neuropathol. Commun.* **2015**, *3*, 32. [CrossRef]
48. Smith, K.L.; Kassem, M.S.; Clarke, D.J.; Kuligowski, M.P.; Bedoya-Perez, M.A.; Todd, S.M.; Lagopoulos, J.; Bennett, M.R.; Arnold, J.C. Microglial cell hyper-ramification and neuronal dendritic spine loss in the hippocampus and medial prefrontal cortex in a mouse model of PTSD. *Brain Behav. Immun.* **2019**, *80*, 889–899. [CrossRef]
49. Streit, W.J.; Sammons, N.W.; Kuhns, A.J.; Sparks, D.L. Dystrophic microglia in the aging human brain. *Glia* **2004**, *45*, 208–212. [CrossRef]
50. Streit, W.J.; Braak, H.; Xue, Q.S.; Bechmann, I. Dystrophic (senescent) rather than activated microglial cells are associated with tau pathology and likely precede neurodegeneration in Alzheimer's disease. *Acta Neuropathol.* **2009**, *118*, 475–485. [CrossRef]
51. Chen, W.; Abud, E.A.; Yeung, S.T.; Lakatos, A.; Nassi, T.; Wang, J.; Blum, D.; Buee, L.; Poon, W.W.; Blurton-Jones, M. Increased tauopathy drives microglia-mediated clearance of beta-amyloid. *Acta Neuropathol. Commun.* **2016**, *4*, 63. [CrossRef] [PubMed]

52. Flynn, C.M.; Yuan, Q. Probiotic supplement as a promising strategy in early tau pathology prevention: Focusing on GSK-3beta? *Front. Neurosci.* **2023**, *17*, 1159314. [CrossRef] [PubMed]
53. Chen, Y.; Yu, Y. Tau and neuroinflammation in Alzheimer's disease: Interplay mechanisms and clinical translation. *J. Neuroinflamm.* **2023**, *20*, 165. [CrossRef] [PubMed]

Disclaimer/Publisher's Note: The statements, opinions and data contained in all publications are solely those of the individual author(s) and contributor(s) and not of MDPI and/or the editor(s). MDPI and/or the editor(s) disclaim responsibility for any injury to people or property resulting from any ideas, methods, instructions or products referred to in the content.

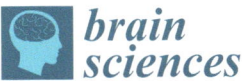

Article

Intranasal Administration of Apelin-13 Ameliorates Cognitive Deficit in Streptozotocin-Induced Alzheimer's Disease Model via Enhancement of Nrf2-HO1 Pathways

Hai Lu [1,2], Ming Chen [1] and Cuiqing Zhu [1,*]

[1] State Key Laboratory of Medical Neurobiology, Institutes of Brain Science, MOE Frontier Center for Brain Science, Fudan University, Shanghai 200032, China; 15111010013@fudan.edu.cn (H.L.); ming_chen@fudan.edu.cn (M.C.)
[2] College of Clinical Medicine, Jining Medical University, Jining 272067, China
* Correspondence: cqzhu@shmu.edu.cn; Tel.: +86-21-54237858

Abstract: Background: The discovery of novel diagnostic methods and therapies for Alzheimer's disease (AD) faces significant challenges. Previous research has shed light on the neuroprotective properties of Apelin-13 in neurodegenerative disorders. However, elucidating the mechanism underlying its efficacy in combating AD-related nerve injury is imperative. In this study, we aimed to investigate Apelin-13's mechanism of action in an in vivo model of AD induced by streptozocin (STZ). Methods: We utilized an STZ-induced nerve injury model of AD in mice to investigate the effects of Apelin-13 administration. Apelin-13 was administered intranasally, and cognitive impairment was assessed using standardized behavioral tests, primarily, behavioral assessment, histological analysis, and biochemical assays, in order to evaluate synaptic plasticity and oxidative stress signaling pathways. Results: Our findings indicate that intranasal administration of Apelin-13 ameliorated cognitive impairment in the STZ-induced AD model. Furthermore, we observed that this effect was potentially mediated by the enhancement of synaptic plasticity and the attenuation of oxidative stress signaling pathways. Conclusions: The results of this study suggest that intranasal administration of Apelin-13 holds promise as a therapeutic strategy for preventing neurodegenerative diseases such as AD. By improving synaptic plasticity and mitigating oxidative stress, Apelin-13 may offer a novel approach to neuroprotection in AD and related conditions.

Keywords: Alzheimer's disease; apelin-13; intranasal administration; oxidative stress; Nrf2-HO-1 signaling pathway

1. Introduction

Alzheimer's disease (AD) presents a formidable challenge in terms of diagnosis and treatment, spurring intensified research efforts. The apelin system has recently garnered attention for its potential involvement in AD pathogenesis, as evidenced by an expanding body of literature [1,2].

Apelin, a biologically active peptide hormone, originates from fat cells [3]. It exists in three active forms, comprising either 13, 17, or 36 amino acids, derived from a 77-amino-acid prepropeptide precursor by an angiotensin-converting enzyme [4,5]. Notably, Apelin-13 demonstrates significantly greater biological potency than Apelin-36 [4]. The apelin system has demonstrated therapeutic potential across various acute and chronic neurological conditions [6]. Studies have shown its efficacy in alleviating acute brain injuries, such as subarachnoid hemorrhage, traumatic brain injury, and ischemic stroke. Additionally, it has been found to have therapeutic effects on chronic neurodegenerative disease models, involving the regulation of neurotrophic factors, neuroendocrine signaling, oxidative stress, neuroinflammation, neuronal apoptosis, and autophagy [1,7,8]. Moreover, apelin exhibits neuroprotective properties by mitigating oxidative damage in neurons. In vivo experiments have shown that apelin's ability to combat reactive oxygen species (ROS) and free radicals is closely related to its neuroprotective effects against neurodegenerative diseases [9].

Apelin-13 and its receptor APJ are widely distributed in the hippocampus and other brain tissues. The intracerebroventricular injection of Apelin-13 improved stress-induced memory function decline in rats [10], indicating that apelin/APJ signaling may be involved in cognitive ability [11,12]. Moreover, apelin has been implicated in enhancing the function of various factors, including GLP-1, eNO, and ACE2, thereby promoting synaptic plasticity and improving learning and memory. Additionally, apelin exerts a neuroprotective effect by attenuating inflammatory responses through the BDNF signaling pathway [13]. Furthermore, apelin can modulate amyloid-beta (Aβ) metabolism by reducing amyloid precursor protein (APP) levels and inhibiting β-secretase activity, leading to decreased Aβ production and increased Aβ clearance mediated by ABCA1 and NEP. Additionally, apelin may mitigate tau protein phosphorylation and accumulation. Studies have reported that apelin can prevent neurodegeneration by reducing levels of inflammatory mediators, particularly TNF-α and IL-1β, and inhibit neuronal apoptosis by modulating the balance of anti-apoptotic and pro-apoptotic factors [14]. These findings underscore the multifaceted neuroprotective effects of apelin, suggesting its potential as a therapeutic target in Alzheimer's disease intervention.

While oxidative stress is recognized as a crucial mechanism underlying Apelin-13's anti-AD effects, the specific oxidative stress pathway through which apelin mitigates AD-related neurological damage requires further investigation. To assess the effectiveness of Apelin-13, we employed STZ-induced AD mice as an in vivo model system and included donepezil, a standard AD therapeutic, as a positive control. By analyzing parameters such as cognitive function, synaptic plasticity, oxidative stress markers, and signaling pathways, we aimed to clarify the therapeutic potential of Apelin-13 and its mechanism of action. Employing a range of methodological approaches, our study aims to elucidate the precise molecular pathways through which Apelin-13 exerts its neuroprotective effects against AD-associated oxidative stress. The novelty and scientific significance of our study lie in the exploration of intranasal Apelin-13 administration as a potential therapeutic strategy for AD, offering insights into its neuroprotective effects and underlying mechanisms.

2. Materials and Methods

2.1. Experimental Animals

Male adult C57BL/6J mice, aged between 8 and 12 weeks, were accommodated in a controlled environment with a 12 h light/dark cycle, ensuring regulated temperature and humidity levels. They had ad libitum access to food and water throughout the study period. All experimental procedures adhered to the ethical guidelines established by Fudan University and international standards for animal research. Approval for the animal study protocol was granted by the Animal Care and Use Committee of the Shanghai Medical College of Fudan University (No. 20170223-098). Every effort was taken to minimize animal discomfort and to optimize the utilization of animals in the study.

2.2. Experimental Protocol

Mice were categorized in a random manner into different groups (10 animals each). Group 1 served as the control group and received ICV saline (0.9%). Group 2 was the STZ-induced AD group, receiving 3 mg/kg STZ (ICV) based on previous studies [15]. Group 3 was the positive control group, treated with donepezil at a dose of 5 mg/kg/day via oral administration. Groups 4 and 5 received a single dose of 3 mg/kg STZ (ICV). Two days later, Group 4 received nasal administration of Apelin-13 at a dose of 1 mg/kg, while Group 5 received nasal administration of Apelin-13 at a dose of 0.2 mg/kg. Behavioral testing was performed sequentially after the injected program ended. Following the final behavioral assessment, the animals were euthanized and sampled. Specifically, three rats from each group were selected for electrophysiological tests, while another three rats were utilized for biochemical analyses and Western blot tests, depending on the specific objectives of the experiment.

2.3. Drug Administration

For nasal administration, the Apelin-13 (0.2 mg/kg, 1 mg/kg) solution (10 µL) was pipetted bilaterally on the rhinarium, i.e., the glabrous skin around the nostrils, and allowed to diffuse in the squamous epithelium. After the drip, the mouse was fixed for 5–10 s to ensure the liquid was fully inhaled. Donepezil (Sigma-Aldrich, St. Louis, MO, USA) were dissolved in 0.9% saline. A freshly prepared solution of donepezil was administered orally daily at a dose of 5 mg/kg [16]. ML385 (Medchem Express, South Brunswick, NJ, USA) is a specific inhibitor of Nrf2. Before each administration of Apelin-13, the mice received an intraperitoneal injection of 30 mg/kg ML385 [17], dissolved in saline containing 50% PEG300, with a 30 min interval. Zn(II)-protoporphyrin IX (ZnPP, Medchem Express, South Brunswick, NJ, USA) is an inhibitor of HO-1. Mice were injected intraperitoneally with 25 mg/kg ZnPP [18] (dissolved in saline) 30 min before each administration of Apelin-13.

2.4. Stereotaxic Surgery

Mice were anesthetized via a mixture of ketamine and xylazine and, then, secured onto a stereotaxic apparatus (Stoelting Apparatus, Wood Dale, IL, USA). To induce an STZ-AD mouse model, STZ (3 mg/kg, ICV) was bilaterally injected into the lateral ventricles. Control mice underwent the same procedure but received a vehicle injection of the citrate buffer 0.05 mol/L, pH 4.5. STZ was freshly diluted in the citrate buffer prior to injection. The injections were administered using a Hamilton syringe (model 705, Hamilton Company, Giarmata, Romania) with the following coordinates relative to the bregma: AP -0.5 mm, ML ±1.1 mm, and DV -2.8 mm. Each lateral ventricle was infused with a total infusion of 1.5 µL of STZ or citrate buffer at a rate of 0.5 µL/min.

2.5. Morris Water Maze Test

The Morris water maze (MWM) test was conducted following previously established protocols [19]. Each group consisted of eight male mice. Throughout the training phase, the platform was located in the same position (one of the four pool quadrants). Each mouse was placed into the pool facing the wall at one of the four starting positions, and its movement was tracked using a digital tracking system. If a mouse reached the platform, it was immediately removed from the water. In case a mouse failed to locate the platform within 60 s during the training trials, it was gently guided to the platform or given an additional 15 s on the platform before being withdrawn from the pool. The animals underwent four daily trials over five consecutive days, with approximately 30 min intervals between trials. On the sixth day following the final training session, a probe trial was conducted. During this trial, the platform was removed from the pool, and each mouse was placed in the pool facing the wall from the diagonally opposite side of the platform. The mice were allowed to swim freely for 2 min while their movements were recorded using EthoVision software (Version XT6.1), after which they were removed from the pool.

2.6. Y-Maze Test

The Y-maze utilized in this study was constructed from opaque and non-reflective materials to ensure consistent testing conditions. Each arm of the maze contained distinct visual cues to facilitate spatial orientation for the mice. During testing, mice were individually placed at the end of one arm with their heads facing the central area of the maze. Two prominent markers were positioned opposite each other within the maze to serve as visual cues. Mice were then allowed to freely explore the maze for a duration of 8 min. Video recordings of the mouse's movement trajectory were captured from above the maze using Anymaze software (Version 4.99). A mouse was considered to have entered an arm when all four of its limbs entered that arm. The three arms of the maze were designated as a, b, and c. If a mouse sequentially entered three different arms, it was deemed to have exhibited spontaneous alternation behavior. The correct rate of spontaneous alternation was calculated by subtracting 2 from the total number of completed alternations and dividing by the total number of arm entries, multiplied by 100. Between each test session, the inner surface of the maze was cleaned with 75% alcohol to eliminate residual olfactory cues and maintain consistent testing conditions for subsequent trials.

2.7. In Vitro Electrophysiology

Electrophysiology procedures were conducted following previously established methods [20]. Upon quick dissection, brains were immersed in artificial cerebrospinal fluid (ACSF) with the following composition: 125 mM NaCl, 2.5 mM KCl, 2 mM $CaCl_2$, 1 mM $MgCl_2$, 25 mM $NaHCO_3$, 1.25 mM NaH_2PO_4, and 10 mM glucose, and then, saturated with 95% O_2 and 5% CO_2 at approximately 0 °C. Coronal brain slices (300 μm thick) were prepared using a vibratome and transferred to a chamber maintained at 31 °C. Slices were allowed to incubate for at least 1 h before commencing patch-clamp recording. Neurons targeted for whole-cell patch-clamp recording were accessed using glass electrodes with a resistance ranging from 5 to 8 MΩ when filled with the patch pipette solution. The internal solution of the electrode comprised 115 mM CsMeSO$_3$, 10 mM HEPES, 2.5 mM $MgCl_2$, 20 mM $CsCl_2$, 0.6 mM EGTA, 10 mM Na phosphocreatine, 0.4 mM Na-GTP, and 4 mM Mg-ATP. Each experimental group included three male mice for long-term potentiation (LTP) recording. Excitatory postsynaptic currents (EPSCs) were recorded in CA1 neurons, with a concentrated stimulating electrode placed in the Schaffer collaterals. LTP was induced using the 3× theta burst stimulation protocol (TBS), involving four pulses at 100 Hz repeated with 200 ms inter-burst intervals. The average EPSC amplitudes 30 min after LTP induction in each group were compared to assess potential differences in LTP magnitude among the groups. Data acquisition and analysis were performed using pClamp10.7 and Clampfit 10.7 (Axopatch 700B, Molecular Devices, San Jose, CA, USA).

2.8. The Detection of Oxidative Stress Levels

Hippocampal tissues were collected from each group for cell disruption using a sonicator (Huxi Company, Shanghai, China), followed by centrifugation at 3500 r/min for 10 min. Supernatants from groups 1–5 were analyzed to measure the activities of the antioxidant enzymes of superoxide dismutase (SOD), glutathione peroxidase (GSH-Px), catalase (CAT), and the concentration of alondialdehyde (MDA). The SOD (A001-1-2), MDA (A00-1-2), CAT (A007-1-1), and GSH-Px (A005-1-2) test kits were acquired from the Nanjing Jiancheng Biological Research Institute, China. Specifically, SOD and CAT were measured using Coomassie brilliant blue and hydroxylamine methods, respectively. MDA levels were determined through the ammonium molybdate method, while GSH-Px levels were analyzed using the thiobarbituric acid colorimetric method.

2.9. Western Blot Analysis

Upon treatment, tissues were rinsed and, then, immersed in PBS before being subjected to centrifugation. Cell lysis was conducted at 4 °C by vigorously shaking for 15 min in RIPA buffer comprising 150 mM NaCl, 1% NP-40, 0.5% sodium deoxycholate, 0.1% SDS, 50 mM Tris–HCl (pH 7.4), 50 mM β-glycerol phosphate, 20 mM NaF, 20 mM EGTA, 1 mM DTT, and 1 mM Na_3VO_4, along with protease inhibitors. Subsequent to centrifugation at 15,000 rpm for 15 min, the supernatant was isolated and stored at −70 °C until further use. Protein concentration was determined utilizing the Bradford method, and the lysates were boiled for 5 min. Denatured proteins were resolved via sodium dodecyl sulfate–polyacrylamide gel electrophoresis on 8% or 10% polyacrylamide gels and, then, transferred onto PVDF membranes (Millipore, Billerica, MA, USA). Following overnight blocking at 4 °C in 5% BSA in Tris-buffered saline/Tween [containing 0.05% (*v/v*) Tween 20], the membranes were incubated with specific antibodies at dilutions of 1:2000 [phospho-ERK1/2 (Thr202/Tyr204) (Abcam, Cambridge, UK, ab278538), ERK (Abcam, ab32537), anti-Nrf2 (MedChemExpress, South Brunswick, NJ, USA, YA895), and anti-HO-1 (Millipore, 374087)]. A subsequent incubation was performed using a horseradish peroxidase-conjugated secondary anti-rabbit IgG antibody (dilutions of 1:5000, Signalway Antibody, L3012). Blots were developed using the ECL Western blotting detection reagent (Santa Cruz Biotechnology, Dallas, TX, USA).

2.10. Statistical Analysis

Numerical data are presented as mean ± SEM. Analysis of offline data was conducted using Clampfit software (Version 10.5, Axon Instruments, San Jose, CA, USA) and GraphPad Prism 6 (GraphPad Software, La Jolla, CA, USA). Statistical significance was assessed by ANOVA followed by Bonferroni post-tests for multiple comparisons among groups. For electrophysiological tests, 'n' represents the number of cells, with each cell group in every experiment sourced from a minimum of four animals. The threshold for statistical significance was set at $p < 0.05$.

3. Results

3.1. Intranasal Administration of Apelin-13 Improves Cognitive Impairment in STZ-Induced Animal Model of AD Mice

The Morris water maze and Y-maze tests were conducted after 30 days of intranasal Apelin-13 treatment in an STZ-induced animal model of AD to determine whether intranasal administration of Apelin-13 improves spatial learning and memory. We designed parallel positive drug control experiments using donepezil as an effective positive control. First, we examined the open-field behavior of the different treatment groups, and the experimental results showed that there were no differences in the total movement distance of the different drug treatment groups within the 15 min test time (Figure 1B, $n = 7$–10, one-way ANOVA, $p > 0.05$). There were no differences between the different treatment groups in terms of movement time or proportion of edge movement (Figure 1C,D, $n = 7$–10, one-way ANOVA, $p > 0.05$). Trace records (Figure 1E) showed that the swimming trajectory of the STZ-induced AD mice in the target quadrant was shorter than that of the control mice and Apelin-13-treated mice. There was no significant difference in swimming speed between the groups (Figure 1F). The STZ-induced AD mice required more time to find the target quadrant and performed fewer platform crossings. Furthermore, both parameters significantly improved after Apelin-13 treatment in the STZ-induced animal model of AD (Figure 1G, H, $n = 7$–10, one-way ANOVA, $p < 0.05$).

In the Y-maze test (Figure 1I), there was no significant difference in the total number of entries between the different groups (Figure 1J, $n = 7$–10, one-way ANOVA, $p > 0.05$). No significant difference in the alternation ratio between the control and high-Apelin-13 treatment group existed. However, the alternation rate of the high-Apelin-13 treatment group was higher than that of the STZ-induced AD group (Figure 1K, $n = 7$–10, one-way ANOVA, $p < 0.05$). In summary, our data indicate that the intranasal administration of Apelin-13 effectively improves cognitive impairment in an STZ-induced animal model of AD.

3.2. Intranasal Administration of Apelin-13 Restores LTP in CA1 Neurons of STZ-Induced AD Mice

We measured evoked EPSC and LTP in hippocampal slices to investigate the effect of intranasal Apelin-13 administration on synaptic plasticity in the CA1 region of the hippocampus. Figure 2A shows representative EPSC traces before and after TBS stimulation in the four groups of mice used in this study. The ratio of LTP was significantly reduced in the STZ-induced animal model of AD compared to that in control mice. The depression of LTP 30 min after TBS in the STZ-induced animal model of AD treated with Apelin-13 confirmed that Apelin-13 significantly enhances the magnitude of LTP (Figure 2B,C, $n = 8$, one-way ANOVA, $p < 0.05$). These data confirm that intranasal administration of Apelin-13 can rescue impaired LTP in APP/PS1 mice.

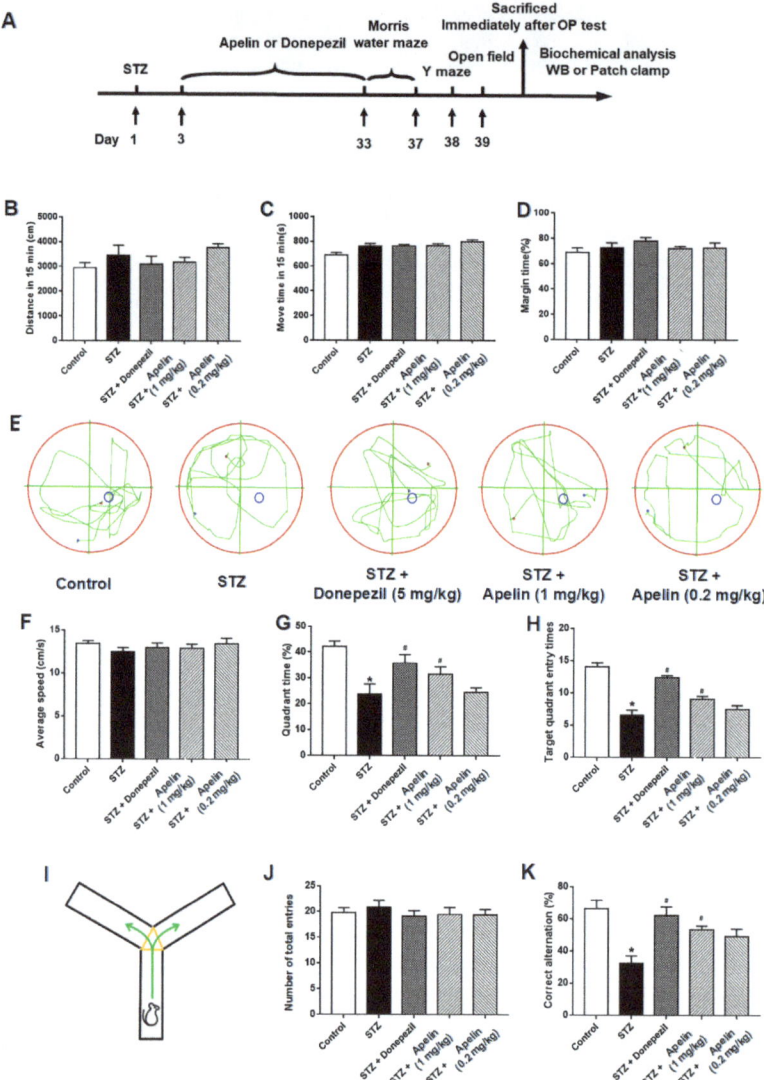

Figure 1. Effect of intranasal administration of Apelin-13 on cognitive impairment in STZ-induced animal model of AD mice. (**A**) Experimental timeline. (**B**) Distance of mouse movement during the 15 min test period for different groups (one-way ANOVA, $p > 0.05$). (**C**) Movement time during the 15 min test period for different groups (one-way ANOVA, $p > 0.05$). (**D**) Percentage of time spent in the margin area for different groups (one-way ANOVA, $p > 0.05$). (**E**) The swimming trajectory of mice during the probe test, Blue and red dots represent the starting and ending points of the mouse trajectories, respectively. Blue circles indicate the location of the platform. (**F**) Average speed of different groups (one-way ANOVA, $p > 0.05$). (**G**) Quadrant time of different groups (one-way ANOVA, * $p < 0.05$ compared to the control group, # $p < 0.05$ compared to the STZ treatment group). (**H**) Target quadrant entry times of different groups (one-way ANOVA, * $p < 0.05$ compared to the control group, # $p < 0.05$ compared to the STZ treatment group). (**I**) Y-maze test. (**J**) Number of arm entrances of different groups (one-way ANOVA, $p > 0.05$). (**K**) Alternation ratio of different groups (one-way ANOVA, * $p < 0.05$ compared to control group, # $p < 0.05$ compared to STZ treatment group). Data are shown as the mean ± s.e.m.

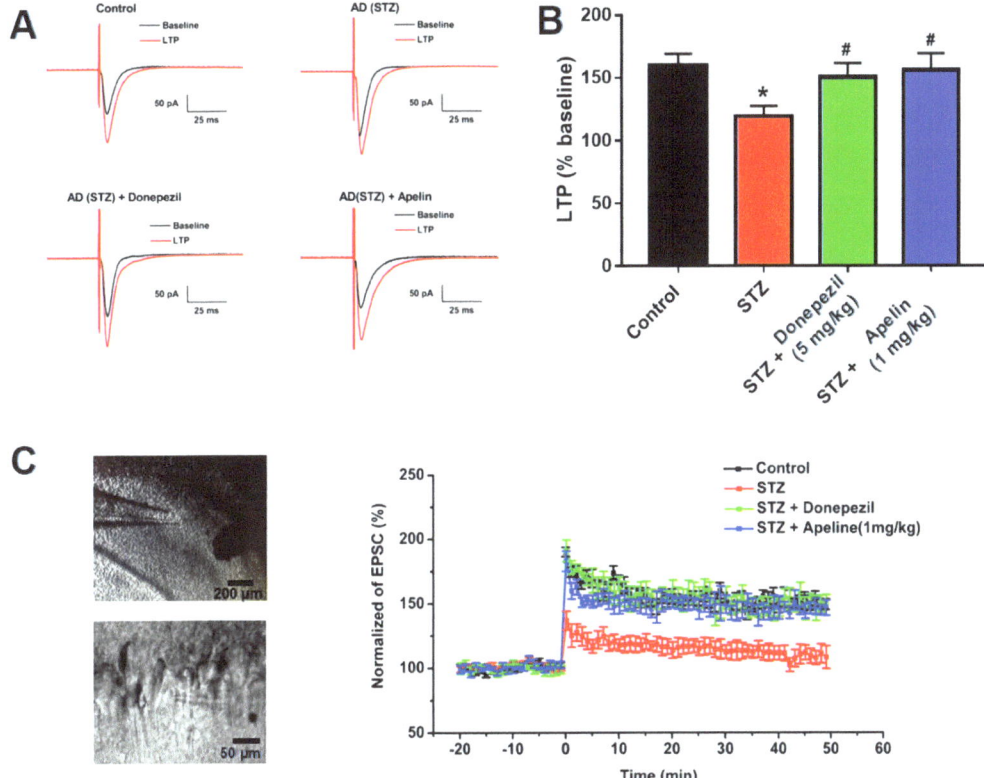

Figure 2. Effect of intranasal administration of Apelin-13 on LTP in CA1 neurons of STZ-induced AD mice. (**A**) Typical traces in different treatment groups. (**B**) Bar graphs showing changes in LTP for different treatment groups ($n = 6$, one-way ANOVA, * $p < 0.05$ compared to control, # $p < 0.05$ compared to STZ treatment group). (**C**) Left: Typical recording cell images (upper panel: bar = 200 μm, lower panel: bar = 50 μm). Right: Time course of the LTP in different treatment groups ($n = 6$). Data are shown as the mean ± s.e.m.

3.3. Intranasal Administration of Apelin-13 Reduces the Oxidative Stress of the Hippocampus in STZ-Induced AD Mice

Many in vivo experiments have shown that Apelin-13 can improve oxidative stress-related indicators in animal models of AD [13]. Therefore, we used biochemical methods to observe the performance of a series of oxidative-stress-related systems in the different treatment groups. After the behavioral tests were performed for each group, we measured the activity of superoxide dismutase (SOD), glutathione peroxidase (GSH-Px), catalase (CAT), and the level of malondialdehyde (MDA) in the hippocampal tissue. The results showed that the activities of SOD, GSH, and CAT in the STZ-induced AD mouse model were significantly lower than those in the control group, and the level of MDA was increased, which was consistent with previous reports [21,22]. Donepezil treatment improved these oxidative stress indicators in an animal model of STZ-induced AD. High and low doses of Apelin-13 also improved these oxidative stress indicators in the STZ-induced AD mice (Figure 3, $n = 3$, one-way ANOVA, $p < 0.05$). These results indicate that intranasal administration of Apelin-13 can reduce oxidative stress by improving the free radical scavenging capacity in vivo.

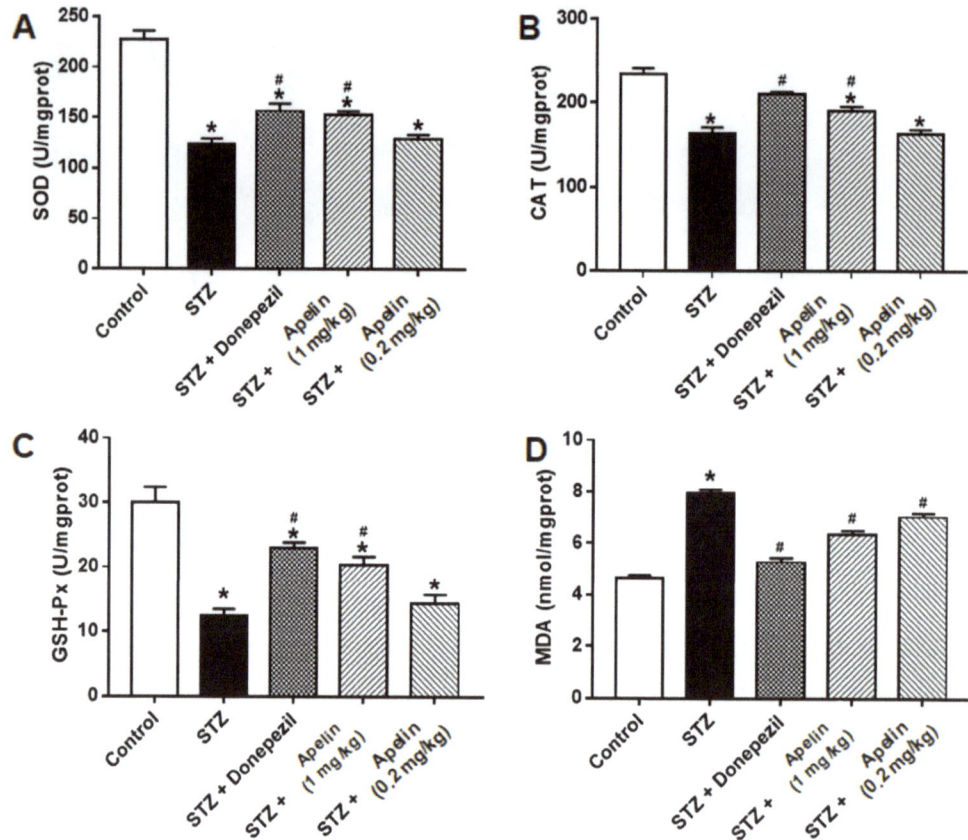

Figure 3. Effect of intranasal administration of Apelin-13 on STZ-induced oxidative stress in the hippocampus. (**A**) Specific activity (U/mg) of SOD in each treatment group (n = 3, one-way ANOVA, * $p < 0.05$ compared to control, # $p < 0.05$ compared to STZ treatment group). (**B**) Specific activity (U/mg) of CAT in each treatment group (n = 3, one-way ANOVA, * $p < 0.05$ compared to control, # $p < 0.05$ compared to STZ treatment group). (**C**) Specific activity (U/mg) of GSH in each treatment group (n = 3, one-way ANOVA, * $p < 0.05$ compared to control, # $p < 0.05$ compared to STZ treatment group). (**D**) The level (nmol/mg) of MDA in each treatment group (n = 3, one-way ANOVA, * $p < 0.05$ compared to control, # $p < 0.05$ compared to STZ treatment group). Data are shown as the mean ± s.e.m.

3.4. Effect of Intranasal Administration of Apelin-13 on the Expression of ERK-Nrf2-HO-1 in STZ-Induced AD Mice

After confirming that the intranasal administration of apelin could improve oxidative stress factors in the hippocampus, we further verified the signaling pathway through which apelin exerts its anti-oxidative stress effect. Previous studies have shown that Aβ25-35 treatment can inhibit the expression of Nrf2 and HO-1 in SH-SY5Y cells [20]. These findings indicate that Apelin-13 may exert anti-neural-injury effects in AD cell models by activating the Nrf2-HO-1 pathway.

First, we examined whether ERK, the classic upstream molecule of the Nrf2-HO-1 signaling pathway, changes in hippocampal tissue. The results showed that STZ caused an increase in the expression of phosphorylated ERK and that this increase was not altered by the positive control drugs donepezil and Apelin-13 (Figure 4A, n = 3, one-way ANOVA,

$p < 0.05$). These results suggest that phosphorylated ERK protein may not be involved in the anti-AD damage mechanism of Apelin-13 administered intranasally.

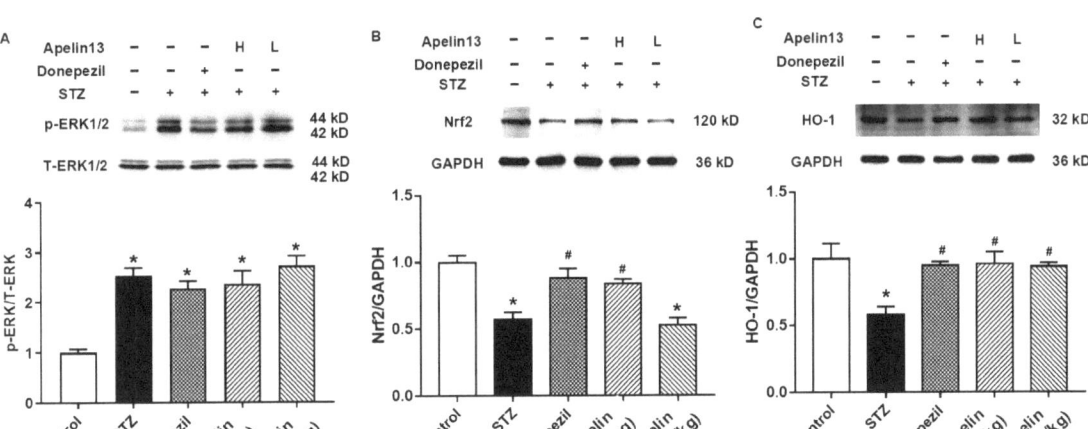

Figure 4. Effect of intranasal administration of Apelin-13 on the expression of ERK-Nrf2-HO-1 in STZ-induced AD mice. (**A**) Representative image of immunoblots and densitometric analysis of changes in levels of ERK family proteins in different treatment groups ($n = 3$, one-way ANOVA, * $p < 0.05$ compared to control). (**B**) Representative image of immunoblots and densitometric analysis of changes in levels of Nrf2 proteins in different treatment groups ($n = 3$, one-way ANOVA, * $p < 0.05$ compared to control, # $p < 0.05$ compared to STZ treatment group). (**C**) Representative image of immunoblots and densitometric analysis of changes in levels of HO-1 proteins in different treatment groups ($n = 3$, one-way ANOVA, * $p < 0.05$ compared to control, # $p < 0.05$ compared to STZ treatment group). Data are shown as the mean ± s.e.m.

We then observed the expression of Nrf2 and HO-1 proteins in the different treatment groups. The results showed that both proteins decreased in the STZ-induced animal model of AD. This effect can be altered by donepezil and high-dose Apelin-13. There was no difference in Nrf2 and HO-1 expression between the donepezil and high-dose Apelin-13 treatment groups and the control group (Figure 4B,C, $n = 3$, one-way ANOVA, $p < 0.05$). These results indicate that the Nrf2-HO-1 signaling pathway may be one of the mechanisms of action of Apelin-13 against STZ-induced nerve injury.

3.5. Inhibition of Nrf2 and HO-1 Pathways Attenuates Cognitive Benefits of Intranasal Apelin-13 Administration in STZ-Induced AD Mice

Furthermore, to elucidate the involvement of the Nrf2-HO-1 pathway in the behavioral effects of Apelin-13, we investigated the involvement of the Nrf2-HO-1 pathway in mediating the cognitive effects of Apelin-13. Mice were treated with the Nrf2 (ML385, 30 mg/kg) or HO-1 inhibitors (ZnPP, 25 mg/kg) before receiving high-dose Apelin-13, followed by an assessment of spatial learning and memory in the Morris water maze and Y-maze tests (Figure 5A).

The Morris water maze test revealed that mice treated with high-dose Apelin-13 exhibited significantly improved spatial learning compared to the control group. However, pretreatment with the Nrf2 inhibitor or the HO-1 inhibitor attenuated these improvements, as evidenced by the shorter time in the target quadrant and the fewer platform crossings compared to the Apelin-13-treated group (Figure 5B–D, $n = 8$, one-way ANOVA, $p < 0.05$).

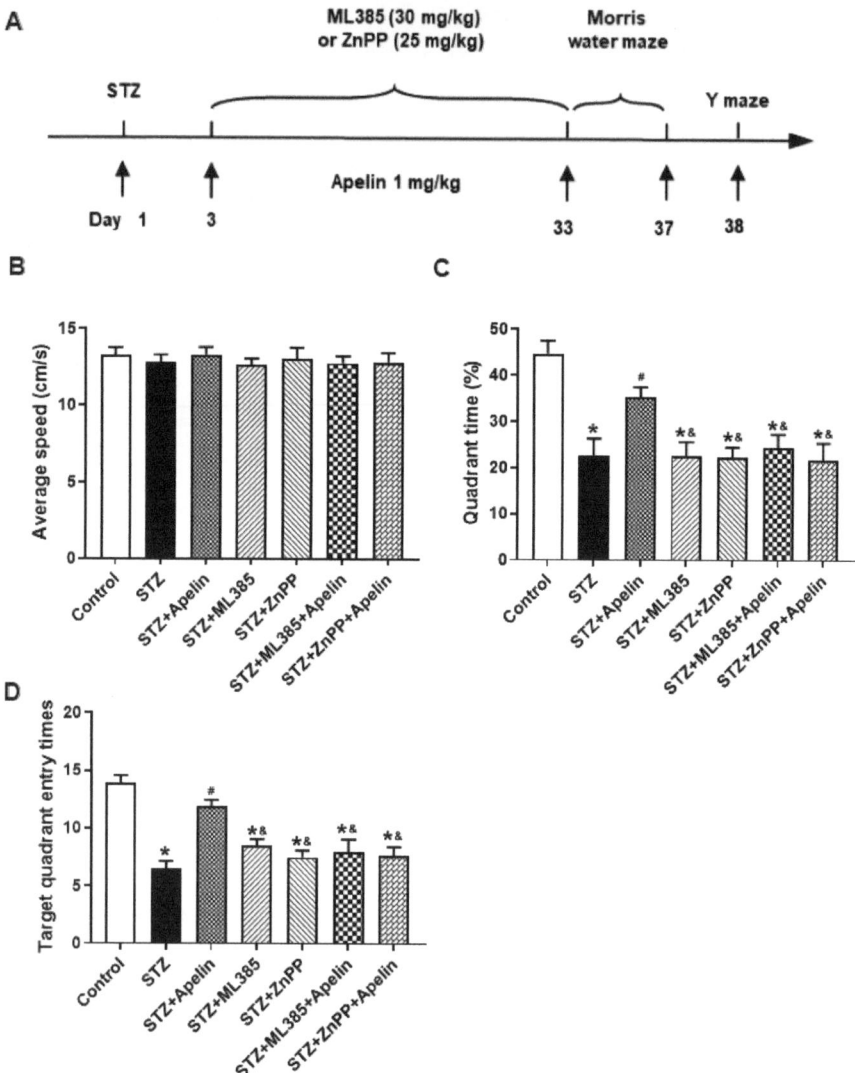

Figure 5. Effect of Nrf2-HO-1 pathway blockade on Apelin-13-mediated improvement of Morris maze performance in STZ-induced AD mice. (**A**) Experimental timeline. (**B**) Average speed of different groups (one-way ANOVA, $p > 0.05$). (**C**) Quadrant time of different groups ($n = 8$, one-way ANOVA, * $p < 0.05$ compared to the control group, # $p < 0.05$ compared to STZ treatment group, & $p < 0.05$ compared to STZ+Apelin-13 treatment group). (**D**) Target quadrant entry times in different groups ($n = 8$, one-way ANOVA, * $p < 0.05$ compared to the control group, # $p < 0.05$ compared to STZ treatment group, & $p < 0.05$ compared to STZ+Apelin-13 treatment group). Data are shown as the mean ± s.e.m.

In the Y-maze test, mice administered high-dose Apelin-13 demonstrated enhanced alternation behavior, indicative of improved spatial working memory, compared to the control group. Conversely, pretreatment with the Nrf2 inhibitor or the HO-1 inhibitor reversed this effect, resulting in a significant decrease in alternation behavior compared to the Apelin-13-treated group (Figure 6B,C, $n = 8$, one-way ANOVA, $p < 0.05$). The results revealed that pretreatment with the Nrf2 inhibitor or the HO-1 inhibitor abolished the cognitive improvement induced by Apelin-13, suggesting that the Nrf2-HO-1 pathway may play a crucial role in mediating the behavioral effects of Apelin-13 in AD mice.

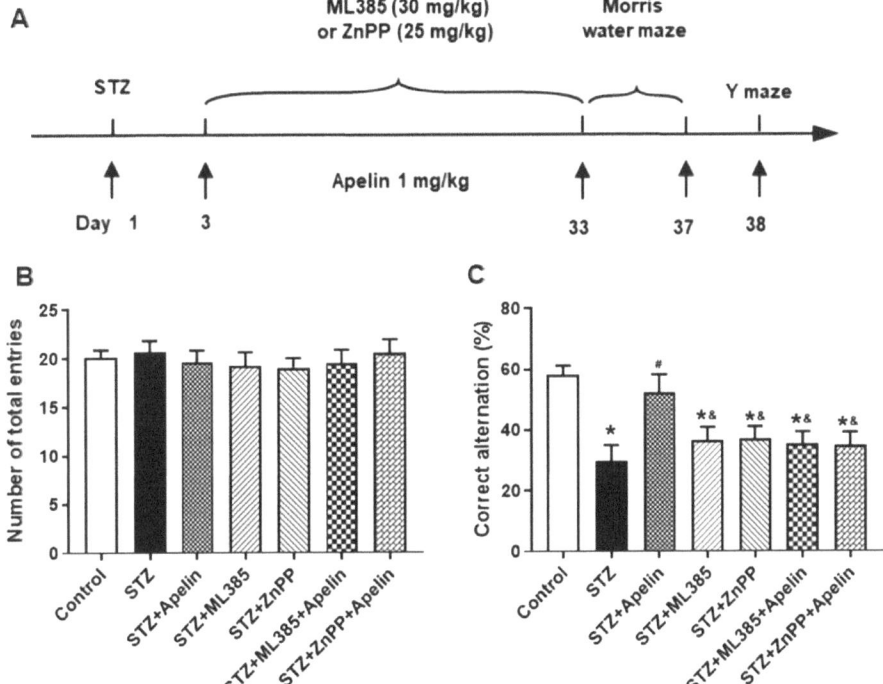

Figure 6. Effect of Nrf2-HO-1 pathway blockade on Apelin-13-mediated improvement of Y-maze performance in STZ-induced animal model of AD mice. (**A**) Experimental timeline. (**B**) Number of arm entrances of different groups (one-way ANOVA, $p > 0.05$). (**C**) Alternation ratio of different groups ($n = 8$, one-way ANOVA, * $p < 0.05$ compared to the control group, # $p < 0.05$ compared to STZ treatment group, & $p < 0.05$ compared to STZ+Apelin-13 treatment group). Data are shown as the mean ± s.e.m.

4. Discussion

The main findings of the present study were that (1) the intranasal administration of Apelin-13 improves cognitive impairment in an STZ-induced animal model of AD, and (2) the anti-STZ-induced-nerve-injury effect of this administration may be achieved by improving synaptic plasticity and anti-oxidative stress signaling pathways.

An innovation of this study is a new exploration of Apelin-13 drug delivery methods. Previous studies have shown that Apelin-13, as a short peptide, cannot be administered intraperitoneally or subcutaneously, similar to conventional drugs, and mostly can only be administered intraventricularly. Many studies have reported that insulin administered through the nasal cavity can be directly absorbed by the nasal mucosa without passing through the peripheral blood circulation and can enter the brain through the blood–brain barrier to treat neurodegenerative diseases such as AD and cognitive impairment [23–25]. Therefore, we used the intranasal administration of Apelin-13 in mice to explore the feasibility of its drug effects.

After a series of behavioral tests in the open field, Y-maze, and water maze, we found that the intranasal administration of Apelin-13 can improve cognitive dysfunction in mice with STZ-induced nerve injury. Our behavioral results are consistent with the latest research reports [13,26,27], although in these studies, Apelin-13 was administrated using the previous ventricular cannula method. Our experimental results confirmed that nasal administration of Apelin-13 treatment can improve the behavioral performance of animal models of nerve injury, indicating that intranasal administration of Apelin-13 is effective and feasible. In future studies, we will explore the effects of the drug at multiple concentrations and time points.

After confirming the validity of the behavioral results, we focused on specific brain regions. It has been reported that apelin and its receptors are expressed in the whole brain, but the hippocampus is one of the regions with relatively high expression [28–30]; this region is also strongly associated with AD. Therefore, we focused on changes that occurred in the hippocampus.

We first observed the long-term potentiation of hippocampal synaptic plasticity, which is closely related to learning and memory functions, in different treatment groups. The results showed that LTP was significantly impaired in the STZ-induced nerve injury group, and high-dose Apelin-13 treatment could improve the LTP impairment caused by STZ-induced nerve injury.

Many in vivo experiments have shown that Apelin-13 can improve oxidative stress-related indicators in STZ-induced nerve injury models [13]. Our experiments showed that the activities of SOD, GSH, and CAT in STZ-induced nerve injury mice were significantly lower than those in the control group, and the activity of MDA was increased, which is consistent with previous reports. These results indicate that the free radical scavenging ability of mice with nerve injuries was decreased, leading to oxidative damage. High and low doses of Apelin-13 also improved oxidative stress indicators in mice with nerve injuries to a certain extent.

Next, we explored the mechanism by which Apelin-13 improves STZ-induced nerve injury. Studies have reported that Apelin-13 exerts neuroprotective effects through anti-inflammatory factors, BDNF/TrkB, PGC-1α/PPARγ, and other signaling pathways [8,13,31–33], and that GLP-1 can improve the learning and memory functions of STZ-injured rats and inhibit tau protein hyperphosphorylation [34–36]. Apelin-13 protects neurons by strengthening autophagy and attenuating early-stage postspinal cord injury apoptosis in vitro [8]. In this study, we investigated whether the ERK-Nrf2-HO-1 pathway, which is related to oxidative stress, plays a role in the Apelin-13 anti-AD cell model of nerve injury. Certainly, the role of ERK in AD pathology is complex and multifaceted. Previous studies have reported conflicting findings regarding the involvement of ERK phosphorylation in the development of AD [37]. Activation of the Ras/ERK pathway has been implicated in predisposing to AD pathogenesis [38], while inhibition of this pathway has been suggested to have a protective effect [39]. Our results suggest that phosphorylated ERK protein may not be directly involved in the anti-AD mechanism of intranasally administered Apelin-13. While our study observed alterations in phosphorylated ERK levels following STZ-induced nerve injury and subsequent Apelin-13 treatment, the exact role of ERK signaling in mediating the therapeutic effects of Apelin-13 remains unclear. Further investigations are warranted to fully elucidate the specific molecular pathways through which Apelin-13 exerts its neuroprotective effects and to determine the interplay between ERK signaling and these pathways in the context of AD.

A recent report confirmed that Aβ25-35 treatment can inhibit the expression of Nrf2 and HO-1 in SH-SY5Y cells [40]. Some studies have reported that Apelin-13 reduces the number of Aβ plaques in the hippocampus [41], and this needs to be further investigated in our future studies to clarify whether the anti-AD effect of Apelin-13 is related to the reduction in Aβ plaques. Our study demonstrated that STZ treatment increases phosphorylated ERK levels and decreases Nrf2 and HO-1 expression. However, the Nrf2 and HO-1 proteins were increased compared with the STZ group after treatment with Apelin-13. The additional behavioral results further corroborate the notion that Apelin-13 exerts an ameliorative effect on cognitive impairment through the Nrf2-HO1 pathway. These findings provide additional support for the involvement of the Nrf2-HO1 pathway in mediating the cognitive-enhancing effects of Apelin-13. Our data support the finding that Apelin-13 regulates antioxidant signaling to ameliorate inflammation-induced AD symptoms, and it remains to be thoroughly investigated whether others, such as inflammatory factors, neurotransmitter signaling, etc., are also involved and whether this pathway still plays a role in Apelin-13's treatment of other causes of AD.

Initially, we explored the protective mechanism of the intranasal administration of Apelin-13 against STZ-induced nerve injury. Importantly, it was confirmed for the first time that the administration of Apelin-13 through the nose can produce effective drug effects, similar to the effects of previous intraventricular administration techniques. Overall, these behavioral findings provide important insights into the mechanisms underlying the cognitive-enhancing effects of Apelin-13 and underscore the therapeutic potential of targeting the Nrf2-HO1 pathway for the treatment of Alzheimer's disease. This study has several limitations that need to be considered. First, the AD model used in this study was relatively homogeneous, and further investigation is needed to confirm whether similar mechanisms operate in other animal models of AD. Second, the upstream and downstream molecules regulated by Apelin-13 in the Nrf2-HO1 pathway need to be explored in depth to provide a stronger basis for target development. These limitations highlight areas for future research aimed at expanding our understanding of the therapeutic potential of Apelin-13 in AD.

5. Conclusions

In summary, our study demonstrates that intranasal administration of Apelin-13 effectively improves cognitive impairment in an STZ-induced AD model by enhancing synaptic plasticity and modulating the Nrf2-HO1 pathway to reduce oxidative stress. These findings underscore the therapeutic potential of Apelin-13 in AD treatment, highlighting its innovative drug delivery method and providing valuable insights into its neuroprotective mechanisms.

Author Contributions: Conceptualization, H.L., M.C. and C.Z.; methodology, H.L. and M.C.; formal analysis, H.L. and M.C.; resources, C.Z.; writing—original draft preparation, H.L., M.C. and C.Z.; supervision, C.Z.; project administration, C.Z. All authors have read and agreed to the published version of the manuscript.

Funding: This research received no external funding.

Institutional Review Board Statement: The animal study protocol was approved by the Animal Care and Use Committee of the Shanghai Medical College of Fudan University (No. 20170223-098, 23 February 2017).

Informed Consent Statement: Not applicable.

Data Availability Statement: The datasets used and analyzed in this study are available from the corresponding author upon request. The data are not publicly available due to institutional copyright policy.

Conflicts of Interest: The authors declare no conflict of interest.

References

1. Luo, H.; Han, L.; Xu, J. Apelin/APJ system: A novel promising target for neurodegenerative diseases. *J. Cell. Physiol.* **2020**, *235*, 638–657. [CrossRef] [PubMed]
2. Wan, T.; Fu, M.; Jiang, Y.; Jiang, W.; Li, P.; Zhou, S. Research progress on mechanism of neuroprotective roles of Apelin-13 in prevention and treatment of Alzheimer's disease. *Neurochem. Res.* **2022**, *47*, 205–217. [CrossRef] [PubMed]
3. Tatemoto, K.; Hosoya, M.; Habata, Y.; Fujii, R.; Kakegawa, T.; Zou, M.-X.; Kawamata, Y.; Fukusumi, S.; Hinuma, S.; Kitada, C. Isolation and characterization of a novel endogenous peptide ligand for the human APJ receptor. *Biochem. Biophys. Res. Commun.* **1998**, *251*, 471–476. [CrossRef] [PubMed]
4. Simpkin, J.C.; Yellon, D.M.; Davidson, S.M.; Lim, S.Y.; Wynne, A.M.; Smith, C.C. Apelin-13 and apelin-36 exhibit direct cardioprotective activity against ischemiareperfusion injury. *Basic Res. Cardiol.* **2007**, *102*, 518–528. [CrossRef] [PubMed]

5. Hosoya, M.; Kawamata, Y.; Fukusumi, S.; Fujii, R.; Habata, Y.; Hinuma, S.; Kitada, C.; Honda, S.; Kurokawa, T.; Onda, H. Molecular and functional characteristics of APJ: Tissue distribution of mRNA and interaction with the endogenous ligand apelin. *J. Biol. Chem.* **2000**, *275*, 21061–21067. [CrossRef] [PubMed]
6. Falcão-Pires, I.; Ladeiras-Lopes, R.; Leite-Moreira, A.F. The apelinergic system: A promising therapeutic target. *Expert Opin. Ther. Targets* **2010**, *14*, 633–645. [CrossRef] [PubMed]
7. Li, A.; Zhao, Q.; Chen, L.; Li, Z. Apelin/APJ system: An emerging therapeutic target for neurological diseases. *Mol. Biol. Rep.* **2023**, *50*, 1639–1653. [CrossRef]
8. Lin, T.; Zhao, Y.; Guo, S.; Wu, Z.; Li, W.; Wu, R.; Wang, Z.; Liu, W. Apelin-13 protects neurons by attenuating early-stage postspinal cord injury apoptosis in vitro. *Brain Sci.* **2022**, *12*, 1515. [CrossRef]
9. Zhang, Y.; Jiang, W.; Sun, W.; Guo, W.; Xia, B.; Shen, X.; Fu, M.; Wan, T.; Yuan, M. Neuroprotective roles of Apelin-13 in neurological diseases. *Neurochem. Res.* **2023**, *48*, 1648–1662. [CrossRef]
10. Dai, T.-T.; Wang, B.; Xiao, Z.-Y.; You, Y.; Tian, S.-W. Apelin-13 upregulates BDNF against chronic stress-induced depression-like phenotypes by ameliorating HPA axis and hippocampal glucocorticoid receptor dysfunctions. *Neuroscience* **2018**, *390*, 151–159. [CrossRef]
11. Han, R.-w.; Xu, H.-j.; Wang, R. The role of apelin-13 in novel object recognition memory. *Peptides* **2014**, *62*, 155–158. [CrossRef]
12. Haghparast, E.; Esmaeili-Mahani, S.; Abbasnejad, M.; Sheibani, V. Apelin-13 ameliorates cognitive impairments in 6-hydroxydopamine-induced substantia nigra lesion in rats. *Neuropeptides* **2018**, *68*, 28–35. [CrossRef]
13. Luo, H.; Xiang, Y.; Qu, X.; Liu, H.; Liu, C.; Li, G.; Han, L.; Qin, X. Apelin-13 suppresses neuroinflammation against cognitive deficit in a streptozotocin-induced rat model of Alzheimer's disease through activation of BDNF-TrkB signaling pathway. *Front. Pharmacol.* **2019**, *10*, 395. [CrossRef]
14. Masoumi, J.; Abbasloui, M.; Parvan, R.; Mohammadnejad, D.; Pavon-Djavid, G.; Barzegari, A.; Abdolalizadeh, J. Apelin, a promising target for Alzheimer disease prevention and treatment. *Neuropeptides* **2018**, *70*, 76–86. [CrossRef]
15. Sirwi, A.; El Sayed, N.S.; Abdallah, H.M.; Ibrahim, S.R.; Mohamed, G.A.; El-Halawany, A.M.; Safo, M.K.; Abdel Rasheed, N.O. Umuhengerin neuroprotective effects in streptozotocin-induced Alzheimer's disease mouse model via targeting Nrf2 and NF-Kβ Signaling cascades. *Antioxidants* **2021**, *10*, 2011. [CrossRef]
16. Saxena, G.; Singh, S.P.; Agrawal, R.; Nath, C. Effect of donepezil and tacrine on oxidative stress in intracerebral streptozotocin-induced model of dementia in mice. *Eur. J. Pharmacol.* **2008**, *581*, 283–289. [CrossRef]
17. Liu, Y.; Gong, Z.; Zhai, D.; Yang, C.; Lu, G.; Wang, S.; Xiao, S.; Li, C.; Chen, L.; Lin, X. Unveiling the therapeutic potential of Dl-3-n-butylphthalide in NTG-induced migraine mouse: Activating the Nrf2 pathway to alleviate oxidative stress and neuroinflammation. *J. Headache Pain* **2024**, *25*, 50. [CrossRef]
18. Lee, T.-S.; Chau, L.-Y. Heme oxygenase-1 mediates the anti-inflammatory effect of interleukin-10 in mice. *Nat. Med.* **2002**, *8*, 240–246. [CrossRef]
19. Zhou, X.; Wang, L.; Xiao, W.; Su, Z.; Zheng, C.; Zhang, Z.; Wang, Y.; Xu, B.; Yang, X.; Hoi, M.P.M. Memantine improves cognitive function and alters hippocampal and cortical proteome in triple transgenic mouse model of Alzheimer's disease. *Exp. Neurobiol.* **2019**, *28*, 390–403. [CrossRef]
20. Wei, H.; Dobkin, C.; Sheikh, A.M.; Malik, M.; Brown, W.T.; Li, X. The therapeutic effect of memantine through the stimulation of synapse formation and dendritic spine maturation in autism and fragile X syndrome. *PLoS ONE* **2012**, *7*, e36981. [CrossRef]
21. Xiang, X.; Wang, X.; Wu, Y.; Hu, J.; Li, Y.; Jin, S.; Wu, X. Activation of GPR55 attenuates cognitive impairment, oxidative stress, neuroinflammation, and synaptic dysfunction in a streptozotocin-induced Alzheimer's mouse model. *Pharmacol. Biochem. Behav.* **2022**, *214*, 173340. [CrossRef]
22. Hira, S.; Saleem, U.; Anwar, F.; Sohail, M.F.; Raza, Z.; Ahmad, B. β-Carotene: A natural compound improves cognitive impairment and oxidative stress in a mouse model of streptozotocin-induced Alzheimer's disease. *Biomolecules* **2019**, *9*, 441. [CrossRef]
23. Benedict, C.; Frey, W.H., II; Schiöth, H.B.; Schultes, B.; Born, J.; Hallschmid, M. Intranasal insulin as a therapeutic option in the treatment of cognitive impairments. *Exp. Gerontol.* **2011**, *46*, 112–115. [CrossRef]
24. Freiherr, J.; Hallschmid, M.; Frey, W.H.; Brünner, Y.F.; Chapman, C.D.; Hölscher, C.; Craft, S.; De Felice, F.G.; Benedict, C. Intranasal insulin as a treatment for Alzheimer's disease: A review of basic research and clinical evidence. *CNS Drugs* **2013**, *27*, 505–514. [CrossRef]
25. Reger, M.A.; Watson, G.S.; Green, P.S.; Wilkinson, C.W.; Baker, L.D.; Cholerton, B.; Fishel, M.A.; Plymate, S.; Breitner, J.; DeGroodt, W. Intranasal insulin improves cognition and modulates β-amyloid in early AD. *Neurology* **2008**, *70*, 440–448. [CrossRef]
26. Nasseri, B.; Zareian, P.; Alizade, H. Apelin attenuates streptozotocin-induced learning and memory impairment by modulating necroptosis signaling pathway. *Int. Immunopharmacol.* **2020**, *84*, 106546. [CrossRef]
27. Aminyavari, S.; Zahmatkesh, M.; Farahmandfar, M.; Khodagholi, F.; Dargahi, L.; Zarrindast, M.-R. Protective role of Apelin-13 on amyloid β25–35-induced memory deficit; Involvement of autophagy and apoptosis process. *Prog. Neuro-Psychopharmacol. Biol. Psychiatry* **2019**, *89*, 322–334. [CrossRef]
28. Reaux, A.; De Mota, N.; Skultetyova, I.; Lenkei, Z.; El Messari, S.; Gallatz, K.; Corvol, P.; Palkovits, M.; Llorens-Cortès, C. Physiological role of a novel neuropeptide, apelin, and its receptor in the rat brain. *J. Neurochem.* **2001**, *77*, 1085–1096. [CrossRef]
29. Reaux, A.; Gallatz, K.; Palkovits, M.; Llorens-Cortes, C. Distribution of apelin-synthesizing neurons in the adult rat brain. *Neuroscience* **2002**, *113*, 653–662. [CrossRef]

30. O'Carroll, A.-M.; Selby, T.L.; Palkovits, M.; Lolait, S.J. Distribution of mRNA encoding B78/apj, the rat homologue of the human APJ receptor, and its endogenous ligand apelin in brain and peripheral tissues. *Biochim. Biophys. Acta (BBA)-Gene Struct. Expr.* **2000**, *1492*, 72–80. [CrossRef]
31. Shen, P.; Yue, Q.; Fu, W.; Tian, S.-W.; You, Y. Apelin-13 ameliorates chronic water-immersion restraint stress-induced memory performance deficit through upregulation of BDNF in rats. *Neurosci. Lett.* **2019**, *696*, 151–155. [CrossRef]
32. Cheng, B.; Chen, J.; Bai, B.; Xin, Q. Neuroprotection of apelin and its signaling pathway. *Peptides* **2012**, *37*, 171–173. [CrossRef]
33. Chen, B.; Wu, J.; Hu, S.; Liu, Q.; Yang, H.; You, Y. Apelin-13 improves cognitive impairment and repairs hippocampal neuronal damage by activating PGC-1α/PPARγ signaling. *Neurochem. Res.* **2023**, *48*, 1504–1515. [CrossRef]
34. Li, Y.; Duffy, K.B.; Ottinger, M.A.; Ray, B.; Bailey, J.A.; Holloway, H.W.; Tweedie, D.; Perry, T.; Mattson, M.P.; Kapogiannis, D. GLP-1 receptor stimulation reduces amyloid-β peptide accumulation and cytotoxicity in cellular and animal models of Alzheimer's disease. *J. Alzheimer's Dis.* **2010**, *19*, 1205–1219. [CrossRef]
35. Hölscher, C. Potential role of glucagon-like peptide-1 (GLP-1) in neuroprotection. *CNS Drugs* **2012**, *26*, 871–882. [CrossRef]
36. Perry, T.A.; Greig, N.H. A new Alzheimer's disease interventive strategy: GLP-1. *Curr. Drug Targets* **2004**, *5*, 565–571. [CrossRef]
37. Zhu, X.; Castellani, R.J.; Takeda, A.; Nunomura, A.; Atwood, C.S.; Perry, G.; Smith, M.A. Differential activation of neuronal ERK, JNK/SAPK and p38 in Alzheimer disease: The 'two hit' hypothesis. *Mech. Ageing Dev.* **2001**, *123*, 39–46. [CrossRef]
38. Kirouac, L.; Rajic, A.J.; Cribbs, D.H.; Padmanabhan, J. Activation of Ras-ERK signaling and GSK-3 by amyloid precursor protein and amyloid beta facilitates neurodegeneration in Alzheimer's disease. *eNeuro* **2017**, *4*. [CrossRef]
39. Wang, X.; Wang, Y.; Zhu, Y.; Yan, L.; Zhao, L. Neuroprotective Effect of S-trans, Trans-farnesylthiosalicylic Acid via Inhibition of RAS/ERK Pathway for the Treatment of Alzheimer's Disease. *Drug Des. Dev. Ther.* **2019**, *13*, 4053–4063. [CrossRef]
40. Zhang, L.; Guo, Y.; Wang, H.; Zhao, L.; Ma, Z.; Li, T.; Liu, J.; Sun, M.; Jian, Y.; Yao, L. Edaravone reduces Aβ-induced oxidative damage in SH-SY5Y cells by activating the Nrf2/ARE signaling pathway. *Life Sci.* **2019**, *221*, 259–266. [CrossRef]
41. Azhir, M.; Gazmeh, S.; Elyasi, L.; Jahanshahi, M.; Bazrafshan, B. The effect of apelin-13 on memory of scopolamine-treated rats and accumulation of amyloid-beta plaques in the hippocampus. *J. Clin. Basic Res.* **2023**, *7*, 15–19.

Disclaimer/Publisher's Note: The statements, opinions and data contained in all publications are solely those of the individual author(s) and contributor(s) and not of MDPI and/or the editor(s). MDPI and/or the editor(s) disclaim responsibility for any injury to people or property resulting from any ideas, methods, instructions or products referred to in the content.

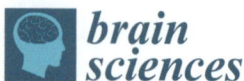

Review

The Interrelated Multifactorial Actions of Cortisol and Klotho: Potential Implications in the Pathogenesis of Parkinson's Disease

Nijee S. Luthra [1],*, Angela Clow [2] and Daniel M. Corcos [3]

[1] Department of Neurology, University of California San Francisco, San Francisco, CA 94127, USA
[2] Department of Psychology, School of Social Sciences, University of Westminster, London W1B 2HW, UK
[3] Department of Physical Therapy & Human Movement Sciences, Feinberg School of Medicine, Northwestern University, Chicago, IL 60208, USA
* Correspondence: nijee.luthra@ucsf.edu

Abstract: The pathogenesis of Parkinson's disease (PD) is complex, multilayered, and not fully understood, resulting in a lack of effective disease-modifying treatments for this prevalent neurodegenerative condition. Symptoms of PD are heterogenous, including motor impairment as well as non-motor symptoms such as depression, cognitive impairment, and circadian disruption. Aging and stress are important risk factors for PD, leading us to explore pathways that may either accelerate or protect against cellular aging and the detrimental effects of stress. Cortisol is a much-studied hormone that can disrupt mitochondrial function and increase oxidative stress and neuroinflammation, which are recognized as key underlying disease mechanisms in PD. The more recently discovered klotho protein, considered a general aging-suppressor, has a similarly wide range of actions but in the opposite direction to cortisol: promoting mitochondrial function while reducing oxidative stress and inflammation. Both hormones also converge on pathways of vitamin D metabolism and insulin resistance, also implicated to play a role in PD. Interestingly, aging, stress and PD associate with an increase in cortisol and decrease in klotho, while physical exercise and certain genetic variations lead to a decrease in cortisol response and increased klotho. Here, we review the interrelated opposite actions of cortisol and klotho in the pathogenesis of PD. Together they impact powerful and divergent mechanisms that may go on to influence PD-related symptoms. Better understanding of these hormones in PD would facilitate the design of effective interventions that can simultaneously impact the multiple systems involved in the pathogenesis of PD.

Keywords: cortisol; klotho; Parkinson's disease; aging; stress

1. Introduction

Parkinson's disease (PD) is the fastest growing neurological disorder globally [1,2]. Fueled by aging, the number of people with PD is expected to exceed 12 million by 2040 [1]. PD is characterized as a movement disorder, resultant from progressive neurodegeneration of dopamine neurons in the substantia nigra pars compacta and its projections. However, it is increasingly apparent that other brain regions are affected, e.g., decreased metabolism in the prefrontal, occipital, and parietal cortices as well as changes in the lentiform nucleus, thalamus, pons and cerebellum [3]. Dopaminergic and non-dopaminergic pathology contribute to a wide range of non-motor symptoms (NMS), including cognitive impairment, mood disorder, circadian disruption, autonomic dysfunction, fatigue, and apathy [4–6]. Despite the heterogeneity in pathogenesis and symptomatology, aging remains the single most important risk factor for development of PD and of NMSs that disrupt the quality of life [7–9].

Mechanisms of aging and neurodegeneration are thought to be interrelated with chronic stress. Both aging and chronic stress are pertinent to the pathogenesis of PD and impact mitochondrial dysfunction, oxidative stress, inflammation, and changes in metabolism [10]. These pathways result in changes in cellular function such as decreased ATP synthesis, increase production of reactive oxygen species (ROS) and Ca+ accumulation, microglia response, and increased proinflammatory cytokines and infiltrating immune cells, all contributing to cell apoptosis. These processes occur in vulnerable brain regions and interplay with genetic and environmental risk factors to contribute to the development and progression of PD [8,10,11]. Here, we review the actions of two hormones known to be implicated in the aging and stress processes and discuss their potential roles in PD pathophysiology. Cortisol is a critical hormone involved in normal stress responsivity, physiological homeostasis, and circadian function. Excess secretion is associated with a wide range of maladaptive correlates of aging and chronic stress [12–15]. Relatively newly discovered, klotho is a longevity hormone that delays aging and enhances cognition [16–18]. In this review, we highlight the yin-yang roles of cortisol and klotho in key aging and stress pathways and how this may associate with progression and symptoms of PD.

2. Function of Cortisol and Klotho
2.1. Cortisol

Cortisol secretion is the product of hypothalamic-pituitary-adrenal (HPA) axis activation. It is a powerful steroid hormone that can pass into every cell of the body, with genomic and non-genomic actions affecting mitochondrial, immune, and metabolic function [19]. The brain is a prominent target for cortisol and thus a central structure for adaptation to stress. A wide brain network involving the hippocampus, amygdala, prefrontal cortex and brainstem nuclei are involved in HPA axis activation in response to acute or chronic stress [20]. The underlying basal secretory activity of the HPA axis is regulated by the hypothalamic central pacemaker: the suprachiasmatic nucleus (SCN). The SCN transmits its circadian signal to peripheral clock genes via neural and hormonal mechanisms, with cortisol secretion playing a significant role, synchronizing circadian oscillations throughout the body [21].

Cortisol has pleiotropic effects on the brain, affecting mood, behavior, cognition, and programming of the stress response [22]. Cortisol is necessary for neuronal differentiation, integrity, and growth, as well as synaptic and dendritic plasticity [23,24]. These processes in turn support brain functions such as decision-making, reward-based behavior, motor control, visual information processing, learning and memory, and energy regulation. Cortisol actions are mediated by the glucocorticoid receptors (GRs) and mineralocorticoid receptors (MRs). In addition to rapid non-genomic mechanisms, cortisol influences brain functions by activating GR-mediated gene transcription [25]. Some of these target genes code for neurotrophic factors and their receptors, anti- and pro-inflammatory markers, signal transduction, neurotransmitter catabolism, energy metabolism, and cell adhesion [25–27]. Stress-induced shifts in cortisol associate with time- and region-dependent changes in neuronal activity to promote the brain's adaptation to the continuously changing environment in the short and long-term [28]. A dysfunctional HPA axis is thought to occur in PD, leading to GR desensitization and high circulating cortisol concentrations [29].

2.2. Klotho

KLOTHO (KL) is a serendipitously discovered gene on chromosome 13 found to have profound effects on lifespan [30]. Deficiency of klotho protein in mice severely shortens lifespan and prompts signs of premature aging while overexpression of klotho increases lifespan by ~30%. Since its initial discovery, increased levels of klotho have been associated with longevity in several populations and decreased levels of klotho have been associated with aging-related diseases including cancer, cardiovascular disease, kidney disease, and recently neurodegenerative diseases [31–37].

Klotho is expressed primarily in the kidneys and choroid plexus [30,38,39]. Klotho mRNA is also detectable in many other brain regions, including cortex, hippocampus, cerebellum, striatum, substantia nigra, olfactory bulb, and medulla [38–41]. Klotho's actions are complex and multidimensional—it suppresses insulin and *Wnt* signaling [42,43], regulates ion channel clustering and transport [44], modulates *N*-methyl-D-aspartate receptor (NMDAR) signaling [18] and promotes fibroblast growth factor (FGF) function [45]. Klotho, linked with FGF23, is important for regulation of calcium, phosphate, and vitamin D homeostasis [46–51]. Klotho linked with FGF21 is involved in stimulation of the starvation response, activating the HPA axis and sympathetic nervous system, as well as increasing intracellular klotho expression in the SCN within the hypothalamus [52].

3. Cortisol and Klotho in Neurodegenerative Disease

Cortisol and klotho have relevance to various neuropsychiatric and neurodegenerative disorders. Cortisol levels are increased in individuals with depression, sleep disturbances, and neurodegenerative diseases like AD and PD [53–58]. Conversely, lower circulating klotho levels are reported in bipolar disorder, depression, multiple sclerosis, temporal lobe epilepsy, AD and recently, PD [36,37,59–62].

Accumulating evidence suggests that the HPA axis is dysregulated in PD. Cortisol levels are found to be increased in toxin animal models of PD [63]. Elevated cortisol levels also induce impairment of motor function and accelerate nigral neuronal loss in rats exposed to chronic stress and subsequent increase in cortisol [64]. Individuals with PD have elevated cortisol secretion in blood and saliva, especially in the morning [58,65,66]. More recently, glucocorticoid concentrations measured in the hair of PD patients showed an excess of cortisone, the main cortisol metabolite, but not cortisol itself [67].

Klotho was initially linked to neurodegenerative diseases in studies of AD. Klotho is decreased in the CSF of AD patients [36]. Higher klotho is also associated with reduced amyloid-beta (Aβ) burden and improved cognition in populations at risk for AD [68]. Emerging studies are now connecting klotho with PD. Klotho-insufficient mice develop neurodegeneration of mesencephalic dopaminergic neurons in substantia nigra and ventral tegmentum area, while klotho overexpression protects dopaminergic neurons against oxidative injury [40,69,70]. Exogenous klotho administration demonstrates neuroprotective potential in toxin rat models of PD through alleviation of astrogliosis, apoptosis, and oxidative stress [71]. One study reported that while plasma klotho levels were not significantly different between people with PD and healthy controls, klotho levels were lower in men compared to women with PD [72]. This is interesting since sex is an important biological factor in development and phenotype of PD as well as hormonal regulation in general. Another study looking at two independent cohorts of people with PD found that CSF levels of klotho were lower in people with PD compared to healthy controls [37]. A recent perspective by Grillo et al. (2022) also points out that enteric cells express klotho, and both blood and enteric levels of klotho are altered in the setting of gut disease or inflammation [73]. The authors go on to suggest that since PD pathology is hypothesized to start in the enteric nervous system, this poses an important need to assess klotho in the gastrointestinal tract of people with PD and evaluate whether modulation of klotho in the gut may serve as a disease-modifying strategy.

Lastly, it is important to note how the main PD symptomatic treatment, levodopa, is associated with cortisol and klotho. Administration of levodopa decreases HPA axis activity, thereby decreasing cortisol levels [74,75]. It is currently unclear if levodopa affects klotho levels or vice versa and future studies should take this into account.

4. Factors Modulating Cortisol and Klotho Regulation

4.1. Aging

Aging is the most critical risk factor for PD [7,76], yet the relationship between molecular/cellular processes of healthy aging and those of PD pathogenesis remain unclear. It can be hypothesized that specific regions of the PD brain (e.g., dopaminergic neurons in substantia nigra pars compacta) undergo localized, accelerated aging [77]. Aging links together several pathological mechanisms known to play a significant role in PD—from increased inflammation and oxidative stress to mitochondrial dysfunction and dysregulation of lysosomal, proteasomal and autophagic functions– and all likely to contribute to neurodegeneration. The concept of "inflammaging" has been proposed as a principal mechanism in PD [78] and describes the sustained systemic inflammatory state that develops with advanced age [79]. This chronic inflammation is thought to result from exposure to chronic stressors and/or imbalance between inflammatory and anti-inflammatory networks.

The convergence of cortisol and klotho along the pathways of aging has notable implications for PD. Cortisol levels decrease in decades 20s–30s, are relatively stable in 40-50s, and increase after age 60 [80]. Elevated cortisol has been reported in age-related illnesses such as cardiovascular disease, type II diabetes mellitus, osteoporosis, and cognitive impairment [81–84]. In contrast, klotho levels are highest at birth in humans, with levels 7-fold higher than adulthood levels, and decline after age 40 [85,86]. Several studies link klotho to increased lifespan and better health outcomes, including decreased risk for cardiovascular disease and stroke, decreased macrovascular complications in patients with type 2 diabetes, and improved grip strength [33,86,87]. Klotho has also recently been included in a panel of biomarkers that may predict frailty in the elderly [88].

4.2. Stress

The notion that chronic stress, in addition to aging, may play a role in the pathogenesis of PD has been controversial over the years but, despite some inconsistencies in the literature, is now generally recognized [29]. In one population-based cohort study of over 2 million males, higher job demands and expectations increased PD risk [89]. In another study, the risk of PD significantly increased with the number of exposures to stressful events [90]. Post-traumatic stress disorder and adjustment disorder, both indicating occurrence of significant stressors, also associated with increased risk of PD, independent of comorbid depression or anxiety [91,92].

Stress is known to affect functions of the limbic system such as learning, memory and emotions [93]. The hippocampus has extensive distribution of GRs and plays a crucial role in the biological effects of chronic stress [94,95]. Stress and hypercortisolemia also disrupt sleep [96], which exerts powerful effects on the hippocampus and affects initial learning and memory consolidation [97]. Recent evidence shows that stress also modulates motor system function [98]. Since most parts of the motor system express GRs, their circuits are susceptible to the influence of cortisol. Stress can modulate movement through activation of the HPA axis and via stress-associated emotional changes. In PD mouse models, chronic stress exposure worsens motor deficits, aggravates the neurodegeneration of the nigrostriatal system, and completely blocks compensatory recovery of motor tasks [64]. A recent viewpoint by van der Heide et al. (2020) proposes a model of how chronic stress in patients with PD, resulting in higher cortisol levels, can lead to both higher susceptibility for depressive and anxiety disorders and a more rapid progression of the disease [99]. The authors review evidence on how chronic stress reduces levels of brain derived neurotrophic factor (BDNF), inducing atrophy in key brain regions of mood and behavior, and creates a proinflammatory environment that increases nigrostriatal cell loss.

Given klotho's role in healthy aging, it is no wonder that it too has been linked to stress. Klotho levels are reported to be lower in caregivers with chronic high stress and show an age-related decline [60]. Klotho genetic variations that alter klotho levels influence the effects of stress on cellular aging, as evidenced by changes in multiple biomarkers of aging, including telomere length, CRP levels, metabolic dysfunction and white matter microstructural integrity [100]. Mice with chronic stress demonstrate downregulation of klotho in the nucleus accumbens (NAc) and depressive-like behavior [101], responses modulated by Klotho regulation of NMDARs.

4.3. Genetics

PD pathogenesis is mediated by an interaction between multiple environmental and genetic factors. The role of cortisol and klotho in PD may also be dependent on genetic variations that dictate levels or function of these two hormones.

As discussed previously, cortisol functions by binding to GRs and MRs. Genetic variation in GR has been postulated to play a role in the physiological response to endogenous cortisol. Over 3000 single nucleotide polymorphisms (SNPs) in the GR gene have been documented. Most studies show that *BclI* and N363S gene variants are associated with clinical measures of increased glucocorticoid sensitivity, while the ER22/23EK and GR-9β are associated with decreased glucocorticoid sensitivity [102]. The ER22/23EK polymorphism links with improved survival and lower levels of the inflammatory marker C-reactive protein (CRP) [103]. *BclI* has consistently been shown to be associated with a higher susceptibility to major depression [104]. It is currently unclear if and how these genotypes impact PD. Lastly, polymorphisms in the catechol-O-methyl-transferase (COMT) gene have also been associated with glucocorticoid responsivity and cortisol levels. In particular, individuals with the Met/Met COMT homozygote polymorphisms are more sensitive to stressful events and have higher cortisol responses [105]. Interestingly in people with PD, Met/Met COMT homozygote polymorphism associates with lower IQ score and greater motor severity of disease [106].

Genetic variations in the *KL* gene may influence systemic klotho levels or its function. *KL* variant *rs9315202* downregulates klotho mRNA expression and associates with advanced epigenetic age and elevated aging markers such as CRP [100,107]. There is also a well-studied protective variant, termed *KL*-VS, that contains two SNPs, rs95536314 and rs9527025, in complete linkage disequilibrium. Carrying one copy of *KL*-VS increases klotho levels [18,108], while carrying two copies, decreases it [108]. *KL*-VS heterozygosity is associated with longer lifespan [31], slowed epigenetic age [100], and higher cognitive function [18,108] in most but not all populations. In a population at risk for dementia, *KL*-VS allele attenuates Aβ burden and associates with reduced risk of conversion to mild cognitive impairment or AD [68]. In PD, *KL*-VS heterozygotes have higher CSF klotho levels; however, the haplotype itself is associated with shorter interval between onset of PD and progression to MCI and worse motor phenotype [37]. Therefore, it remains to be clarified how genetic variations in *KL* gene may affect function of the klotho protein and affect individuals with PD.

It is unknown whether there are direct correlations between cortisol or klotho and the genes linked to PD. However, as both hormones are involved in mechanisms that become aberrant in PD, there may be undiscovered connections. For example, both cortisol and klotho influence mitochondrial function in opposite ways and may interact with genetic variations in genes linked to mitochondrial dysfunction in PD (i.e., Parkin, PINK1, DJ-1, LRRK2).

4.4. Physical Exercise

Just as cortisol and klotho are sensitive to aging and psychological stress, they are also responsive (in the opposite direction) to external stimuli that promote healthy aging, such as physical activity. The past decade has produced much evidence to support that physical exercise is potentially neuroprotective in PD.

Physical exercise can improve dysregulated cortisol levels in healthy individuals and those with major depressive disorder [109]. High intensity exercise (>90% heart rate reserve) decreases fluctuations in salivary cortisol [110]. Another study showed that exercising intensely (70% heart rate reserve) suppresses the subsequent cortisol response to a psychosocial stressor [111]. Smyth et al. have shown that high intensity treadmill exercise in individuals with PD reduces cortisol secretion during the post-awakening period after nocturnal sleep [112]. Yoga and dance movement therapy also lead to decreased cortisol levels [113,114].

Contrarily, klotho levels are amplified by treadmill exercise in both young and aged mice [115,116]. In humans, higher levels of klotho are associated with superior lower extremity strength and functioning [117,118] Klotho levels also tend to be higher in exercise-trained individuals compared to their untrained counter-partners [119]. In healthy adults, various exercise programs (endurance, resistance, high intensity interval training) boost plasma klotho levels either acutely or after a 12–16-week training period [120–124]. Recent study also finds that yoga, consisting of deep breathing exercises, meditation, and postures, upregulates expression of the *KL* gene [125].

5. Candidate Mechanisms of Cortisol and Klotho Interactions in PD

Together cortisol and klotho represent powerful yet complementary mechanisms by which life stress can be internalized and aging can be regulated. We go on to highlight 4 candidate mechanisms where klotho and cortisol may be competing in the life course of PD.

5.1. Mitochondrial Dysfunction and Oxidative Stress

Mitochondrial dysfunction (altered morphology, turnover and transport) plays a fundamental role in the pathogenesis of PD by chronic production of reactive oxygen species and induction of α-synuclein misfolding, promoting neurodegeneration in the substantia nigra [126]. The causes of mitochondrial dysfunction are complex and multipart, including damage to mitochondrial DNA, environmental neurotoxins, and mutations of the PINK1, DJ-1, and Parkin genes linked to PD [127,128]. In addition, mitochondrial function is intimately interlinked with other cell processes including iron, copper, and glutathione metabolism [129]. Dysfunction in any one process impacts the others, leading to a disruptive vicious cycle driving neuronal cell death and pathology. Mitochondrial dysfunction also occurs as a consequence of aging [130] and chronic stress [131,132] with changes linked to increased inflammatory responses. This is because, in addition to their other roles, mitochondria are now considered central hubs in regulating innate immunity and inflammatory responses [133].

The hormone cortisol is intricately coupled with mitochondrial function. Once the HPA axis is activated, it is synthesized within the mitochondria of the zona fasciculata of the adrenal cortex and has potent reciprocal effects on mitochondrial function throughout the body [134]. In this way, mitochondria are both mediators and targets of the main stress axis, with cortisol as a liaison for whole body mitochondria-to-mitochondria communication to regulate energy metabolism. Aging and stress-associated increase in cortisol can reduce the activity of specific mitochondrial electron transport chain complexes and increase mitochondrial oxidative stress [134]. In mouse models of PD, psychological stress diminishes up to 50% of mitochondrial respiration and glycolysis and links to cell death and exacerbation of motor symptoms [135].

Age-related declines in klotho can drive dysfunctional mitochondrial bioenergetics in skeletal muscle and kidney whilst systemic delivery of exogenous klotho rejuvenates and enhances function [136,137]. Mitochondria not only regulate the normal ROS level, but excessive ROS can also directly damage mitochondria and lead to apoptosis and cell death. Klotho induces the expression of the manganese superoxide dismutase (MnSOD) protein, a mitochondrial antioxidant enzyme that detoxifies superoxides, and thus reduces ROS [138]. A study in human stem cells shows that klotho attenuates cellular damage and cell apoptosis induced by oxidative stress by protecting mitochondrial structure [139]. Klotho is also known to play a significant role in brain metabolism as an antioxidant [140,141]. Reduction at these levels result in the inability of astrocytes to rapidly modify their metabolic activity to support adjacent neurons, making them more vulnerable to neurodegeneration [142].

5.2. Neuroinflammation

Several lines of evidence from humans and animal models support the involvement of inflammation in the onset and progression of PD. While inflammation may be a consequence of neuronal loss in PD, the chronic inflammatory response may also contribute to the progression of PD. Neuroinflammation stems from crosstalk between neurons, microglia, astroglia and endothelial cells [133], which are susceptible to α-synuclein aggregates and mitochondrial dysfunction. Under disease conditions, the homeostatic functions of the microglia and astroglia are disrupted, leading to reduced secretion of neurotrophic factors, increased secretion of proinflammatory cytokines (interleukin (IL)-6, IL1β, Tumor Necrosis Factor α (TNFα), interferon (IFN)-γ, etc.)) and chemokines (CCL2, CXCL1, etc.) and increased receptor expression for proinflammatory markers and major histocompatibility complex (MHC-I) in microglial cells [143]. Additionally, peripheral immune cells (such as CD4+ T cells) are recruited to the brain parenchyma, further augmenting the proinflammatory environment.

Cortisol plays a significant and beneficial role in regulation of inflammation, but old age and chronic stress are associated with dysregulation of the HPA axis and cortisol secretion [144]. Cortisol and pro-inflammatory cytokines interact on multiple levels. Under normal conditions, cortisol inhibits the immune system cells that produce peripheral cytokines. It also inhibits transcription and action of many of the pro-inflammatory cytokines including IL-1β, IL-6, and TNFα [145–147]. In a reciprocal relationship, cytokines can also influence glucocorticoid secretion, availability, and signaling. IL-1β and IL-6 can activate the HPA axis directly, while IL-1 and TNFα can impair cortisol signaling by interfering with GR phosphorylation [148,149]. In settings of chronic stress, excessive cortisol secretion leads to compensatory down-regulation or resistance of the GR and its anti-inflammatory actions, resulting instead in a pro-inflammatory milieu facilitating a wide range of disease risks including neurotoxicity [12,13]. In this scenario, increased levels of cortisol are associated with an increase in pro-inflammatory cytokines such as IL-6 [150]. Therefore, cortisol can have dual effects—it can limit inflammation under normal conditions but promote inflammation under conditions of chronic stress.

Recent studies suggest that klotho could also play a role in mediating the interface between the brain and immune system in the choroid plexus. Selectively reducing klotho within the choroid plexus of mice triggers inflammation and enhances activation of innate immune cells [151]. As a separate pathway, klotho suppresses activation of macrophages by enhancing FGF23 signaling [151]. Klotho also decreases activation of NF-κB and influences expression of the pro-inflammatory cytokines, IFNγ and TNFα [152,153], the latter being a 'master regulator' of production of pro-inflammatory cytokines. To counter inflammation, klotho increases production of IL-10, which is responsible for inhibiting the expression of pro-inflammatory cytokines such as TNFα [154].

A key event in the neuroinflammatory processes is the activation of inflammasomes, multiprotein complexes that mediate pro-inflammatory cytokine secretion and maturation. The inflammasome component NLRP3 is strongly linked to neuroinflammation. Klotho overexpression inhibits the NLRP3/caspase signaling pathways and enhances cognition in animal models of neurodegenerative disease [155]. In contrast, high cortisol levels activate NLRP1 and NLRP3 inflammasomes and promote neuroinflammation and neuronal injury [156,157].

5.3. Insulin Resistance

Insulin and insulin-like growth factor 1 (IGF-1) signaling represent an evolutionary conserved pathway of longevity. Oxidative stress is implicated in the onset and progression of insulin resistance and type 2 diabetes [158], which is a prominent feature of normal aging and a preclinical indicator in many neurodegenerative disorders [159]. Peripheral insulin resistance is related to impairment of central insulin signaling and reported to be an early etiological factor in development of PD [160,161]. It is also associated with more rapid progression of PD disease and related cognitive impairment and dementia [162]. Functional brain imaging in PD further shows hypometabolism in the inferior parietal cortex and the caudate nucleus, which correlate with cognitive deficits and motor symptoms, respectively [163]. In PD, insulin resistance is proposed to lead to a state of bioenergetic failure and hypometabolism in the brain that may promote neurotoxicity [164].

Elevated cortisol is a major causal candidate for the development of insulin resistance with aging. It is well-known that while insulin exerts anabolic actions, cortisol exerts catabolic actions and the two hormones counteract each other in many metabolic functions, from glucose utilization to lipid storage [165]. On the other hand, klotho deficiency decreases insulin production and increases insulin sensitivity [141,166]. While the mechanisms of this are not entirely clear, it is known that klotho suppresses the downstream signaling pathway of the IGF-1 reception and insulin receptor substrate without directly binding to these receptors. Insulin also increases shedding of klotho, thereby increasing circulating klotho [167].

5.4. Vitamin D Metabolism

Another route by which cortisol and klotho may contribute to the multifactorial toxic cycle implicated in PD is via their actions on the neuroprotective hormone vitamin D. Vitamin D is a fat-soluble hormone that can pass the blood–brain barrier, supporting its significance in the central nervous system. Vitamin D insufficiency is associated with an increased risk of several CNS diseases including PD [168,169]. Vitamin D is reported to regulate more than 200 genes, influencing a variety of cellular processes such as neurotransmission neuroprotection, and downregulation of inflammation and oxidative stress [170]. It stimulates expression of many neurotrophic factors including neurotrophin 3 (NT-3), BDNF, glial cell-derived neurotrophic factor (GDNF), ciliary neurotrophic factor (CNTF), and neuroprotective cytokine IL-34 [171].

The vitamin D receptor is found throughout the human brain but crucially, is abundant in the substantia nigra pars compacta, the primary target of neurodegeneration in PD [172]. Additionally, 1α-hydroxylase—the enzyme that converts vitamin D to its active form,1,25(OH)$_2$D$_3$—is highly expressed in the substantia nigra, suggesting that vitamin D may be directly or indirectly related to the pathogenesis of PD via loss of protection for vulnerable dopaminergic neurons in this brain region [173]. In the past two decades, a high prevalence of vitamin D deficiency has been noted in individuals with PD [174]. Vitamin D concentrations also negatively correlate with PD risk and disease severity [175]. A small but significant association between vitamin D status at baseline and disease motor severity at 36 months has been reported [176]. Higher vitamin D concentrations link to better cognitive function and mood in individuals with PD [170,177]. Unfortunately, a (somewhat limited) trial of Vitamin D supplementation did not appear to improve PD symptoms [178].

Vitamin D is now suggested to be a biomarker of healthy aging with a strong association between low levels and higher all-cause mortality with large and significant effect sizes in multiple studies [179]. Cortisol has an antagonist relationship with vitamin D. Higher cortisol levels correlate with lower vitamin D levels [180]. Several studies also suggest that vitamin D may regulate the HPA axis. In hippocampal cell cultures, vitamin D suppresses glucocorticoid-induced transcription and cytotoxicity [181]. In the CNS, the most intense staining for vitamin D receptor and activating enzyme is described to be in the hypothalamus, including in the paraventricular nucleus (PVN) containing the corticotrophin releasing hormone (CRH)-positive neurons [173]. These neurons also stain positive for vitamin D 24-hydroxylase, and therefore are likely vitamin D responsive [182].

The anti-aging protein klotho plays a key role in regulating vitamin D metabolism. Membrane bound klotho is a cofactor for FGF23. Together, they form the receptor complex instrumental in Vitamin D production [183]. The biological functions of Vitamin D and klotho are highly intertwined because vitamin D induces the expression of klotho, and klotho keeps vitamin D levels in check. Klotho inhibits 1α-hydroxylase to decrease the active form of vitamin D—1-25(OH)2 D3, and increases activity of 24-hydroxylase, which converts both vitamin D and 1-25(OH)2 D3 into 24-hydroxylated products targeted for excretion. Lastly, low vitamin D levels are associated with depression and chronic stress, both conditions also linked to decreased klotho and elevated cortisol [60,184,185].

6. Cortisol and Klotho Associations with PD Symptomatology
6.1. Mood and Cognition

Initial studies revealed that cortisol and klotho may influence non-motor symptoms of PD. Cortisol levels have most commonly been correlated with neuropsychiatric symptoms.

A large number of people with Major Depressive Disorder (MDD) show abnormalities in the HPA axis functioning, with coinciding increased plasma levels of cortisol [185]. MDD patients also show neurochemical changes in CRH in the PVN, a structure now known to contain inclusions of α-synuclein, hallmark of PD pathology [186]. In individuals with PD, cortisol has been shown to correlate with the severity of depression [187] and with prevalence of anxiety and anhedonia [67]. In PD patients with impulse control disorders, increased cortisol is associated with more risk-taking behavior [188].

There is a growing body of evidence that increased cortisol is associated with late-life cognitive decline in normal aging in people with pre-clinical or clinical AD [57,189,190]. In non-demented patients, high cortisol correlates with decreased total brain volume, particularly in grey matter, and poorer cognitive function [191,192]. Elevated cortisol has also been linked to hippocampal atrophy, correlating with memory dysfunction [193]. Studies are needed to evaluate the link between cortisol and cognition in PD.

While klotho levels have not been related to psychiatric symptoms in PD itself, low klotho levels have been associated with depression [60]. Interestingly, a small exploratory study also found that CSF klotho levels are increased by electroconvulsive treatment for depression [194]. Lastly, *KL* gene polymorphisms can influence responsiveness to selective serotonin reuptake inhibitors (SSRIs) in people with depression [195].

Klotho has been shown to confer cognitive resilience in healthy aging and neurodegenerative disease. In animal models, klotho overexpression increases long-term potentiation and enhances spatial learning and memory [17]. In normal aging individuals, carrying the *KL* genetic variant (*KL*-VS), resulting in higher system klotho protein levels, links to enhanced cognition and enhanced functional brain connectivity [18,108]. Higher klotho levels also associate with enhanced volume of dorsolateral prefrontal cortex, an area that drives executive function [196]. Clinical studies studying klotho in relation to cognition in PD are lacking but initial studies reveal that acute elevation of klotho by peripheral delivery is sufficient to restore cognition in transgenic mouse models of PD [71].

6.2. Circadian Rhythm

In recent years, it has become increasingly apparent that the circadian rhythm influences PD, with patients experiencing diurnal fluctuations in motor and non-motor symptoms, despite stable pharmacokinetics of dopaminergic medications [197]. While mechanisms behind this remain unclear, it is known that neurodegeneration affects the central structures responsible for sleep and wakefulness, which may in turn affect input to the hypothalamic SCN, housing the molecular clock of the circadian system. This molecular clock consists of core clock genes, and disruption in their function in the pathogenesis of PD has recently gained attention [198]. In people with PD, degeneration of the dopamine containing cells in the retina may further affect input needed for alignment of dark/light cycles [199]. Lastly, dopaminergic therapy has a bidirectional relationship with circadian rhythm—responsiveness of motor symptoms to medication declines later in the day and medication leads to uncoupling of circadian and sleep regulation [200–202].

The circadian pattern of cortisol secretion provides a key signal from the SCN to peripheral clock genes. PD-associated changes in HPA axis function leads to a flatter circadian profile for cortisol and signaling to peripheral clock genes is compromised with resultant circadian disorder [65,198]. It is interesting to note that chronic kidney disease is associated with dysregulation of the SCN [203], and kidney disease is a risk factor for PD.

Unlike the hormone cortisol, there is not much written about klotho and circadian function. An early report in healthy humans found that serum klotho showed a circadian rhythm with falling levels in the evening, a marked nadir at midnight and levels rising again by the morning [204]. No such circadian variation in klotho has been found in human CSF [36] or in the serum of healthy rats [205]. However, a relationship between klotho and sleep appears more robust with subjective sleep quality being positively associated with klotho in sedentary middle-aged adults [206]. Lower levels of klotho are also reported in people with obstructive sleep apnea and associated with overnight markers of hypoxemia [207]. Klotho levels are also decreased with excessive sleep duration [208], which is known to increase the risk of inflammatory diseases.

6.3. Motor Symptoms

When looking at healthy aging populations, cortisol negatively correlates with grip strength [209] while lower levels of klotho associate with decreased grip strength and knee strength [87,117]. In people newly diagnosed with PD, higher cortisol levels correlate with greater motor burden of disease, measured using the Unified Parkinson's Disease Rating Scale (UPDRS) part III [210]. Thus far, only one study reports that lower CSF levels of klotho link to increased UPDRS III scores and higher Hoehn and Yahr disease stage [37]. When mice deficient in klotho were initially described, a parkinsonian phenotype was noted, with development of hypokinesis and decreased stride length along with midbrain dopaminergic neuronal loss at 5 weeks of age [30]. Later studies demonstrated that treatment with klotho, either via intracerebroventricular injection in toxin mouse model of PD or administered intraperitoneally in α-synuclein transgenic mouse model of PD, ameliorates motor deficits [71]. More studies are needed in humans to confirm that changes in cortisol and klotho affect PD motor symptoms.

7. Proposed Model

Evidently there exists a complex interplay between aging and chronic stress in the pathogenesis of PD through mechanisms involving mitochondrial dysfunction and oxidative stress, neuroinflammation, insulin resistance, and vitamin D. It is difficult to extract precise cause and effect in the vicious circle resulting in neurodegeneration; however, there is a case that the hormones cortisol and klotho can contribute to the disease process in a yin-yang manner. Moreover, given their broad effects, these hormones may be key players in both idiopathic and familial PD. Our model proposed in Figure 1 suggests that in PD, there is accelerated aging and increased stress, leading to decrease in circulating klotho and increase in cortisol. As the balanced dualism of these hormones becomes dysregulated, there is resultant pro-inflammatory environment and mitochondrial dysfunction facilitating a wide range of pathways leading to neurotoxicity. Vitamin D metabolism may also be shifted along with increase in insulin resistance, further facilitating disease processes. Interestingly, both cortisol and klotho levels may be amenable to change, with physical activity increasing klotho and decreasing cortisol, and psychological stress/depression decreasing klotho and increasing cortisol.

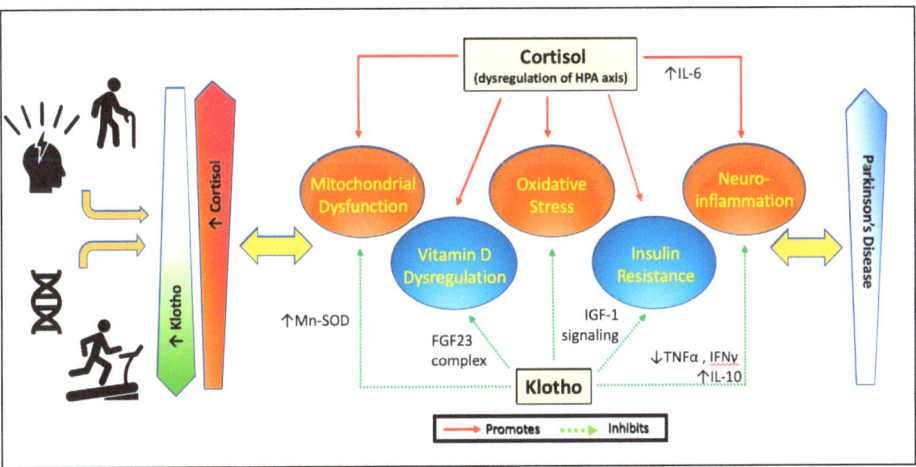

Figure 1. Proposed model for effects of cortisol and klotho on pathways linked to Parkinson's disease. With stress and aging, cortisol levels increase due to dysregulation of the HPA axis and

klotho levels decrease. Exercise decreases cortisol levels and increases klotho levels. Certain genetic variations may further dampen cortisol sensitivity and cellular response to stress or increase klotho levels or change its function. Chronic elevation of cortisol with aging or stress leads to increase in mitochondrial dysfunction, oxidative stress and activation of inflammatory cytokines, while promoting insulin resistance and correlating with lower vitamin D levels. Klotho normally protects mitochondrial structure and function, decreases oxidative stress, decreases inflammatory states, suppresses the downstream signaling pathway that leads to insulin resistance, and downregulates vitamin D metabolizing enzymes to control active vitamin D levels. This dysregulation of cortisol and reduction in klotho with aging and stress, important risk factors for PD, are hypothesized to affect the course of PD. Changes in cortisol and klotho in disease conditions may affects signs, symptoms, or progression of PD.

8. Conclusions

In summary, we have highlighted the multifactorial actions of cortisol and klotho in the pathogenesis of PD. Downstream effects of cortisol and klotho may influence non-motor and motor symptoms of PD. Given that PD is a heterogenous disorder with multiple pathways involved in neurodegeneration, identifying strategies with a broad neuroprotective potential, e.g., via exercise-induced modifications of cortisol and klotho secretion, offers the potential of increasing the brain's overall resilience. Future studies on how these hormones of aging and stress play a role in PD will lend evidence to whether these can be potential biomarkers or novel targets for interventional strategies.

Author Contributions: Conceptualization: N.S.L. and D.M.C.; Writing—Original Draft Preparation: N.S.L. and A.C; Writing—Review and Editing, N.S.L., A.C. and D.M.C. All authors have read and agreed to the published version of the manuscript.

Funding: Research reported in this publication was supported by the National Institute of Neurological Disorders and Stroke of the National Institutes of Health under Award Number U01NS113851. The content is solely the responsibility of the authors and does not necessarily represent the official views of the National Institutes of Health. Research reported in this publication was also supported, in part, by the National Institutes of Health's National Center for Advancing Translational Sciences, Grant Number UL1TR001422. The content is solely the responsibility of the authors and does not necessarily represent the official views of the National Institutes of Health.

Institutional Review Board Statement: Not applicable.

Informed Consent Statement: Not applicable.

Data Availability Statement: Not applicable.

Conflicts of Interest: The authors declare no conflict of interest.

References

1. Dorsey, E.R.; Bloem, B.R. The Parkinson Pandemic-A Call to Action. *JAMA Neurol.* **2018**, *75*, 9–10. [CrossRef]
2. Feigin, V.L.; Abajobir, A.A.; Abate, K.H.; Abd-Allah, F.; Abdulle, A.M.; Abera, S.F.; Abyu, G.Y.; Ahmed, M.B.; Aichour, A.N.; Aichour, I.; et al. Global, regional, and national burden of neurological disorders during 1990–2015: A systematic analysis for the Global Burden of Disease Study 2015. *Lancet Neurol.* **2017**, *16*, 877–897. [CrossRef] [PubMed]
3. Blesa, J.; Foffani, G.; Dehay, B.; Bezard, E.; Obeso, J.A. Motor and non-motor circuit disturbances in early Parkinson disease: Which happens first? *Nat. Rev. Neurosci.* **2022**, *23*, 115–128. [CrossRef] [PubMed]
4. Chaudhuri, K.R.; Sauerbier, A. Parkinson disease. Unravelling the nonmotor mysteries of Parkinson disease. *Nat. Rev. Neurol.* **2016**, *12*, 10–11. [CrossRef] [PubMed]
5. Hughes, K.C.; Gao, X.; Baker, J.M.; Stephen, C.; Kim, I.Y.; Valeri, L.; Schwarzschild, M.A.; Ascherio, A. Non-motor features of Parkinson's disease in a nested case-control study of US men. *J. Neurol. Neurosurg. Psychiatry* **2018**, *89*, 1288–1295. [CrossRef]
6. Schapira, A.H.V.; Chaudhuri, K.R.; Jenner, P. Non-motor features of Parkinson disease. *Nat. Rev. Neurosci.* **2017**, *18*, 509. [CrossRef]
7. Reeve, A.; Simcox, E.; Turnbull, D. Ageing and Parkinson's disease: Why is advancing age the biggest risk factor? *Ageing Res. Rev.* **2014**, *14*, 19–30. [CrossRef]

8. Pang, S.Y.; Ho, P.W.; Liu, H.F.; Leung, C.T.; Li, L.; Chang, E.E.S.; Ramsden, D.B.; Ho, S.L. The interplay of aging, genetics and environmental factors in the pathogenesis of Parkinson's disease. *Transl Neurodegener* **2019**, *8*, 23. [CrossRef]
9. Marinus, J.; Zhu, K.; Marras, C.; Aarsland, D.; van Hilten, J.J. Risk factors for non-motor symptoms in Parkinson's disease. *Lancet Neurol.* **2018**, *17*, 559–568. [CrossRef]
10. Hindle, J.V. Ageing, neurodegeneration and Parkinson's disease. *Age Ageing* **2010**, *39*, 156–161. [CrossRef]
11. Kennedy, B.K.; Berger, S.L.; Brunet, A.; Campisi, J.; Cuervo, A.M.; Epel, E.S.; Franceschi, C.; Lithgow, G.J.; Morimoto, R.I.; Pessin, J.E.; et al. Geroscience: Linking aging to chronic disease. *Cell* **2014**, *159*, 709–713. [CrossRef] [PubMed]
12. Lupien, S.J.; Juster, R.P.; Raymond, C.; Marin, M.F. The effects of chronic stress on the human brain: From neurotoxicity, to vulnerability, to opportunity. *Front. Neuroendocrinol.* **2018**, *49*, 91–105. [CrossRef] [PubMed]
13. Cohen, S.; Janicki-Deverts, D.; Doyle, W.J.; Miller, G.E.; Frank, E.; Rabin, B.S.; Turner, R.B. Chronic stress, glucocorticoid receptor resistance, inflammation and disease risk. *Proc. Natl. Acad. Sci. USA* **2012**, *109*, 5995–5999. [CrossRef] [PubMed]
14. Lupien, S.J.; McEwen, B.S.; Gunnar, M.R.; Heim, C. Effects of stress throughout the lifespan on the brain, behaviour and cognition. *Nat. Rev. Neurosci.* **2009**, *10*, 434–445. [CrossRef] [PubMed]
15. Rackova, L.; Mach, M.; Brnoliakova, Z. An update in toxicology of ageing. *Environ. Toxicol. Pharmacol.* **2021**, *84*, 103611. [CrossRef] [PubMed]
16. Kurosu, H.; Yamamoto, M.; Clark, J.D.; Pastor, J.V.; Nandi, A.; Gurnani, P.; McGuinness, O.P.; Chikuda, H.; Yamaguchi, M.; Kawaguchi, H.; et al. Suppression of aging in mice by the hormone Klotho. *Science* **2005**, *309*, 1829–1833. [CrossRef]
17. Dubal, D.B.; Zhu, L.; Sanchez, P.E.; Worden, K.; Broestl, L.; Johnson, E.; Ho, K.; Yu, G.Q.; Kim, D.; Betourne, A.; et al. Life extension factor klotho prevents mortality and enhances cognition in hAPP transgenic mice. *J. Neurosci.* **2015**, *35*, 2358–2371. [CrossRef]
18. Dubal, D.B.; Yokoyama, J.S.; Zhu, L.; Broestl, L.; Worden, K.; Wang, D.; Sturm, V.E.; Kim, D.; Klein, E.; Yu, G.Q.; et al. Life extension factor klotho enhances cognition. *Cell Rep* **2014**, *7*, 1065–1076. [CrossRef]
19. Dedovic, K.; Duchesne, A.; Andrews, J.; Engert, V.; Pruessner, J.C. The brain and the stress axis: The neural correlates of cortisol regulation in response to stress. *Neuroimage* **2009**, *47*, 864–871. [CrossRef]
20. Hermans, E.J.; Henckens, M.J.; Joels, M.; Fernandez, G. Dynamic adaptation of large-scale brain networks in response to acute stressors. *Trends Neurosci.* **2014**, *37*, 304–314. [CrossRef]
21. Nader, N.; Chrousos, G.P.; Kino, T. Interactions of the circadian CLOCK system and the HPA axis. *Trends Endocrinol Metab* **2010**, *21*, 277–286. [CrossRef] [PubMed]
22. Viho, E.M.G.; Buurstede, J.C.; Mahfouz, A.; Koorneef, L.L.; van Weert, L.; Houtman, R.; Hunt, H.J.; Kroon, J.; Meijer, O.C. Corticosteroid Action in the Brain: The Potential of Selective Receptor Modulation. *Neuroendocrinology* **2019**, *109*, 266–276. [CrossRef] [PubMed]
23. Fietta, P.; Fietta, P.; Delsante, G. Central nervous system effects of natural and synthetic glucocorticoids. *Psychiatry Clin. Neurosci.* **2009**, *63*, 613–622. [CrossRef]
24. Liston, C.; Gan, W.B. Glucocorticoids are critical regulators of dendritic spine development and plasticity in vivo. *Proc. Natl. Acad. Sci. USA* **2011**, *108*, 16074–16079. [CrossRef]
25. Ratman, D.; Vanden Berghe, W.; Dejager, L.; Libert, C.; Tavernier, J.; Beck, I.M.; De Bosscher, K. How glucocorticoid receptors modulate the activity of other transcription factors: A scope beyond tethering. *Mol. Cell. Endocrinol.* **2013**, *380*, 41–54. [CrossRef] [PubMed]
26. Carter, B.S.; Meng, F.; Thompson, R.C. Glucocorticoid treatment of astrocytes results in temporally dynamic transcriptome regulation and astrocyte-enriched mRNA changes in vitro. *Physiol. Genom.* **2012**, *44*, 1188–1200. [CrossRef] [PubMed]
27. Gray, J.D.; Rubin, T.G.; Hunter, R.G.; McEwen, B.S. Hippocampal gene expression changes underlying stress sensitization and recovery. *Mol. Psychiatry* **2014**, *19*, 1171–1178. [CrossRef] [PubMed]
28. Joels, M. Corticosteroids and the brain. *J. Endocrinol.* **2018**, *238*, R121–R130. [CrossRef]
29. Van Wamelen, D.J.; Wan, Y.M.; Ray Chaudhuri, K.; Jenner, P. Stress and cortisol in Parkinson's disease. *Int. Rev. Neurobiol.* **2020**, *152*, 131–156.
30. Kuro-o, M.; Matsumura, Y.; Aizawa, H.; Kawaguchi, H.; Suga, T.; Utsugi, T.; Ohyama, Y.; Kurabayashi, M.; Kaname, T.; Kume, E. Mutation of the mouse klotho gene leads to a syndrome resembling ageing. *Nature* **1997**, *390*, 45–51. [CrossRef]
31. Arking, D.E.; Atzmon, G.; Arking, A.; Barzilai, N.; Dietz, H.C. Association between a functional variant of the KLOTHO gene and high-density lipoprotein cholesterol, blood pressure, stroke and longevity. *Circ. Res.* **2005**, *96*, 412–418. [CrossRef] [PubMed]
32. Arking, D.E.; Becker, D.M.; Yanek, L.R.; Fallin, D.; Judge, D.P.; Moy, T.F.; Becker, L.C.; Dietz, H.C. KLOTHO allele status and the risk of early-onset occult coronary artery disease. *Am. J. Hum. Genet.* **2003**, *72*, 1154–1161. [CrossRef] [PubMed]
33. Semba, R.D.; Cappola, A.R.; Sun, K.; Bandinelli, S.; Dalal, M.; Crasto, C.; Guralnik, J.M.; Ferrucci, L. Plasma klotho and cardiovascular disease in adults. *J. Am. Geriatr. Soc.* **2011**, *59*, 1596–1601. [CrossRef] [PubMed]
34. Drew, D.A.; Katz, R.; Kritchevsky, S.; Ix, J.; Shlipak, M.; Gutierrez, O.M.; Newman, A.; Hoofnagle, A.; Fried, L.; Semba, R.D.; et al. Association between Soluble Klotho and Change in Kidney Function: The Health Aging and Body Composition Study. *J. Am. Soc. Nephrol.* **2017**, *28*, 1859–1866. [CrossRef]
35. Doi, S.; Zou, Y.; Togao, O.; Pastor, J.V.; John, G.B.; Wang, L.; Shiizaki, K.; Gotschall, R.; Schiavi, S.; Yorioka, N.; et al. Klotho inhibits transforming growth factor-beta1 (TGF-beta1) signaling and suppresses renal fibrosis and cancer metastasis in mice. *J. Biol. Chem.* **2011**, *286*, 8655–8665. [CrossRef]

36. Semba, R.D.; Moghekar, A.R.; Hu, J.; Sun, K.; Turner, R.; Ferrucci, L.; O'Brien, R. Klotho in the cerebrospinal fluid of adults with and without Alzheimer's disease. *Neurosci. Lett.* **2014**, *558*, 37–40. [CrossRef]
37. Zimmermann, M.; Kohler, L.; Kovarova, M.; Lerche, S.; Schulte, C.; Wurster, I.; Machetanz, G.; Deuschle, C.; Hauser, A.K.; Gasser, T.; et al. The longevity gene Klotho and its cerebrospinal fluid protein profiles as a modifier for Parkinson's disease. *Eur. J. Neurol.* **2021**, *28*, 1557–1565. [CrossRef]
38. Clinton, S.M.; Glover, M.E.; Maltare, A.; Laszczyk, A.M.; Mehi, S.J.; Simmons, R.K.; King, G.D. Expression of klotho mRNA and protein in rat brain parenchyma from early postnatal development into adulthood. *Brain Res.* **2013**, *1527*, 1–14. [CrossRef]
39. German, D.C.; Khobahy, I.; Pastor, J.; Kuro, O.M.; Liu, X. Nuclear localization of Klotho in brain: An anti-aging protein. *Neurobiol. Aging* **2012**, *33*, 1483.e25–1483.e30. [CrossRef]
40. Brobey, R.K.; German, D.; Sonsalla, P.K.; Gurnani, P.; Pastor, J.; Hsieh, C.C.; Papaconstantinou, J.; Foster, P.P.; Kuro-o, M.; Rosenblatt, K.P. Klotho Protects Dopaminergic Neuron Oxidant-Induced Degeneration by Modulating ASK1 and p38 MAPK Signaling Pathways. *PLoS ONE* **2015**, *10*, e0139914. [CrossRef]
41. Li, S.A.; Watanabe, M.; Yamada, H.; Nagai, A.; Kinuta, M.; Takei, K. Immunohistochemical localization of Klotho protein in brain, kidney, and reproductive organs of mice. *Cell Struct. Funct.* **2004**, *29*, 91–99. [CrossRef] [PubMed]
42. Utsugi, T.; Ohno, T.; Ohyama, Y.; Uchiyama, T.; Saito, Y.; Matsumura, Y.; Aizawa, H.; Itoh, H.; Kurabayashi, M.; Kawazu, S.; et al. Decreased insulin production and increased insulin sensitivity in the klotho mutant mouse, a novel animal model for human aging. *Metabolism* **2000**, *49*, 1118–1123. [CrossRef] [PubMed]
43. Liu, H.; Fergusson, M.M.; Castilho, R.M.; Liu, J.; Cao, L.; Chen, J.; Malide, D.; Rovira, I.I.; Schimel, D.; Kuo, C.J.; et al. Augmented Wnt signaling in a mammalian model of accelerated aging. *Science* **2007**, *317*, 803–806. [CrossRef]
44. Chang, Q.; Hoefs, S.; van der Kemp, A.W.; Topala, C.N.; Bindels, R.J.; Hoenderop, J.G. The beta-glucuronidase Klotho hydrolyzes and activates the TRPV5 channel. *Science* **2005**, *310*, 490–493. [CrossRef]
45. Urakawa, I.; Yamazaki, Y.; Shimada, T.; Iijima, K.; Hasegawa, H.; Okawa, K.; Fujita, T.; Fukumoto, S.; Yamashita, T. Klotho converts canonical FGF receptor into a specific receptor for FGF23. *Nature* **2006**, *444*, 770–774. [CrossRef] [PubMed]
46. Erben, R.G. alpha-Klotho's effects on mineral homeostasis are fibroblast growth factor-23 dependent. *Curr. Opin. Nephrol. Hypertens.* **2018**, *27*, 229–235. [CrossRef] [PubMed]
47. Hum, J.M.; O'Bryan, L.; Smith, R.C.; White, K.E. Novel functions of circulating Klotho. *Bone* **2017**, *100*, 36–40. [CrossRef]
48. Kuro, O.M. Molecular Mechanisms Underlying Accelerated Aging by Defects in the FGF23-Klotho System. *Int. J. Nephrol.* **2018**, *2018*, 9679841. [CrossRef]
49. Razzaque, M.S. The FGF23-Klotho axis: Endocrine regulation of phosphate homeostasis. *Nat. Rev. Endocrinol.* **2009**, *5*, 611–619. [CrossRef]
50. Huang, C.L.; Moe, O.W. Klotho: A novel regulator of calcium and phosphorus homeostasis. *Pflügers Arch.-Eur. J. Physiol.* **2011**, *462*, 185–193. [CrossRef]
51. Tsujikawa, H.; Kurotaki, Y.; Fujimori, T.; Fukuda, K.; Nabeshima, Y. Klotho, a gene related to a syndrome resembling human premature aging, functions in a negative regulatory circuit of vitamin D endocrine system. *Mol. Endocrinol.* **2003**, *17*, 2393–2403. [CrossRef] [PubMed]
52. Bookout, A.L.; de Groot, M.H.; Owen, B.M.; Lee, S.; Gautron, L.; Lawrence, H.L.; Ding, X.; Elmquist, J.K.; Takahashi, J.S.; Mangelsdorf, D.J.; et al. FGF21 regulates metabolism and circadian behavior by acting on the nervous system. *Nat. Med.* **2013**, *19*, 1147–1152. [CrossRef] [PubMed]
53. Jia, Y.; Liu, L.; Sheng, C.; Cheng, Z.; Cui, L.; Li, M.; Zhao, Y.; Shi, T.; Yau, T.O.; Li, F.; et al. Increased Serum Levels of Cortisol and Inflammatory Cytokines in People with Depression. *J. Nerv. Ment. Dis.* **2019**, *207*, 271–276. [CrossRef] [PubMed]
54. Fiksdal, A.; Hanlin, L.; Kuras, Y.; Gianferante, D.; Chen, X.; Thoma, M.V.; Rohleder, N. Associations between symptoms of depression and anxiety and cortisol responses to and recovery from acute stress. *Psychoneuroendocrinology* **2019**, *102*, 44–52. [CrossRef] [PubMed]
55. Vgontzas, A.N.; Bixler, E.O.; Lin, H.M.; Prolo, P.; Mastorakos, G.; Vela-Bueno, A.; Kales, A.; Chrousos, G.P. Chronic insomnia is associated with nyctohemeral activation of the hypothalamic-pituitary-adrenal axis: Clinical implications. *J. Clin. Endocrinol. Metab.* **2001**, *86*, 3787–3794. [CrossRef] [PubMed]
56. Vgontzas, A.N.; Tsigos, C.; Bixler, E.O.; Stratakis, C.A.; Zachman, K.; Kales, A.; Vela-Bueno, A.; Chrousos, G.P. Chronic insomnia and activity of the stress system: A preliminary study. *J Psychosom Res* **1998**, *45*, 21–31. [CrossRef]
57. Ouanes, S.; Popp, J. High Cortisol and the Risk of Dementia and Alzheimer's Disease: A Review of the Literature. *Front. Aging Neurosci.* **2019**, *11*, 43. [CrossRef]
58. Costa, C.M.; Oliveira, G.L.; Fonseca, A.C.S.; Lana, R.C.; Polese, J.C.; Pernambuco, A.P. Levels of cortisol and neurotrophic factor brain-derived in Parkinson's disease. *Neurosci. Lett.* **2019**, *708*, 134359. [CrossRef]
59. Barbosa, I.G.; Rocha, N.P.; Alpak, G.; Vieira, E.L.M.; Huguet, R.B.; Rocha, F.L.; de Oliveira Diniz, B.S.; Teixeira, A.L. Klotho dysfunction: A pathway linking the aging process to bipolar disorder? *J. Psychiatr. Res.* **2017**, *95*, 80–83. [CrossRef]
60. Prather, A.A.; Epel, E.S.; Arenander, J.; Broestl, L.; Garay, B.I.; Wang, D.; Dubal, D.B. Longevity factor klotho and chronic psychological stress. *Transl. Psychiatry* **2015**, *5*, e585. [CrossRef]
61. Emami Aleagha, M.S.; Siroos, B.; Ahmadi, M.; Balood, M.; Palangi, A.; Haghighi, A.N.; Harirchian, M.H. Decreased concentration of Klotho in the cerebrospinal fluid of patients with relapsing-remitting multiple sclerosis. *J. Neuroimmunol.* **2015**, *281*, 5–8. [CrossRef] [PubMed]

62. Teocchi, M.A.; Ferreira, A.E.; da Luz de Oliveira, E.P.; Tedeschi, H.; D'Souza-Li, L. Hippocampal gene expression dysregulation of Klotho, nuclear factor kappa B and tumor necrosis factor in temporal lobe epilepsy patients. *J. Neuroinflammation* **2013**, *10*, 53. [CrossRef] [PubMed]
63. Mizobuchi, M.; Hineno, T.; Kakimoto, Y.; Hiratani, K. Increase of plasma adrenocorticotrophin and cortisol in 1-methyl-4-phenyl-1,2,3,6-tetrahydropyridine (MPTP)-treated dogs. *Brain Res.* **1993**, *612*, 319–321. [CrossRef] [PubMed]
64. Smith, L.K.; Jadavji, N.M.; Colwell, K.L.; Katrina Perehudoff, S.; Metz, G.A. Stress accelerates neural degeneration and exaggerates motor symptoms in a rat model of Parkinson's disease. *Eur. J. Neurosci.* **2008**, *27*, 2133–2146. [CrossRef] [PubMed]
65. Hartmann, A.; Veldhuis, J.D.; Deuschle, M.; Standhardt, H.; Heuser, I. Twenty-four hour cortisol release profiles in patients with Alzheimer's and Parkinson's disease compared to normal controls: Ultradian secretory pulsatility and diurnal variation. *Neurobiol. Aging* **1997**, *18*, 285–289. [CrossRef]
66. Skogar, O.; Fall, P.A.; Hallgren, G.; Lokk, J.; Bringer, B.; Carlsson, M.; Lennartsson, U.; Sandbjork, H.; Tornhage, C.J. Diurnal salivary cortisol concentrations in Parkinson's disease: Increased total secretion and morning cortisol concentrations. *Int. J. Gen. Med.* **2011**, *4*, 561–569. [CrossRef]
67. Van den Heuvel, L.L.; du Plessis, S.; Stalder, T.; Acker, D.; Kirschbaum, C.; Carr, J.; Seedat, S. Hair glucocorticoid levels in Parkinson's disease. *Psychoneuroendocrinology* **2020**, *117*, 104704. [CrossRef]
68. Belloy, M.E.; Napolioni, V.; Han, S.S.; Le Guen, Y.; Greicius, M.D.; Alzheimer's Disease Neuroimaging Initiative. Association of Klotho-VS Heterozygosity with Risk of Alzheimer Disease in Individuals Who Carry APOE4. *JAMA Neurol.* **2020**, *77*, 849–862. [CrossRef]
69. Kosakai, A.; Ito, D.; Nihei, Y.; Yamashita, S.; Okada, Y.; Takahashi, K.; Suzuki, N. Degeneration of mesencephalic dopaminergic neurons in klotho mouse related to vitamin D exposure. *Brain Res.* **2011**, *1382*, 109–117. [CrossRef]
70. Baluchnejadmojarad, T.; Eftekhari, S.M.; Jamali-Raeufy, N.; Haghani, S.; Zeinali, H.; Roghani, M. The anti-aging protein klotho alleviates injury of nigrostriatal dopaminergic pathway in 6-hydroxydopamine rat model of Parkinson's disease: Involvement of PKA/CaMKII/CREB signaling. *Exp. Gerontol.* **2017**, *100*, 70–76. [CrossRef]
71. Leon, J.; Moreno, A.J.; Garay, B.I.; Chalkley, R.J.; Burlingame, A.L.; Wang, D.; Dubal, D.B. Peripheral Elevation of a Klotho Fragment Enhances Brain Function and Resilience in Young, Aging and alpha-Synuclein Transgenic Mice. *Cell Rep* **2017**, *20*, 1360–1371. [CrossRef]
72. Kakar, R.S.; Pastor, J.V.; Moe, O.W.; Ambrosio, F.; Castaldi, D.; Sanders, L.H. Peripheral Klotho and Parkinson's Disease. *Mov. Disord.* **2021**, *36*, 1274–1276. [CrossRef] [PubMed]
73. Grillo, P.; Basilicata, M.; Schirinzi, T. Alpha-Klotho in Parkinson's disease: A perspective on experimental evidence and potential clinical implications. *Neural. Regen. Res.* **2022**, *17*, 2687–2688.
74. Muller, T.; Muhlack, S. Acute levodopa intake and associated cortisol decrease in patients with Parkinson disease. *Clin. Neuropharmacol.* **2007**, *30*, 101–106. [CrossRef] [PubMed]
75. Muller, T.; Welnic, J.; Muhlack, S. Acute levodopa administration reduces cortisol release in patients with Parkinson's disease. *J. Neural. Transm.* **2007**, *114*, 347–350. [CrossRef]
76. Tanner, C.M.; Goldman, S.M. Epidemiology of Parkinson's disease. *Neurol. Clin.* **1996**, *14*, 317–335. [CrossRef] [PubMed]
77. Collier, T.J.; Kanaan, N.M.; Kordower, J.H. Ageing as a primary risk factor for Parkinson's disease: Evidence from studies of non-human primates. *Nat. Rev. Neurosci.* **2011**, *12*, 359–366. [CrossRef]
78. Calabrese, V.; Santoro, A.; Monti, D.; Crupi, R.; Di Paola, R.; Latteri, S.; Cuzzocrea, S.; Zappia, M.; Giordano, J.; Calabrese, E.J.; et al. Aging and Parkinson's Disease: Inflammaging, neuroinflammation and biological remodeling as key factors in pathogenesis. *Free Radic. Biol. Med.* **2018**, *115*, 80–91. [CrossRef]
79. Franceschi, C.; Campisi, J. Chronic inflammation (inflammaging) and its potential contribution to age-associated diseases. *J. Gerontol. Ser. A Biol. Sci. Med. Sci.* **2014**, *69*, S4–S9. [CrossRef]
80. Moffat, S.D.; An, Y.; Resnick, S.M.; Diamond, M.P.; Ferrucci, L. Longitudinal Change in Cortisol Levels Across the Adult Life Span. *J. Gerontol. Ser. A Biol. Sci. Med. Sci.* **2020**, *75*, 394–400. [CrossRef]
81. Iob, E.; Steptoe, A. Cardiovascular Disease and Hair Cortisol: A Novel Biomarker of Chronic Stress. *Curr. Cardiol. Rep.* **2019**, *21*, 116. [CrossRef] [PubMed]
82. Sharma, V.K.; Singh, T.G. Chronic Stress and Diabetes Mellitus: Interwoven Pathologies. *Curr. Diabetes Rev.* **2020**, *16*, 546–556. [PubMed]
83. Al-Rawaf, H.A.; Alghadir, A.H.; Gabr, S.A. Circulating MicroRNA Expression, Vitamin D, and Hypercortisolism as Predictors of Osteoporosis in Elderly Postmenopausal Women. *Dis. Markers* **2021**, *2021*, 3719919. [CrossRef]
84. Lara, V.P.; Caramelli, P.; Teixeira, A.L.; Barbosa, M.T.; Carmona, K.C.; Carvalho, M.G.; Fernandes, A.P.; Gomes, K.B. High cortisol levels are associated with cognitive impairment no-dementia (CIND) and dementia. *Clin. Chim. Acta* **2013**, *423*, 18–22. [CrossRef]
85. Yamazaki, Y.; Imura, A.; Urakawa, I.; Shimada, T.; Murakami, J.; Aono, Y.; Hasegawa, H.; Yamashita, T.; Nakatani, K.; Saito, Y.; et al. Establishment of sandwich ELISA for soluble alpha-Klotho measurement: Age-dependent change of soluble alpha-Klotho levels in healthy subjects. *Biochem. Biophys. Res. Commun.* **2010**, *398*, 513–518. [CrossRef] [PubMed]
86. Semba, R.D.; Cappola, A.R.; Sun, K.; Bandinelli, S.; Dalal, M.; Crasto, C.; Guralnik, J.M.; Ferrucci, L. Plasma klotho and mortality risk in older community-dwelling adults. *J. Gerontol. Ser. A Biol. Sci. Med. Sci.* **2011**, *66*, 794–800. [CrossRef] [PubMed]

87. Semba, R.D.; Cappola, A.R.; Sun, K.; Bandinelli, S.; Dalal, M.; Crasto, C.; Guralnik, J.M.; Ferrucci, L. Relationship of low plasma klotho with poor grip strength in older community-dwelling adults: The InCHIANTI study. *Eur. J. Appl. Physiol.* **2012**, *112*, 1215–1220. [CrossRef]
88. Cardoso, A.L.; Fernandes, A.; Aguilar-Pimentel, J.A.; de Angelis, M.H.; Guedes, J.R.; Brito, M.A.; Ortolano, S.; Pani, G.; Athanasopoulou, S.; Gonos, E.S.; et al. Towards frailty biomarkers: Candidates from genes and pathways regulated in aging and age-related diseases. *Ageing Res. Rev.* **2018**, *47*, 214–277. [CrossRef]
89. Sieurin, J.; Andel, R.; Tillander, A.; Valdes, E.G.; Pedersen, N.L.; Wirdefeldt, K. Occupational stress and risk for Parkinson's disease: A nationwide cohort study. *Mov. Disord.* **2018**, *33*, 1456–1464. [CrossRef]
90. Vlajinac, H.; Sipetic, S.; Marinkovic, J.; Ratkov, I.; Maksimovic, J.; Dzoljic, E.; Kostic, V. The stressful life events and Parkinson's disease: A case-control study. *Stress Health* **2013**, *29*, 50–55. [CrossRef]
91. White, D.L.; Kunik, M.E.; Yu, H.; Lin, H.L.; Richardson, P.A.; Moore, S.; Sarwar, A.I.; Marsh, L.; Jorge, R.E. Post-Traumatic Stress Disorder is Associated with further Increased Parkinson's Disease Risk in Veterans with Traumatic Brain Injury. *Ann. Neurol.* **2020**, *88*, 33–41. [CrossRef] [PubMed]
92. Svensson, E.; Farkas, D.K.; Gradus, J.L.; Lash, T.L.; Sorensen, H.T. Adjustment disorder and risk of Parkinson's disease. *Eur. J. Neurol.* **2016**, *23*, 751–756. [CrossRef]
93. Marin, M.F.; Lord, C.; Andrews, J.; Juster, R.P.; Sindi, S.; Arsenault-Lapierre, G.; Fiocco, A.J.; Lupien, S.J. Chronic stress, cognitive functioning and mental health. *Neurobiol. Learn. Mem.* **2011**, *96*, 583–595. [CrossRef]
94. De Kloet, E.R.; Joels, M.; Holsboer, F. Stress and the brain: From adaptation to disease. *Nat. Rev. Neurosci.* **2005**, *6*, 463–475. [CrossRef]
95. Swaab, D.F.; Bao, A.M.; Lucassen, P.J. The stress system in the human brain in depression and neurodegeneration. *Ageing Res. Rev.* **2005**, *4*, 141–194. [CrossRef] [PubMed]
96. Nollet, M.; Wisden, W.; Franks, N.P. Sleep deprivation and stress: A reciprocal relationship. *Interface Focus* **2020**, *10*, 20190092. [CrossRef]
97. Abel, T.; Havekes, R.; Saletin, J.M.; Walker, M.P. Sleep, plasticity and memory from molecules to whole-brain networks. *Curr. Biol.* **2013**, *23*, R774–R788. [CrossRef] [PubMed]
98. Metz, G.A. Stress as a modulator of motor system function and pathology. *Rev. Neurosci.* **2007**, *18*, 209–222. [CrossRef]
99. Van der Heide, A.; Meinders, M.J.; Speckens, A.E.M.; Peerbolte, T.F.; Bloem, B.R.; Helmich, R.C. Stress and Mindfulness in Parkinson's Disease: Clinical Effects and Potential Underlying Mechanisms. *Mov. Disord.* **2021**, *36*, 64–70. [CrossRef]
100. Wolf, E.J.; Morrison, F.G.; Sullivan, D.R.; Logue, M.W.; Guetta, R.E.; Stone, A.; Schichman, S.A.; McGlinchey, R.E.; Milberg, W.P.; Miller, M.W. The goddess who spins the thread of life: Klotho, psychiatric stress, and accelerated aging. *Brain Behav. Immun.* **2019**, *80*, 193–203. [CrossRef]
101. Wu, H.J.; Wu, W.N.; Fan, H.; Liu, L.E.; Zhan, J.Q.; Li, Y.H.; Chen, C.N.; Jiang, S.Z.; Xiong, J.W.; Yu, Z.M.; et al. Life extension factor klotho regulates behavioral responses to stress via modulation of GluN2B function in the nucleus accumbens. *Neuropsychopharmacology* **2022**, *47*, 1710–1720. [CrossRef] [PubMed]
102. Koper, J.W.; van Rossum, E.F.; van den Akker, E.L. Glucocorticoid receptor polymorphisms and haplotypes and their expression in health and disease. *Steroids* **2014**, *92*, 62–73. [CrossRef] [PubMed]
103. Van Rossum, E.F.; Feelders, R.A.; van den Beld, A.W.; Uitterlinden, A.G.; Janssen, J.A.; Ester, W.; Brinkmann, A.O.; Grobbee, D.E.; de Jong, F.H.; Pols, H.A.; et al. Association of the ER22/23EK polymorphism in the glucocorticoid receptor gene with survival and C-reactive protein levels in elderly men. *Am. J. Med.* **2004**, *117*, 158–162. [CrossRef] [PubMed]
104. Van Rossum, E.F.; Binder, E.B.; Majer, M.; Koper, J.W.; Ising, M.; Modell, S.; Salyakina, D.; Lamberts, S.W.; Holsboer, F. Polymorphisms of the glucocorticoid receptor gene and major depression. *Biol. Psychiatry* **2006**, *59*, 681–688. [CrossRef] [PubMed]
105. Lovallo, W.R.; Enoch, M.A.; Sorocco, K.H.; Vincent, A.S.; Acheson, A.; Cohoon, A.J.; Hodgkinson, C.A.; Goldman, D. Joint Impact of Early Life Adversity and COMT Val158Met (rs4680) Genotypes on the Adult Cortisol Response to Psychological Stress. *Psychosom. Med.* **2017**, *79*, 631–637. [CrossRef] [PubMed]
106. Wang, Y.C.; Zou, Y.B.; Xiao, J.; Pan, C.D.; Jiang, S.D.; Zheng, Z.J.; Yan, Z.R.; Tang, K.Y.; Tan, L.M.; Tang, M.S. COMT Val158Met polymorphism and Parkinson's disease risk: A pooled analysis in different populations. *Neurol. Res.* **2019**, *41*, 319–325. [CrossRef]
107. Wolf, E.J.; Chen, C.D.; Zhao, X.; Zhou, Z.; Morrison, F.G.; Daskalakis, N.P.; Stone, A.; Schichman, S.; Grenier, J.G.; Fein-Schaffer, D.; et al. Klotho, PTSD and advanced epigenetic age in cortical tissue. *Neuropsychopharmacology* **2021**, *46*, 721–730. [CrossRef]
108. Yokoyama, J.S.; Sturm, V.E.; Bonham, L.W.; Klein, E.; Arfanakis, K.; Yu, L.; Coppola, G.; Kramer, J.H.; Bennett, D.A.; Miller, B.L.; et al. Variation in longevity gene KLOTHO is associated with greater cortical volumes. *Ann. Clin. Transl. Neurol.* **2015**, *2*, 215–230. [CrossRef]
109. Beserra, A.H.N.; Kameda, P.; Deslandes, A.C.; Schuch, F.B.; Laks, J.; Moraes, H.S. Can physical exercise modulate cortisol level in subjects with depression? A systematic review and meta-analysis. *Trends Psychiatry Psychother.* **2018**, *40*, 360–368. [CrossRef]
110. Gottschall, J.S.; Davis, J.J.; Hastings, B.; Porter, H.J. Exercise Time and Intensity: How Much Is Too Much? *Int. J. Sports Physiol. Perform.* **2020**, *15*, 808–815. [CrossRef]
111. Caplin, A.; Chen, F.S.; Beauchamp, M.R.; Puterman, E. The effects of exercise intensity on the cortisol response to a subsequent acute psychosocial stressor. *Psychoneuroendocrinology* **2021**, *131*, 105336. [CrossRef] [PubMed]

112. Smyth, N.; Skender, E.; David, F.J.; Munoz, M.J.; Fantuzzi, G.; Clow, A.; Goldman, J.G.; Corcos, D.M. Endurance exercise reduces cortisol in Parkinson's disease with mild cognitive impairment. *Mov. Disord.* **2019**, *34*, 1238–1239. [CrossRef] [PubMed]
113. Pascoe, M.C.; Thompson, D.R.; Ski, C.F. Yoga, mindfulness-based stress reduction and stress-related physiological measures: A meta-analysis. *Psychoneuroendocrinology* **2017**, *86*, 152–168. [CrossRef]
114. Ho, R.T.H.; Fong, T.C.T.; Chan, W.C.; Kwan, J.S.K.; Chiu, P.K.C.; Yau, J.C.Y.; Lam, L.C.W. Psychophysiological Effects of Dance Movement Therapy and Physical Exercise on Older Adults with Mild Dementia: A Randomized Controlled Trial. *J. Gerontol. Ser. B Psychol. Sci. Soc. Sci.* **2020**, *75*, 560–570. [CrossRef] [PubMed]
115. Ji, N.; Luan, J.; Hu, F.; Zhao, Y.; Lv, B.; Wang, W.; Xia, M.; Zhao, X.; Lao, K. Aerobic exercise-stimulated Klotho upregulation extends life span by attenuating the excess production of reactive oxygen species in the brain and kidney. *Exp. Ther. Med.* **2018**, *16*, 3511–3517. [CrossRef] [PubMed]
116. Rao, Z.; Zheng, L.; Huang, H.; Feng, Y.; Shi, R. α-Klotho Expression in Mouse Tissues Following Acute Exhaustive Exercise. *Front. Physiol.* **2019**, *10*, 1498. [CrossRef] [PubMed]
117. Semba, R.D.; Ferrucci, L.; Sun, K.; Simonsick, E.; Turner, R.; Miljkovic, I.; Harris, T.; Schwartz, A.V.; Asao, K.; Kritchevsky, S.; et al. Low Plasma Klotho Concentrations and Decline of Knee Strength in Older Adults. *J. Gerontol. Ser. A Biol. Sci. Med. Sci.* **2016**, *71*, 103–108. [CrossRef]
118. Crasto, C.L.; Semba, R.D.; Sun, K.; Cappola, A.R.; Bandinelli, S.; Ferrucci, L. Relationship of low-circulating "anti-aging" klotho hormone with disability in activities of daily living among older community-dwelling adults. *Rejuvenation Res.* **2012**, *15*, 295–301. [CrossRef]
119. Saghiv, M.S.; Sira, D.B.; Goldhammer, E.; Sagiv, M. The effects of aerobic and anaerobic exercises on circulating soluble-Klotho and IGF-I in young and elderly adults and in CAD patients. *J. Circ. Biomark.* **2017**, *6*, 1849454417733388. [CrossRef]
120. Matsubara, T.; Miyaki, A.; Akazawa, N.; Choi, Y.; Ra, S.G.; Tanahashi, K.; Kumagai, H.; Oikawa, S.; Maeda, S. Aerobic exercise training increases plasma Klotho levels and reduces arterial stiffness in postmenopausal women. *Am. J. Physiol. Heart Circ. Physiol.* **2014**, *306*, H348–H355. [CrossRef]
121. Amaro-Gahete, F.J.; De-la, O.A.; Jurado-Fasoli, L.; Espuch-Oliver, A.; de Haro, T.; Gutierrez, A.; Ruiz, J.R.; Castillo, M.J. Exercise training increases the S-Klotho plasma levels in sedentary middle-aged adults: A randomised controlled trial. The FIT-AGEING study. *J. Sports. Sci.* **2019**, *37*, 2175–2183. [CrossRef] [PubMed]
122. Amaro-Gahete, F.J.; de-la-O, A.; Jurado-Fasoli, L.; Gutierrez, A.; Ruiz, J.R.; Castillo, M.J. Association of physical activity and fitness with S-Klotho plasma levels in middle-aged sedentary adults: The FIT-AGEING study. *Maturitas* **2019**, *123*, 25–31. [CrossRef] [PubMed]
123. Santos-Dias, A.; MacKenzie, B.; Oliveira-Junior, M.C.; Moyses, R.M.; Consolim-Colombo, F.M.; Vieira, R.P. Longevity protein klotho is induced by a single bout of exercise. *Br. J. Sports Med.* **2017**, *51*, 549–550. [CrossRef]
124. Tan, S.J.; Chu, M.M.; Toussaint, N.D.; Cai, M.M.; Hewitson, T.D.; Holt, S.G. High-intensity physical exercise increases serum α-klotho levels in healthy volunteers. *J. Circ. Biomark.* **2018**, *7*, 1849454418794582. [CrossRef]
125. Gautam, S.; Kumar, U.; Kumar, M.; Rana, D.; Dada, R. Yoga improves mitochondrial health and reduces severity of autoimmune inflammatory arthritis: A randomized controlled trial. *Mitochondrion* **2021**, *58*, 147–159. [CrossRef] [PubMed]
126. Bose, A.; Beal, M.F. Mitochondrial dysfunction in Parkinson's disease. *J. Neurochem.* **2016**, *139*, 216–231. [CrossRef]
127. Subramaniam, S.R.; Chesselet, M.F. Mitochondrial dysfunction and oxidative stress in Parkinson's disease. *Prog. Neurobiol.* **2013**, *106–107*, 17–32. [CrossRef] [PubMed]
128. Pickrell, A.M.; Youle, R.J. The roles of PINK1, parkin, and mitochondrial fidelity in Parkinson's disease. *Neuron* **2015**, *85*, 257–273. [CrossRef]
129. Liddell, J.R.; White, A.R. Nexus between mitochondrial function, iron, copper and glutathione in Parkinson's disease. *Neurochem. Int.* **2018**, *117*, 126–138. [CrossRef]
130. Currais, A. Ageing and inflammation—A central role for mitochondria in brain health and disease. *Ageing Res. Rev.* **2015**, *21*, 30–42. [CrossRef]
131. Madrigal, J.L.; Olivenza, R.; Moro, M.A.; Lizasoain, I.; Lorenzo, P.; Rodrigo, J.; Leza, J.C. Glutathione depletion, lipid peroxidation and mitochondrial dysfunction are induced by chronic stress in rat brain. *Neuropsychopharmacology* **2001**, *24*, 420–429. [CrossRef] [PubMed]
132. Allen, J.; Caruncho, H.J.; Kalynchuk, L.E. Severe life stress, mitochondrial dysfunction, and depressive behavior: A pathophysiological and therapeutic perspective. *Mitochondrion* **2021**, *56*, 111–117. [CrossRef] [PubMed]
133. Pajares, M.; Rojo, A.I.; Manda, G.; Bosca, L.; Cuadrado, A. Inflammation in Parkinson's Disease: Mechanisms and Therapeutic Implications. *Cells* **2020**, *9*, 1687. [CrossRef] [PubMed]
134. Picard, M.; McEwen, B.S.; Epel, E.S.; Sandi, C. An energetic view of stress: Focus on mitochondria. *Front. Neuroendocrinol.* **2018**, *49*, 72–85. [CrossRef] [PubMed]
135. Grigoruta, M.; Martinez-Martinez, A.; Dagda, R.Y.; Dagda, R.K. Psychological Stress Phenocopies Brain Mitochondrial Dysfunction and Motor Deficits as Observed in a Parkinsonian Rat Model. *Mol. Neurobiol.* **2020**, *57*, 1781–1798. [CrossRef]
136. Sahu, A.; Mamiya, H.; Shinde, S.N.; Cheikhi, A.; Winter, L.L.; Vo, N.V.; Stolz, D.; Roginskaya, V.; Tang, W.Y.; St Croix, C.; et al. Age-related declines in alpha-Klotho drive progenitor cell mitochondrial dysfunction and impaired muscle regeneration. *Nat. Commun.* **2018**, *9*, 4859. [CrossRef]

137. Miao, J.; Huang, J.; Luo, C.; Ye, H.; Ling, X.; Wu, Q.; Shen, W.; Zhou, L. Klotho retards renal fibrosis through targeting mitochondrial dysfunction and cellular senescence in renal tubular cells. *Physiol. Rep.* **2021**, *9*, e14696. [CrossRef]
138. Lim, S.W.; Jin, L.; Luo, K.; Jin, J.; Shin, Y.J.; Hong, S.Y.; Yang, C.W. Klotho enhances FoxO3-mediated manganese superoxide dismutase expression by negatively regulating PI3K/AKT pathway during tacrolimus-induced oxidative stress. *Cell Death Dis.* **2017**, *8*, e2972. [CrossRef]
139. Chen, H.; Huang, X.; Fu, C.; Wu, X.; Peng, Y.; Lin, X.; Wang, Y. Recombinant Klotho Protects Human Periodontal Ligament Stem Cells by Regulating Mitochondrial Function and the Antioxidant System during H_2O_2-Induced Oxidative Stress. *Oxid. Med. Cell. Longev.* **2019**, *2019*, 9261565. [CrossRef]
140. Emami Aleagha, M.S.; Harirchian, M.H.; Lavasani, S.; Javan, M.; Allameh, A. Differential Expression of Klotho in the Brain and Spinal Cord is Associated with Total Antioxidant Capacity in Mice with Experimental Autoimmune Encephalomyelitis. *J. Mol. Neurosci.* **2018**, *64*, 543–550. [CrossRef]
141. Typiak, M.; Piwkowska, A. Antiinflammatory Actions of Klotho: Implications for Therapy of Diabetic Nephropathy. *Int. J. Mol. Sci.* **2021**, *22*, 956. [CrossRef] [PubMed]
142. Mazucanti, C.H.; Kawamoto, E.M.; Mattson, M.P.; Scavone, C.; Camandola, S. Activity-dependent neuronal Klotho enhances astrocytic aerobic glycolysis. *J. Cereb. Blood Flow Metab.* **2019**, *39*, 1544–1556. [CrossRef] [PubMed]
143. Marogianni, C.; Sokratous, M.; Dardiotis, E.; Hadjigeorgiou, G.M.; Bogdanos, D.; Xiromerisiou, G. Neurodegeneration and Inflammation-An Interesting Interplay in Parkinson's Disease. *Int. J. Mol. Sci.* **2020**, *21*, 8421. [CrossRef] [PubMed]
144. Diniz, B.S.; Vieira, E.M. Stress, Inflammation and Aging: An Association Beyond Chance. *Am. J. Geriatr. Psychiatry* **2018**, *26*, 964–965. [CrossRef]
145. Tracey, K.J. The inflammatory reflex. *Nature* **2002**, *420*, 853–859. [CrossRef]
146. Elenkov, I.J.; Chrousos, G.P. Stress Hormones, Th1/Th2 patterns, Pro/Anti-inflammatory Cytokines and Susceptibility to Disease. *Trends Endocrinol. Metab.* **1999**, *10*, 359–368. [CrossRef]
147. Swolin-Eide, D.; Ohlsson, C. Effects of cortisol on the expression of interleukin-6 and interleukin-1 beta in human osteoblast-like cells. *J. Endocrinol.* **1998**, *156*, 107–114. [CrossRef]
148. Mastorakos, G.; Chrousos, G.P.; Weber, J.S. Recombinant interleukin-6 activates the hypothalamic-pituitary-adrenal axis in humans. *J. Clin. Endocrinol. Metab.* **1993**, *77*, 1690–1694.
149. Turnbull, A.V.; Rivier, C. Regulation of the HPA axis by cytokines. *Brain Behav. Immun.* **1995**, *9*, 253–275. [CrossRef]
150. Chen, X.; Gianferante, D.; Hanlin, L.; Fiksdal, A.; Breines, J.G.; Thoma, M.V.; Rohleder, N. HPA-axis and inflammatory reactivity to acute stress is related with basal HPA-axis activity. *Psychoneuroendocrinology* **2017**, *78*, 168–176. [CrossRef]
151. Zhu, L.; Stein, L.R.; Kim, D.; Ho, K.; Yu, G.Q.; Zhan, L.; Larsson, T.E.; Mucke, L. Klotho controls the brain-immune system interface in the choroid plexus. *Proc. Natl. Acad. Sci. USA* **2018**, *115*, E11388–E11396. [CrossRef] [PubMed]
152. Urabe, A.; Doi, S.; Nakashima, A.; Ike, T.; Morii, K.; Sasaki, K.; Doi, T.; Arihiro, K.; Masaki, T. Klotho deficiency intensifies hypoxia-induced expression of IFN-α/β through upregulation of RIG-I in kidneys. *PLoS ONE* **2021**, *16*, e0258856. [CrossRef] [PubMed]
153. Hui, H.; Zhai, Y.; Ao, L.; Cleveland, J.C.; Liu, H., Jr.; Fullerton, D.A.; Meng, X. Klotho suppresses the inflammatory responses and ameliorates cardiac dysfunction in aging endotoxemic mice. *Oncotarget* **2017**, *8*, 15663–15676. [CrossRef]
154. Mytych, J.; Romerowicz-Misielak, M.; Koziorowski, M. Klotho protects human monocytes from LPS-induced immune impairment associated with immunosenescent-like phenotype. *Mol. Cell. Endocrinol.* **2018**, *470*, 1–13. [CrossRef]
155. Xiang, T.; Luo, X.; Ye, L.; Huang, H.; Wu, Y. Klotho alleviates NLRP3 inflammasome-mediated neuroinflammation in a temporal lobe epilepsy rat model by activating the Nrf2 signaling pathway. *Epilepsy Behav.* **2022**, *128*, 108509. [CrossRef]
156. Zhang, B.; Zhang, Y.; Xu, T.; Yin, Y.; Huang, R.; Wang, Y.; Zhang, J.; Huang, D.; Li, W. Chronic dexamethasone treatment results in hippocampal neurons injury due to activate NLRP1 inflammasome in vitro. *Int. Immunopharmacol.* **2017**, *49*, 222–230. [CrossRef] [PubMed]
157. Feng, X.; Zhao, Y.; Yang, T.; Song, M.; Wang, C.; Yao, Y.; Fan, H. Glucocorticoid-Driven NLRP3 Inflammasome Activation in Hippocampal Microglia Mediates Chronic Stress-Induced Depressive-Like Behaviors. *Front. Mol. Neurosci.* **2019**, *12*, 210. [CrossRef]
158. Rains, J.L.; Jain, S.K. Oxidative stress, insulin signaling, and diabetes. *Free Radic. Biol. Med.* **2011**, *50*, 567–575. [CrossRef] [PubMed]
159. Camandola, S.; Mattson, M.P. Brain metabolism in health, aging, and neurodegeneration. *EMBO J.* **2017**, *36*, 1474–1492. [CrossRef]
160. Liu, W.; Tang, J. Association between diabetes mellitus and risk of Parkinson's disease: A prisma-compliant meta-analysis. *Brain Behav.* **2021**, *11*, e02082. [CrossRef]
161. Deischinger, C.; Dervic, E.; Kaleta, M.; Klimek, P.; Kautzky-Willer, A. Diabetes Mellitus is Associated with a Higher Relative Risk for Parkinson's Disease in Women than in Men. *J. Parkinson's Dis.* **2021**, *11*, 793–800. [CrossRef] [PubMed]
162. Bosco, D.; Plastino, M.; Cristiano, D.; Colica, C.; Ermio, C.; De Bartolo, M.; Mungari, P.; Fonte, G.; Consoli, D.; Consoli, A.; et al. Dementia is associated with insulin resistance in patients with Parkinson's disease. *J. Neurol. Sci.* **2012**, *315*, 39–43. [CrossRef] [PubMed]
163. Albrecht, F.; Ballarini, T.; Neumann, J.; Schroeter, M.L. FDG-PET hypometabolism is more sensitive than MRI atrophy in Parkinson's disease: A whole-brain multimodal imaging meta-analysis. *Neuroimage Clin.* **2019**, *21*, 101594. [CrossRef] [PubMed]

164. Nguyen, T.T.; Ta, Q.T.H.; Nguyen, T.T.D.; Le, T.T.; Vo, V.G. Role of Insulin Resistance in the Alzheimer's Disease Progression. *Neurochem. Res.* **2020**, *45*, 1481–1491. [CrossRef]
165. Stalder, T.; Kirschbaum, C.; Alexander, N.; Bornstein, S.R.; Gao, W.; Miller, R.; Stark, S.; Bosch, J.A.; Fischer, J.E. Cortisol in hair and the metabolic syndrome. *J. Clin. Endocrinol. Metab.* **2013**, *98*, 2573–2580. [CrossRef]
166. Kim, H.J.; Lee, J.; Chae, D.W.; Lee, K.B.; Sung, S.A.; Yoo, T.H.; Han, S.H.; Ahn, C.; Oh, K.H. Serum klotho is inversely associated with metabolic syndrome in chronic kidney disease: Results from the KNOW-CKD study. *BMC Nephrol.* **2019**, *20*, 119. [CrossRef]
167. Chen, C.D.; Podvin, S.; Gillespie, E.; Leeman, S.E.; Abraham, C.R. Insulin stimulates the cleavage and release of the extracellular domain of Klotho by ADAM10 and ADAM17. *Proc. Natl. Acad. Sci. USA* **2007**, *104*, 19796–19801. [CrossRef]
168. Tuohimaa, P.; Keisala, T.; Minasyan, A.; Cachat, J.; Kalueff, A. Vitamin D, nervous system and aging. *Psychoneuroendocrinology* **2009**, *34*, S278–S286. [CrossRef]
169. Knekt, P.; Kilkkinen, A.; Rissanen, H.; Marniemi, J.; Saaksjarvi, K.; Heliovaara, M. Serum vitamin D and the risk of Parkinson disease. *Arch. Neurol.* **2010**, *67*, 808–811. [CrossRef]
170. Lv, L.; Tan, X.; Peng, X.; Bai, R.; Xiao, Q.; Zou, T.; Tan, J.; Zhang, H.; Wang, C. The relationships of vitamin D, vitamin D receptor gene polymorphisms, and vitamin D supplementation with Parkinson's disease. *Transl. Neurodegener.* **2020**, *9*, 34. [CrossRef]
171. DeLuca, G.C.; Kimball, S.M.; Kolasinski, J.; Ramagopalan, S.V.; Ebers, G.C. Review: The role of vitamin D in nervous system health and disease. *Neuropathol. Appl. Neurobiol.* **2013**, *39*, 458–484. [CrossRef] [PubMed]
172. Cui, X.; Pelekanos, M.; Liu, P.Y.; Burne, T.H.; McGrath, J.J.; Eyles, D.W. The vitamin D receptor in dopamine neurons; its presence in human substantia nigra and its ontogenesis in rat midbrain. *Neuroscience* **2013**, *236*, 77–87. [CrossRef] [PubMed]
173. Eyles, D.W.; Smith, S.; Kinobe, R.; Hewison, M.; McGrath, J.J. Distribution of the vitamin D receptor and 1 alpha-hydroxylase in human brain. *J. Chem. Neuroanat.* **2005**, *29*, 21–30. [CrossRef] [PubMed]
174. Evatt, M.L.; DeLong, M.R.; Kumari, M.; Auinger, P.; McDermott, M.P.; Tangpricha, V.; Parkinson Study Group DATATOP Investigators. High prevalence of hypovitaminosis D status in patients with early Parkinson disease. *Arch. Neurol.* **2011**, *68*, 314–319. [CrossRef] [PubMed]
175. Sleeman, I.; Aspray, T.; Lawson, R.; Coleman, S.; Duncan, G.; Khoo, T.K.; Schoenmakers, I.; Rochester, L.; Burn, D.; Yarnall, A. The Role of Vitamin D in Disease Progression in Early Parkinson's Disease. *J. Parkinson's Dis.* **2017**, *7*, 669–675. [CrossRef] [PubMed]
176. Newmark, H.L.; Newmark, J. Vitamin D and Parkinson's disease—A hypothesis. *Mov. Disord.* **2007**, *22*, 461–468. [CrossRef]
177. Peterson, A.L.; Murchison, C.; Zabetian, C.; Leverenz, J.B.; Watson, G.S.; Montine, T.; Carney, N.; Bowman, G.L.; Edwards, K.; Quinn, J.F. Memory, mood and vitamin D in persons with Parkinson's disease. *J. Parkinson's Dis.* **2013**, *3*, 547–555. [CrossRef]
178. Hiller, A.L.; Murchison, C.F.; Lobb, B.M.; O'Connor, S.; O'Connor, M.; Quinn, J.F. A randomized, controlled pilot study of the effects of vitamin D supplementation on balance in Parkinson's disease: Does age matter? *PLoS ONE* **2018**, *13*, e0203637. [CrossRef]
179. Caristia, S.; Filigheddu, N.; Barone-Adesi, F.; Sarro, A.; Testa, T.; Magnani, C.; Aimaretti, G.; Faggiano, F.; Marzullo, P. Vitamin D as a Biomarker of Ill Health among the Over-50s: A Systematic Review of Cohort Studies. *Nutrients* **2019**, *11*, 2384. [CrossRef]
180. Guarnotta, V.; Di Gaudio, F.; Giordano, C. Vitamin D Deficiency in Cushing's Disease: Before and after Its Supplementation. *Nutrients* **2022**, *14*, 973. [CrossRef]
181. Obradovic, D.; Gronemeyer, H.; Lutz, B.; Rein, T. Cross-talk of vitamin D and glucocorticoids in hippocampal cells. *J. Neurochem.* **2006**, *96*, 500–509. [CrossRef] [PubMed]
182. Smolders, J.; Schuurman, K.G.; van Strien, M.E.; Melief, J.; Hendrickx, D.; Hol, E.M.; van Eden, C.; Luchetti, S.; Huitinga, I. Expression of vitamin D receptor and metabolizing enzymes in multiple sclerosis-affected brain tissue. *J. Neuropathol. Exp. Neurol.* **2013**, *72*, 91–105. [CrossRef] [PubMed]
183. Dermaku-Sopjani, M.; Kurti, F.; Xuan, N.T.; Sopjani, M. Klotho-Dependent Role of 1,25(OH)$_2$D$_3$ in the Brain. *Neurosignals* **2021**, *29*, 14–23. [PubMed]
184. Hoogendijk, W.J.; Lips, P.; Dik, M.G.; Deeg, D.J.; Beekman, A.T.; Penninx, B.W. Depression is associated with decreased 25-hydroxyvitamin D and increased parathyroid hormone levels in older adults. *Arch. Gen. Psychiatry* **2008**, *65*, 508–512. [CrossRef] [PubMed]
185. Vreeburg, S.A.; Hoogendijk, W.J.; van Pelt, J.; Derijk, R.H.; Verhagen, J.C.; van Dyck, R.; Smit, J.H.; Zitman, F.G.; Penninx, B.W. Major depressive disorder and hypothalamic-pituitary-adrenal axis activity: Results from a large cohort study. *Arch. Gen. Psychiatry* **2009**, *66*, 617–626. [CrossRef]
186. Lucassen, P.J.; Pruessner, J.; Sousa, N.; Almeida, O.F.; Van Dam, A.M.; Rajkowska, G.; Swaab, D.F.; Czeh, B. Neuropathology of stress. *Acta Neuropathol.* **2014**, *127*, 109–135. [CrossRef]
187. Seifried, C.; Boehncke, S.; Heinzmann, J.; Baudrexel, S.; Weise, L.; Gasser, T.; Eggert, K.; Fogel, W.; Baas, H.; Badenhoop, K.; et al. Diurnal variation of hypothalamic function and chronic subthalamic nucleus stimulation in Parkinson's disease. *Neuroendocrinology* **2013**, *97*, 283–290. [CrossRef]
188. Djamshidian, A.; O'Sullivan, S.S.; Papadopoulos, A.; Bassett, P.; Shaw, K.; Averbeck, B.B.; Lees, A. Salivary cortisol levels in Parkinson's disease and its correlation to risk behaviour. *J. Neurol. Neurosurg. Psychiatry* **2011**, *82*, 1107–1111. [CrossRef]
189. Sang, Y.M.; Wang, L.J.; Mao, H.X.; Lou, X.Y.; Zhu, Y.J. The association of short-term memory and cognitive impairment with ghrelin, leptin and cortisol levels in non-diabetic and diabetic elderly individuals. *Acta Diabetol.* **2018**, *55*, 531–539. [CrossRef]
190. Ouanes, S.; Castelao, E.; Gebreab, S.; von Gunten, A.; Preisig, M.; Popp, J. Life events, salivary cortisol and cognitive performance in nondemented subjects: A population-based study. *Neurobiol. Aging* **2017**, *51*, 1–8. [CrossRef]

191. Geerlings, M.I.; Sigurdsson, S.; Eiriksdottir, G.; Garcia, M.E.; Harris, T.B.; Gudnason, V.; Launer, L.J. Salivary cortisol, brain volumes and cognition in community-dwelling elderly without dementia. *Neurology* **2015**, *85*, 976–983. [CrossRef] [PubMed]
192. Echouffo-Tcheugui, J.B.; Conner, S.C.; Himali, J.J.; Maillard, P.; DeCarli, C.S.; Beiser, A.S.; Vasan, R.S.; Seshadri, S. Circulating cortisol and cognitive and structural brain measures: The Framingham Heart Study. *Neurology* **2018**, *91*, e1961–e1970. [CrossRef] [PubMed]
193. Tatomir, A.; Micu, C.; Crivii, C. The impact of stress and glucocorticoids on memory. *Clujul Med.* **2014**, *87*, 3. [CrossRef] [PubMed]
194. Hoyer, C.; Sartorius, A.; Aksay, S.S.; Bumb, J.M.; Janke, C.; Thiel, M.; Haffner, D.; Leifheit-Nestler, M.; Kranaster, L. Electroconvulsive therapy enhances the anti-ageing hormone Klotho in the cerebrospinal fluid of geriatric patients with major depression. *Eur. Neuropsychopharmacol.* **2018**, *28*, 428–435. [CrossRef]
195. Paroni, G.; Seripa, D.; Fontana, A.; D'Onofrio, G.; Gravina, C.; Urbano, M.; Addante, F.; Lozupone, M.; Copetti, M.; Pilotto, A.; et al. Klotho Gene and Selective Serotonin Reuptake Inhibitors: Response to Treatment in Late-Life Major Depressive Disorder. *Mol. Neurobiol.* **2017**, *54*, 1340–1351. [CrossRef]
196. Yokoyama, J.S.; Marx, G.; Brown, J.A.; Bonham, L.W.; Wang, D.; Coppola, G.; Seeley, W.W.; Rosen, H.J.; Miller, B.L.; Kramer, J.H.; et al. Systemic klotho is associated with KLOTHO variation and predicts intrinsic cortical connectivity in healthy human aging. *Brain Imaging Behav.* **2017**, *11*, 391–400. [CrossRef]
197. Li, S.; Wang, Y.; Wang, F.; Hu, L.F.; Liu, C.F. A New Perspective for Parkinson's Disease: Circadian Rhythm. *Neurosci. Bull.* **2017**, *33*, 62–72. [CrossRef]
198. Shkodina, A.D.; Tan, S.C.; Hasan, M.M.; Abdelgawad, M.; Chopra, H.; Bilal, M.; Boiko, D.I.; Tarianyk, K.A.; Alexiou, A. Roles of clock genes in the pathogenesis of Parkinson's disease. *Ageing Res. Rev.* **2022**, *74*, 101554. [CrossRef]
199. Witkovsky, P. Dopamine and retinal function. *Doc. Ophthalmol.* **2004**, *108*, 17–39. [CrossRef]
200. Bonuccelli, U.; Del Dotto, P.; Lucetti, C.; Petrozzi, L.; Bernardini, S.; Gambaccini, G.; Rossi, G.; Piccini, P. Diurnal motor variations to repeated doses of levodopa in Parkinson's disease. *Clin. Neuropharmacol.* **2000**, *23*, 28–33. [CrossRef]
201. Nyholm, D.; Lennernas, H.; Johansson, A.; Estrada, M.; Aquilonius, S.M. Circadian rhythmicity in levodopa pharmacokinetics in patients with Parkinson disease. *Clin. Neuropharmacol.* **2010**, *33*, 181–185. [CrossRef] [PubMed]
202. Bolitho, S.J.; Naismith, S.L.; Rajaratnam, S.M.; Grunstein, R.R.; Hodges, J.R.; Terpening, Z.; Rogers, N.; Lewis, S.J. Disturbances in melatonin secretion and circadian sleep-wake regulation in Parkinson disease. *Sleep Med.* **2014**, *15*, 342–347. [CrossRef] [PubMed]
203. Egstrand, S.; Olgaard, K.; Lewin, E. Circadian rhythms of mineral metabolism in chronic kidney disease-mineral bone disorder. *Curr. Opin. Nephrol. Hypertens* **2020**, *29*, 367–377. [CrossRef] [PubMed]
204. Carpenter, T.O.; Insogna, K.L.; Zhang, J.H.; Ellis, B.; Nieman, S.; Simpson, C.; Olear, E.; Gundberg, C.M. Circulating levels of soluble klotho and FGF23 in X-linked hypophosphatemia: Circadian variance, effects of treatment and relationship to parathyroid status. *J. Clin. Endocrinol. Metab.* **2010**, *95*, E352–E357. [CrossRef]
205. Nordholm, A.; Egstrand, S.; Gravesen, E.; Mace, M.L.; Morevati, M.; Olgaard, K.; Lewin, E. Circadian rhythm of activin A and related parameters of mineral metabolism in normal and uremic rats. *Pflügers Arch. Eur. J. Physiol.* **2019**, *471*, 1079–1094. [CrossRef]
206. Mochon-Benguigui, S.; Carneiro-Barrera, A.; Castillo, M.J.; Amaro-Gahete, F.J. Is Sleep Associated with the S-Klotho Anti-Aging Protein in Sedentary Middle-Aged Adults? The FIT-AGEING Study. *Antioxidants* **2020**, *9*, 738. [CrossRef]
207. Khurana, S.; Soda, N.; Shiddiky, M.J.A.; Nayak, R.; Bose, S. Current and future strategies for diagnostic and management of obstructive sleep apnea. *Expert Rev. Mol. Diagn.* **2021**, *21*, 1287–1301. [CrossRef]
208. Huang, D.; Wang, S. Association between the Anti-Aging Protein Klotho and Sleep Duration in General Population. *Int. J. Gen. Med.* **2021**, *14*, 10023–10030. [CrossRef]
209. Katsuhara, S.; Yokomoto-Umakoshi, M.; Umakoshi, H.; Matsuda, Y.; Iwahashi, N.; Kaneko, H.; Ogata, M.; Fukumoto, T.; Terada, E.; Sakamoto, R.; et al. Impact of Cortisol on Reduction in Muscle Strength and Mass: A Mendelian Randomization Study. *J. Clin. Endocrinol. Metab.* **2022**, *107*, e1477–e1487. [CrossRef]
210. Haglin, L.; Backman, L. Covariation between plasma phosphate and daytime cortisol in early Parkinson's disease. *Brain Behav.* **2016**, *6*, e00556. [CrossRef]

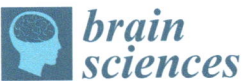

Article

Olfactory Impairment Is the Main Predictor of Higher Scores at REM Sleep Behavior Disorder (RBD) Screening Questionnaire in Parkinson's Disease Patients

Paolo Solla [1,*], Qian Wang [2], Claudia Frau [1,2], Valentina Floris [1], Francesco Loy [3], Leonardo Antonio Sechi [2] and Carla Masala [3]

1. Neurological Unit, AOU Sassari, University of Sassari, Viale S. Pietro 10, 07100 Sassari, Italy
2. Department of Biomedical Sciences, University of Sassari, Viale S. Pietro 10, 07100 Sassari, Italy
3. Department of Biomedical Sciences, University of Cagliari, SP 8 Cittadella Universitaria, 09042 Monserrato, Italy
* Correspondence: psolla@uniss.it

Abstract: Introduction: Olfactory impairment and REM sleep behavior disorder (RBD) are common non-motor symptoms in Parkinson's disease (PD) patients, often preceding the onset of the specific motor symptoms and, thus, crucial for strategies directed to anticipate PD diagnosis. In this context, the specific interaction between olfactory impairment and RBD has not been clearly defined. Objective: The aim of this study was to determine the possible role of olfactory impairment and other clinical characteristics as possible predictors of higher scores at RBD screening questionnaire (RBDSQ) in a large population of PD patients. Methods: In this study, 590 PD patients were included from the Parkinson's Progression Markers Initiative. Demographic and clinical features were registered. All participants completed motor and non-motor evaluations at the baseline visit. For motor assessments, the disease severity was evaluated by the Movement Disorder Society-Unified Parkinson's Disease Rating Scale (MDS-UPDRS) pars III. Regarding non-motor symptoms assessment, Montreal Cognitive Assessments (MoCA), University of Pennsylvania Smell Identification Test (UPSIT) and RBD screening questionnaire (RBDSQ) were registered. Results: Among 590 PD patients included in this study, 111 patients with possible RBD were found (18.8%). RBD was less frequent in female PD patients ($p \leq 0.011$). Among patients with or without possible RBD diagnosis, statistically significant differences in MDS-UPDRS III (23.3 ± 11.4 vs. 19.7 ± 9.1, respectively, $p \leq 0.002$) and in UPSIT score (19.7 ± 8.3 vs. 22.6 ± 8.0, respectively, $p \leq 0.001$) were found. Moreover, significant correlations between RBDSQ versus UPDRS III score and versus UPSIT score were observed. Multivariate linear regression analysis showed that UPSIT was the most significant predictor of higher scores at RBDSQ, while the other significant predictors were UPDRS III and age. Conclusions: The severity of olfactory impairment appears tightly correlated to RBD symptoms, highlighting the role of these biomarkers for PD patients. Additionally, according to this large study, our data confirmed that RBD in PD patients exhibits peculiar gender differences.

Keywords: Parkinson's disease; olfactory dysfunction; REM sleep behavior disorder

1. Introduction

Parkinson's disease is the second most common neurodegenerative disease after Alzheimer's disease and is characterized by motor symptoms (such as resting tremor, rigidity, postural instability, and bradykinesia), and non-motor symptoms including olfactory dysfunctions, sleep disorders, cognitive impairment, autonomic dysregulation, etc. [1]. Among non-motor symptoms, olfactory impairment represents the most common disturbance affecting 96% of PD patients, often preceding the onset of the specific motor symptoms [2,3], and deteriorating more rapidly in the early phase of the disease [4] or in association with non-tremor dominant PD subtypes [5–7]. Olfactory impairment as a prodromal non-motor symptom is crucial for strategies directed to anticipate the diagnosis of PD, bearing in mind that motor symptoms appear only after a loss of a conspicuous number of neurons due to nigral degeneration with consequent striatal dopamine depletion [8]. In this process of progressive neurodegeneration, Braak and colleagues have identified a peculiar spreading pattern of aggregated and misfolded α-synuclein proteins, which are the major constituents of Lewy bodies, starting in the caudal brainstem and advancing rostrally through the upper brainstem, limbic regions, and finally the neocortex [9]. The prodromal phase of PD corresponds to a disease stage where neurodegeneration processes, described as Braak stages 1–3, involve extranigral sites, such as the olfactory bulb and tracts, the lower brainstem, and the peripheral autonomic nervous system [9]. Interestingly, regarding the impact on the olfactory structures of the neuroinflammatory processes in PD and neurodegenerative diseases, it would be valuable to elaborate on the neuroinflammatory pathogenesis [10,11].

Moreover, in addition to olfactory disturbances, other non-motor symptoms in PD patients such as REM sleep behavior disorder (RBD), constipation, and depression may precede the movement disorders for years [12]. These symptoms are often associated, and the relationship between olfactory impairment and other non-motor symptoms such as depression and constipation is well-known [13,14]. Among them, RBD has been defined as a complex multidimensional parasomnia characterized by dream enactment and complex motor behaviors during REM sleep, which may cause injury and loss of muscle atonia during REM sleep, known as REM sleep without atonia [15]. This peculiar sleep disorder is strongly associated with synucleinopathy neurodegeneration, as most patients with RBD develop signs and symptoms relative to a synucleinopathy, such as PD, Lewy body disease or multiple system atrophy within approximately 10 years [16,17]. Indeed, there are converging proofs substantiating that idiopathic RBD is often a prodromal form of synucleinopathy [16]. These findings include neurodegenerative biomarker research, longitudinal cohort outcome investigations, and pathological confirmation from both autopsy series and demonstration of extranigral α-synuclein pathology in living patients with RBD [16]. Furthermore, a recent review has highlighted that RBD, which has been primarily described in synucleinopathies, has also been found to be present in other atypical parkinsonisms such as progressive supranuclear palsy syndrome (PSPS) and corticobasal syndrome (CBS) [18]. Among RBD patients, it was observed that 74% of subjects met Movement Disorders Society criteria for a diagnosis of prodromal PD [19]. Moreover, the presence of a probable RBD was associated with a faster progression of motor symptoms in PD patients with a postural instability and gait dysfunction (PIGD) phenotype in comparison with those presenting with a tremor dominant subtype [20].

Identification of prodromal symptoms constitutes an even greater unmet need given that new potential disease-modifying drugs will have their greatest possibility for success at these initial manifestations. In this context, the identification of olfactory disorders and RBD as early as possible would probably be useful both in clinical practice and in clinical trials of potentially neuroprotective treatments.

While olfactory impairment may be assessed and diagnosed using validated clinical instruments such as the University of Pennsylvania Smell Identification Test (UPSIT) [21] and the Sniffin' Sticks Extended test [22], establishing a RBD diagnosis commonly required a polysomnography (PSG), which represents the gold standard [23]. However, in studies evaluating a large population of patients, the RBD screening questionnaire represents a validated diagnostic instrument consisting of a 10-item patient self-rating questionnaire (maximum total score: 13 points) covering the clinical features of RBD [24] and representing a useful tool for the screening of RBD in PD patients [25]. In this context, the specific interaction between motor and non-motor symptoms, such as olfactory impairment and RBD in PD patients have not been evaluated, especially in a large population [25–27]. In fact, the assessment of olfactory impairment, and especially odor identification, may help to predict the onset of a Lewy body disease in patients with idiopathic RBD over a relatively short time period [28]. Furthermore, in RBD patients, anosmia predicts a higher short-term risk of transition to Lewy body disease, although it cannot distinguish between PD and Lewy body disease [29]. In the current study, we aim to determine the potential role of olfactory impairment and other factors (age at the onset, disease duration, sex, cognitive abilities, and motor impairment) as possible predictors of higher scores at the RBD screening questionnaire (RBDSQ) in a large population of PD patients.

2. Materials and Methods

2.1. Study Population

A total of 590 PD patients (235 women and 355 men) with a mean age of 61.4 ± 10.1 years were included in this study from Parkinson's Progression Markers Initiative (PPMI). PPMI is an ongoing comprehensive observational, multicenter, international project started in June 2010 and designed to identify biomarkers relative to PD progression. Indeed, the primary aim of PPMI is to identify genomic, biochemical, or imaging biomarkers of clinical progression finalized both to improve the understanding of PD etiology and course and to provide crucial tools to enhance the likelihood of success of PD modifying therapeutic trials [30,31]. PPMI data are publicly available (www.ppmi-info.org/data), accessed on 9 January 2023, and updated in real-time, and rely on a partnership of government, PD foundations, academics and industry working cooperatively. The detailed study protocol, manuals, and storage processes are available at www.ppmi-info.org/study-design, accessed on 9 January 2023. This project has been approved by the institutional review board at each site, with written informed consent obtained from all subjects before enrolment of PD patients in the project. The study was performed in agreement with relevant guidelines and regulations.

According to PPMI protocol, inclusion criteria for PD patients were: (1) at least two of the following signs: bradykinesia, resting tremor, and rigidity or an asymmetric bradykinesia or asymmetric resting tremor; (2) diagnosis for 2 years or less; (3) Hoehn and Yahr stage I or II at observation; (4) striatal dopamine transporter deficits on (123I)IFP-CIT SPECT imaging, greater in the contralateral to the most clinically affected side; (5) PD drug naivety; and (6) male or female age 30 years or older at time of PD diagnosis. Exclusion criteria were the following: (1) receiving any of the following drugs: neuroleptics, alpha methyldopa, methylphenidate, reserpine, metoclopramide, or amphetamine derivative, within 6 months of age at observation; and (2) use of investigational drugs or devices within 60 days prior to observation (dietary supplements taken outside of a clinical trial are not exclusionary, e.g., coenzyme Q10).

2.2. Assessments

Demographic and clinical features were registered. All participants completed motor and non-motor evaluations at the baseline visit. For motor assessments, disease severity was evaluated by the Movement Disorder Society-Unified Parkinson's Disease Rating Scale (MDS-UPDRS) part III [32].

Regarding non-motor symptoms, cognitive abilities were assessed using the Montreal Cognitive Assessments (MoCA) [33]. The used version of the MoCA is a one-page 30-point test (available at www.mocatest.org) that evaluates different domains (visual-constructional skills, executive functions, attention and concentration, memory, language, conceptual thinking, calculations, and spatial orientation) and should be administered approximately in ten minutes. The total score of MoCA is 30, and any score ≥26 is considered as normal [33].

Instead, olfactory function was evaluated using UPSIT, a smell identification test with 40 items at a suprathreshold level, which provides an indication of quantitative smell loss as anosmia and different levels of hyposmia. The UPSIT test consists of 40 questions with 4 diverse 10-page booklets. The number of items out of 40 that were perceived correctly served as the dependent measure [21]. As previously described in a systematic review, PD patients were defined as anosmic if their score was ≤18/40, whereas they were considered normosmic if their scores were >33 in men or >34 in women [34].

The REM sleep behavior disorder was registered using RBD screening questionnaire (RBDSQ) [24]. This questionnaire consists of 10 items and is a patient self-rating instrument assessing the subject's sleep. The bed partner's input may be useful but not necessary, because patients do not always have a long-time companion. The maximum total score of the RBDSQ is 13 points [24].

In agreement with a previous study revealing the best cut-off value for RBD using the RBDSQ [25], a score superior to 6 points was set as the cut-off value for a possible RBD diagnosis.

2.3. Statistical Analysis

The SPSS software, version 26 (IBM Corporation, Armonk, NY, USA), was used for statistical analysis. All data were presented as mean values ± standard deviation (SD). Variables normality was checked with the Kolmogorov–Smirnov test. For comparison of the demographic and clinical features between PD with or without diagnosis of possible RBD, all variables were assessed by means of independent sample t test or the Yates-corrected chi-square test, as appropriate.

Bivariate correlations among demographic data, clinical, motor, and non-motor assessments were performed using Pearson's correlation coefficient (r). Moreover, a multivariate linear regression analysis was performed to assess the potential contribution of each significant variable on RBD severity in PD patients. The multivariate linear regression analysis was performed using age at observation, gender, PD duration, MDS-UPDRS III, UPSIT score and MoCA score as independent variables, while RBDSQ score was considered the dependent variable. A p value < 0.05 was considered statistically significant.

3. Results

Demographic and clinical features of all PD patients, also differentiated in patients with or without possible RBD diagnosis, were reported in Table 1.

Table 1. Demographic and clinical information of PD patients.

	Total PD Patients	PD Patients without RBD	PD Patients with Possible RBD	p Value
Demographics	n = 590	n = 479 (81.2%)	n = 111 (18.8%)	
Age at observation	61.4 (10.1)	61.7 (10.1)	60.1 (10.2)	0.135
PD duration (years)	2.7 (3.3)	2.7 (3.5)	2.7 (2.2)	0.948
Sex n, female (%)	235 (39.8%)	203 (42.3%)	32 (28.8%)	**0.011**
MDS-UPDRS-III	20.4 (9.7)	19.7 (9.1)	23.3 (11.4)	**0.002**
RBDSQ	4.1 (2.8)	3.0 (1.6)	8.7 (1.6)	**0.0001**
UPSIT	22.0 (8.1)	22.6 (8.0)	19.7 (8.3)	**0.001**
MoCA	26.7 (2.9)	26.8 (2.8)	26.7 (2.9)	0.387

PD = Parkinson's disease; SD = standard deviation; MDS-UPDRS-III = Movement Disorder Society Revision of the Unified Parkinson's disease rating scale part III; RBDSQ = Rapid Eye Movement Sleep Behavior Disorder Screening Questionnaire; n = number; UPSIT = University of Pennsylvania Smell Identification Test; MoCA = Montreal Cognitive Assessment. Significant p values are highlighted in bold. Data are expressed as mean (SD) or mean (percentage).

Among 590 PD patients included in this study, 235 were women (39.8%), while patients with possible RBD were 111 (18.8%). PD patients with or without possible RBD diagnosis were similar for age and PD duration, with mean age at observation equal to 61.4 ± 10.1 years, while mean PD duration was 2.7 (SD 3.3) years. Prevalence on female PD patients with possible RBD was minor in comparison with those without RBD (28.8% versus 42.3%, respectively; $p \leq 0.011$). Among patients with or without possible RBD diagnosis, statistically significant differences in MDS-UPDRS III (23.3 ± 11.4 vs. 19.7 ± 9.1, respectively; $p \leq 0.002$) and in UPSIT score (19.7 ± 8.3 vs. 22.6 ± 8.0, respectively;

$p \leq 0.001$) were found. PD patients with or without RBD did not show a significant impairment in MoCA scores (26.7 ± 2.9 vs. 26.8 ± 2.8, respectively).

At the olfactory assessment, among 590 PD patients, 213 were defined as anosmic (36%), whereas 62 patients were considered as normosmic. Among PD patients with anosmia, 67 (28.5%) were women and 146 (41.5%) were men. Thus, a gender difference in olfactory impairment was found, with the prevalence on PD patients affected by anosmia significantly lower in the female gender in comparison with males (chi-square with Yates correction: 9.2169; $p \leq 0.0025$).

In Table 2, significant correlations among demographic data, clinical, motor, and non-motor assessments in patients affected by PD were reported.

Table 2. Correlations among demographic data, clinical, motor, and non-motor assessments in patients affected by Parkinson's disease.

		RBDSQ	Age	UPDRS-III	MoCA	UPSIT	PD Duration
RBDSQ	r	1	−0.072	0.150	−0.004	−0.179	−0.006
	p		0.081	**0.001**	0.921	**0.001**	0.883
Age	r	−0.072	1	0.129	−0.189	−0.204	0.023
	p	0.081		**0.002**	**0.001**	**0.001**	0.577
UPDRS-III	r	0.150	0.129	1	−0.147	−0.180	0.183
	p	**0.001**	**0.002**		**0.001**	**0.001**	**0.001**
MoCA	r	−0.004	−0.189	−0.147	1	0.121	−0.086
	p	0.921	**0.001**	**0.001**		**0.003**	**0.037**
UPSIT	r	−0.179	−0.204	−0.180	0.121	1	−0.016
	p	**0.001**	**0.001**	**0.001**	**0.003**		0.702
PD duration	r	−0.006	0.023	0.183	−0.086	−0.016	1
	p	0.883	0.577	**0.001**	**0.037**	0.702	

RBDSQ = Rapid Eye Movement Sleep Behavior Disorder Screening Questionnaire; UPDRS-III = Movement Disorder Society Revision of the Unified Parkinson's disease rating scale part III; MoCA = Montreal Cognitive Assessment; UPSIT = University of Pennsylvania Smell Identification Test; PD = Parkinson's disease; r = Pearson's correlation coefficient. Significant *p* values are highlighted in bold.

In particular, we found statistically significant correlations between RBDSQ versus UPDRS-III score (r = 0.150, $p < 0.001$) and versus UPSIT score (r = −0.179, $p < 0.001$). Other statistically significant correlations were found between UPSIT score versus age at observation (r = 0.204, $p < 0.001$), versus UPDRS-III score (r = 0.180, $p < 0.001$), and versus MoCA score (r = 0.121, $p < 0.003$).

Furthermore, to better clarify the impact of bivariate correlations related to RBDSQ score, a multivariate linear regression analysis was performed to predict higher scores at RBDSQ in PD patients in relation to demographic/clinical data (age at observation, sex, disease duration), motor (UPDRS III) and non-motor symptoms (UPSIT and MoCA) as independent variables (Table 3). In the multivariate linear regression analyses, the RBDSQ was set as a dependent variable, while age at observation, sex, PD duration, UPDRS-III, UPSIT score, and MoCA score were independent variables.

Multivariate linear regression analysis showed that the mean value of the UPSIT test (Figure 1A), which indicated the olfactory function of the patients, was the most significant predictor for higher scores in the RBDSQ [$F_{(6,589)}$ = 6.634, $p < 0.0001$], while other significant predictors were UPDRS-III (Figure 1B) and age ($p < 0.001$ and $p < 0.003$, respectively) (Figure 1C). The model explained around 25% of the variance ($R^2 = 0.253$).

Table 3. Multivariate linear regression analyses using RBDSQ as a dependent variable and age at observation, gender, PD duration, UPDRS-III, UPSIT score and MoCA score as independent variables.

	Unstandardized Coefficients		Standardized Coefficients		
	B	Std Error	β	t	p
(Costant)	6.276	1.455		4.314	0.000
UPSIT	−0.060	0.014	−0.175	−4.183	**0.0001**
UPDRS-III	0.039	0.012	0.137	3.269	**0.001**
Age	−0.034	0.011	−0.124	−2.974	**0.003**
Gender	0.221	0.232	0.039	0.955	0.340
MoCA	0.012	0.039	0.012	0.294	0.769
PD duration	−0.021	0.035	−0.025	−0.603	0.547

RBDSQ = Rapid Eye Movement Sleep Behavior Disorder Screening Questionnaire; UPDRS-III = Unified Parkinson's disease rating scale part III; MoCA = Montreal Cognitive Assessment; UPSIT = University of Pennsylvania Smell Identification Test; PD = Parkinson's disease; Std Error: Standard error of the mean. Significant p values are highlighted in bold.

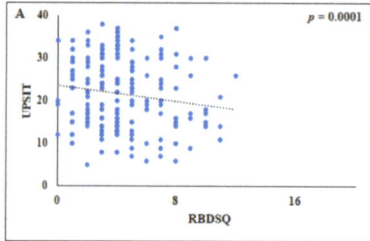
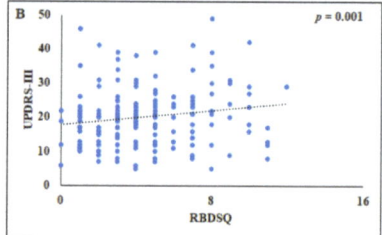
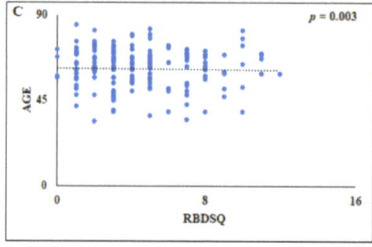

Figure 1. Scatterplots of the relationship between Rapid Eye Movement Sleep Behavior Disorder Screening Questionnaire (RBDSQ) versus University of Pennsylvania Smell Identification Test (UPSIT) (**A**), between RBDSQ versus Unified Parkinson's disease rating scale part III (UPDRS) (**B**), and between RBDSQ versus age (**C**).

4. Discussion

The aim of this study was to determine the potential role of olfactory dysfunction and other factors (such as age at the onset, sex, cognitive abilities, and motor symptoms) as potential predictors of higher scores at the RBDSQ in PD patients, investigating a large population of PD patients. RBD is tightly associated with PD and other synucleinopathies such as dementia with Lewy bodies and multiple system atrophy, often starting before the onset of any clear specific signs or symptoms of these neurodegenerative diseases, proposing that RBD may be one of the most important prodromal manifestations [16].

From a general point of view, we found a frequency of possible RBD near to 19% in all enrolled PD patients. This finding appears in line with other previous studies identifying a presumptive prevalence of RBD in 15–40% of PD patients using RBD screening scales, quite different from the frequency of confirmed RBD in up to 62.5% in studies using video polysomnography [25,35–37]. At the same time, we found that a large group of parkinsonian patients from the same population presented an evident olfactory disorder (anosmia) with frequency higher than 35%, confirming anosmia as a well-documented marker of PD [2,3]. Thus, comparing RBD and smell disturbances, it emerges that the presence of anosmia in PD patients was more frequent than RBD. This finding is line with previous studies suggesting that olfactory dysfunction is reported in 96% of PD patients [2,3].

Interestingly, we also found that patients with possible RBD presented with a greater impairment at the motor assessment with MDS-UPDRS-III. This finding appears to be in agreement with previous studies reporting that RBD presence in individuals with PD was associated with a severe clinical form of the disease [36] documenting a risk factor for PD forms with greater severity of motor symptoms [35].

However, the main finding of our study was the demonstration that olfaction impairment and RBD were strongly associated. In this context, we found that the decrease of the UPSIT score was the most significant predictor of higher scores at RBDSQ, while other predictors such as UPDRS-III and age at observation were less significant. Thus, according to our data, the presence of a more severe olfactory impairment is strongly correlated with a more symptomatic expression of this specific parasomnia.

A probable reason of this association between RBD and impaired olfactory function is likely due to the proximity of the specific brainstem nuclei involved in these pathologies, as well documented by the anatomopathological studies of Braak and colleagues [9].

Indeed, it is well-known that physiological sleep atonia during REM sleep is modulated by the subcoeruleus nucleus, together with the amygdala [38]. The main pathways of these structures are involved in the inhibitory inputs to the neurons of the spinal anterior horns, determining the loss of skeletal muscular tone [39,40]. In this scenario, the loss of physiological atonia during sleep in PD patients with RBD is related to the reduction of signal intensity in the locus coeruleus/subcoeruleus [38]. Moreover, structural and functional neuroimaging abnormalities in the brainstem, and more precisely with involvement in the dorsal pons, likely impacts REM sleep atonia control [41]. It is interesting to notice that damage in the forebrain cholinergic system is considered a strong candidate for explaining the marked olfactory impairment among neurological disorders, often with significant destruction of the nucleus basalis of Meynert or ascending basolateral cholinergic circuits [42].

In this regard, previous investigations have suggested an association between RBD and olfactory impairment [26,43,44]. For example, Stiasny-Kolster et al. found that almost all the RBD patients (97%) showed an impairment of the olfactory threshold, while 63% of these patients had lost the skill to differentiate odors [43]. However, in our opinion, the present study provides more defined evidence due to the large number of PD patients included.

Interestingly, we observed a significant gender difference in PD patients with possible RBD, with more men affected by this peculiar sleep disorder in comparisons with women. In this regard, it is remarkable to note that previous research has shown conflicting results. Indeed, although previous reports in RBD suggested the presence of a gender difference [45,46], one of the most important epidemiological investigations carried out in a middle-to-older age population-based sample did not show any difference between men and women [47]. The findings of our study, which has the advantage of having been conducted in a large population of parkinsonian patients, indicate the effective presence of a gender difference in the frequency of this sleep disorder, with a greater impact on male gender.

In fact, gender differences are not uncommon in PD, particularly among the wide spectrum of non-motor symptoms [48,49], and especially in a specific prodromal disturbance such as olfactory impairment [50]. Furthermore, the present study also confirmed the presence of gender differences regarding the olfactory impairment, with male PD patients more anosmic when compared to females, supporting the hypothesis that men may show an increased risk to develop these non-motor symptoms.

This evidence strongly suggests that future investigations on PD patients should be more focused on sex differences since the necessity to develop gender-tailored management in PD is more and more evident. In this context, the gender may provide insights into mechanisms of neurodegeneration and improve epidemiologic and therapeutic clinical trial designs. In fact, the possibility to focus PD patients on specific subtypes appears as a key resource for drug development and understanding of the clinical and biological features of PD progression milestones. Moreover, the full definition of gender-related differences may play an important role to improve the precision medicine approach in PD.

Regarding this issue, for example, there is also a lack of data on sex differences in response to antiparkinsonian drugs and adverse events. The same issue is widely underestimated in the investigations related to the prodromal symptoms of PD, and the present study provides interesting data in this regard. Forthcoming studies are therefore needed to elaborate on gender-tailored management in PD [51].

As a limitation, it should be noted that the study presented with a cross-sectional design, without investigating possible correlations over time and measure longitudinal changes. Another limitation was the lack of REM sleep confirmation by video PSG, which is mandatory for a definite RBD diagnosis. However, since this study was designed as an investigation in a large population, PSG was not performed because the examination is time- and labor-consuming, while an appropriate questionnaire for RBD screening in clinical settings was used. In this context, the use of RBDSQ in this large population appears reasonable for the screening of this complex parasomnia, and this study should be considered as a pilot study. As a further limitation, we did not explore the relationship of olfactory impairment and RBD in less severe tremor-dominant PD compared to the severe PIGD motor subtype. We retain that future investigations focused on this relationship may give further insight into disease mechanisms.

5. Conclusions

In conclusion, this study showed that the presence of olfactory dysfunction appears to be tightly correlated with RBD symptoms, highlighting the role of these biomarkers for PD patients. Additionally, according to this large study, our data confirmed that RBD in PD patients exhibits peculiar gender differences. The evaluation of olfactory dysfunction and RBD may play a key role both in clinical practice and in the application of potentially neuroprotective treatments in PD patients. Further studies are required to confirm the presence and progression of this relationship between these PD biomarkers also using video-PSG and with longitudinal follow-up.

Author Contributions: Conceptualization, P.S. and C.M.; methodology, P.S.; software, P.S. and Q.W.; validation, P.S. and Q.W.; formal analysis, P.S. and Q.W.; data curation, P.S., Q.W., F.L. and C.M.; writing—original draft preparation, P.S.; writing—review and editing, P.S., Q.W., V.F., C.M., F.L., C.F. and L.A.S.; supervision, P.S., L.A.S and C.M. All authors have read and agreed to the published version of the manuscript.

Funding: This research received no external funding.

Institutional Review Board Statement: This study was conducted using PPMI data. The PPMI study is ethically approved and conducted in accordance with the Declaration of Helsinki, 1964. WCG IRB has reviewed all PPMI research protocols, including patient recruitment, retention, informed consent documents, and in-study instructions (online platform name ClinicalTrials.gov (NCT01141023)).

Informed Consent Statement: WCG IRB has reviewed all PPMI research protocols, including patient recruitment, retention, informed consent documents, and in-study instructions (ClinicalTrials.gov (NCT01141023)).

Data Availability Statement: Not applicable.

Acknowledgments: Data used in the preparation of this study were obtained from the Parkinson's Progression Markers Initiative (PPMI) database (www.ppmi-info.org/access-dataspecimens/download-data) accessed on 9 January 2023. PPMI—a public-private partnerships funded by the Michael J. Fox Foundation for Parkinson's Research and funding partners 4D Pharma, Abbvie, Acurex Therapeutics, Allergan, Amathus Therapeutics, ASAP, Avid Radiopharmaceuticals, Bial Biotech, Biogen, BioLegend, Bristol-Myers Squibb, Calico, Celgene, Dacapo Brain Science, Denali, The Edmond J. Safra Foundation, GE Healthcare, Genentech, GlaxoSmithKline, Golub Capital, Handl Therapeutics, Insitro, Janssen Neuroscience, Lilly, Lundbeck, Merck, Meso Scale Discovery, Neurocrine Biosciences, Pfizer, Piramal, Prevail, Roche, Sanofi Genzyme, Servier, Takeda, Teva, UCB, Verily, and Voyager Therapeutics.

Conflicts of Interest: The authors declare no conflict of interest.

References

1. Schapira, A.H.V.; Chaudhuri, K.R.; Jenner, P. Non-motor features of Parkinson disease. *Nat. Rev. Neurosci.* **2017**, *18*, 435–450. [CrossRef] [PubMed]
2. Haehner, A.; Boesveldt, S.; Berendse, H.W.; Mackay-Sim, A.; Fleischmann, J.; Silburn, P.A.; Johnston, A.N.; Mellick, G.D.; Herting, B.; Reichmann, H.; et al. Prevalence of smell loss in Parkinson's disease—A multicenter study. *Park. Relat. Disord.* **2009**, *15*, 490–494. [CrossRef] [PubMed]
3. Haehner, A.; Hummel, T.; Hummel, C.; Sommer, U.; Junghanns, S.; Reichmann, H. Olfactory loss may be a first sign of idiopathic Parkinson's disease. *Mov. Disord.* **2007**, *22*, 839–842. [CrossRef] [PubMed]
4. Ercoli, T.; Masala, C.; Cadeddu, G.; Mascia, M.M.; Orofino, G.; Gigante, A.F.; Solla, P.; Defazio, G.; Rocchi, L. Does Olfactory Dysfunction Correlate with Disease Progression in Parkinson's Disease? A Systematic Review of the Current Literature. *Brain Sci.* **2022**, *12*, 513. [CrossRef] [PubMed]
5. Stern, M.B.; Doty, R.L.; Dotti, M.; Corcoran, P.; Crawford, D.; McKeown, D.A.; Adler, C.; Gollomp, S.; Hurtig, H. Olfactory function in Parkinson's disease subtypes. *Neurology* **1994**, *44*, 266–268. [CrossRef]
6. Iijima, M.; Kobayakawa, T.; Saito, S.; Osawa, M.; Tsutsumi, Y.; Hashimoto, S.; Uchiyama, S. Differences in odor identification among clinical subtypes of Parkinson's disease. *Eur. J. Neurol.* **2011**, *18*, 425–429. [CrossRef]
7. Solla, P.; Masala, C.; Ercoli, T.; Orofino, G.; Loy, F.; Pinna, I.; Fadda, L.; Defazio, G. Olfactory Impairment in Parkinson's Disease Patients with Tremor Dominant Subtype Compared to Those with Akinetic Rigid Dominant Subtype: A Pilot Study. *Brain Sci.* **2022**, *12*, 196. [CrossRef]
8. Gelpi, E.; Navarro-Otano, J.; Tolosa, E.; Gaig, C.; Compta, Y.; Rey, M.J.; Marti, M.J.; Hernandez, I.; Valldeoriola, F.; Rene, R.; et al. Multiple organ involvement by alpha-synuclein pathology in Lewy body disorders. *Mov. Disord.* **2014**, *29*, 1010–1018. [CrossRef]
9. Braak, H.; Del Tredici, K.; Bratzke, H.; Hamm-Clement, J.; Sandmann-Keil, D.; Rüb, U. Staging of the intracerebral inclusion body pathology associated with idiopathic Parkinson's disease (preclinical and clinical stages). *J. Neurol.* **2002**, *249* (Suppl. 3), III/1–III/5. [CrossRef]
10. Madetko, N.; Migda, B.; Alster, P.; Turski, P.; Koziorowski, D.; Friedman, A. Platelet-to-lymphocyte ratio and neutrophil-tolymphocyte ratio may reflect differences in PD and MSA-P neuroinflammation patterns. *Neurol. Neurochir. Pol.* **2022**, *56*, 148–155. [CrossRef]
11. Morbelli, S.; Chiola, S.; Donegani, M.I.; Arnaldi, D.; Pardini, M.; Mancini, R.; Lanfranchi, F.; D'amico, F.; Bauckneht, M.; Miceli, A.; et al. Metabolic correlates of olfactory dysfunction in COVID-19 and Parkinson's disease (PD) do not overlap. *Eur. J. Nucl. Med. Mol. Imaging* **2022**, *49*, 1939–1950. [CrossRef] [PubMed]
12. Siderowf, A.; Jennings, D.; Eberly, S.; Oakes, D.; Hawkins, K.A.; Ascherio, A.; Stern, M.B.; Marek, K.; PARS Investigators. Impaired olfaction and other prodromal features in the Parkinson At-Risk Syndrome Study. *Mov. Disord.* **2012**, *27*, 406–412. [CrossRef] [PubMed]
13. Baumgartner, A.; Press, D.; Simon, D. The relationship between olfactory dysfunction and constipation in early Parkinson's disease. *Mov. Disord.* **2021**, *36*, 781–782. [CrossRef] [PubMed]
14. Reichmann, H. Premotor Diagnosis of Parkinson's Disease. *Neurosci. Bull.* **2017**, *33*, 526–534. [CrossRef] [PubMed]
15. American Academy of Sleep Medicine. *International Classification of Sleep Disorders: Diagnostic and Coding Manual*, 2nd ed.; American Academy of Sleep Medicine: Westchester, IL, USA, 2005.
16. Iranzo, A.; Lomena, F.; Stockner, H.; Valldeoriola, F.; Vilaseca, I.; Salamero, M.; Molinuevo, J.L.; Sarradell, M.; Duch, J.; Pavia, J.; et al. Decreased striatal dopamine transporter uptake and substantia nigra hyperechogenicity as risk markers of synucleinopathy in patients with idiopathic rapid-eye-movement sleep behaviour disorder: A prospective study. *Lancet Neurol.* **2010**, *9*, 1070–1077. [CrossRef]
17. Dauvilliers, Y.; Schenck, C.H.; Postuma, R.B.; Iranzo, A.; Luppi, P.H.; Plazzi, G.; Montplaisir, J.; Boeve, B. REM sleep behaviour disorder. *Nat. Rev. Dis. Primers* **2018**, *4*, 19. [CrossRef]
18. Alster, P.; Madetko-Alster, N.; Migda, A.; Migda, B.; Kutyłowski, M.; Królicki, L.; Friedman, A. Sleep disturbances in progressive supranuclear palsy syndrome (PSPS) and corticobasal syndrome (CBS). *Neurol. Neurochir. Pol.* **2023**, *ahead of print*. [CrossRef]

19. Barber, T.R.; Lawton, M.; Rolinski, M.; Evetts, S.; Baig, F.; Ruffmann, C.; Gornall, A.; Klein, J.C.; Lo, C.; Dennis, G.; et al. Prodromal Parkinsonism and Neurodegenerative Risk Stratification in REM Sleep Behavior Disorder. *Sleep* **2017**, *40*, zsx071. [CrossRef]
20. Duarte Folle, A.; Paul, K.C.; Bronstein, J.M.; Keener, A.M.; Ritz, B. Clinical progression in Parkinson's disease with features of REM sleep behavior disorder: A population-based longitudinal study. *Park. Relat. Disord.* **2019**, *62*, 105–111. [CrossRef]
21. Doty, R.L.; Bromley, S.M.; Stern, M.B. Olfactory testing as an aid in the diagnosis of Parkinson's disease: Development of optimal discrimination criteria. *Neurodegeneration* **1995**, *4*, 93–97. [CrossRef]
22. Hummel, T.; Kobal, G.; Gudziol, H.; Mackay-Sim, A. Normative data for the "Sniffin' Sticks" including tests of odor identification, odor discrimination, and olfactory thresholds: An upgrade based on a group of more than 3000 subjects. *Eur. Arch. Otorhinolaryngol.* **2007**, *264*, 237–243. [CrossRef] [PubMed]
23. St Louis, E.K.; Boeve, B.F. REM Sleep Behavior Disorder: Diagnosis, Clinical Implications, and Future Directions. *Mayo Clin. Proc.* **2017**, *92*, 1723–1736. [CrossRef]
24. Stiasny-Kolster, K.; Mayer, G.; Schäfer, S.; Möller, J.C.; Heinzel-Gutenbrunner, M.; Oertel, W.H. The REM sleep behavior disorder screening questionnaire—A new diagnostic instrument. *Mov. Disord.* **2007**, *22*, 2386–2393. [CrossRef]
25. Nomura, T.; Inoue, Y.; Kagimura, T.; Uemura, Y.; Nakashima, K. Utility of the REM sleep behavior disorder screening questionnaire (RBDSQ) in Parkinson's disease patients. *Sleep Med.* **2011**, *12*, 711–713. [CrossRef] [PubMed]
26. Iijima, M.; Okuma, Y.; Suzuki, K.; Yoshii, F.; Nogawa, S.; Osada, T.; Hirata, K.; Kitagawa, K.; Hattori, N. Associations between probable REM sleep behavior disorder, olfactory disturbance, and clinical symptoms in Parkinson's disease: A multicenter cross-sectional study. *PLoS ONE* **2021**, *16*, e0247443. [CrossRef] [PubMed]
27. Kang, S.H.; Lee, H.M.; Seo, W.K.; Kim, J.H.; Koh, S.B. The combined effect of REM sleep behavior disorder and hyposmia on cognition and motor phenotype in Parkinson's disease. *J. Neurol. Sci.* **2016**, *368*, 374–378. [CrossRef]
28. Mahlknecht, P.; Iranzo, A.; Högl, B.; Frauscher, B.; Müller, C.; Santamaría, J.; Tolosa, E.; Serradell, M.; Mitterling, T.; Gschliesser, V.; et al. Sleep Innsbruck Barcelona Group. Olfactory dysfunction predicts early transition to a Lewy body disease in idiopathic RBD. *Neurology* **2015**, *84*, 654–658. [CrossRef]
29. Miyamoto, T.; Miyamoto, M. Odor identification predicts the transition of patients with isolated RBD: A retrospective study. *Ann. Clin. Transl. Neurol.* **2022**, *9*, 1177–1185. [CrossRef]
30. Marek, K.; Jennings, D.; Lasch, S.; Siderowf, A.; Tanner, C.; Simuni, T.; Coffey, C.; Kieburtz, K.; Flagg, E.; Chowdhury, S.; et al. The Parkinson progression marker initiative (PPMI). *Prog. Neurobiol.* **2011**, *95*, 629–635.
31. Marek, K.; Chowdhury, S.; Siderowf, A.; Lasch, S.; Coffey, C.S.; Caspell-Garcia, C.; Simuni, T.; Jennings, D.; Tanner, C.M.; Trojanowski, J.Q.; et al. The Parkinson's progression markers initiative (PPMI)—Establishing a PD biomarker cohort. *Ann. Clin. Transl. Neurol.* **2018**, *5*, 1460–1477. [CrossRef]
32. Goetz, C.G.; Tilley, B.C.; Shaftman, S.R.; Stebbins, G.T.; Fahn, S.; Martinez-Martin, P.; Poewe, W.; Sampaio, C.; Stern, M.B.; Dodel, R.; et al. Movement Disorder Society UPDRS Revision Task Force. Movement Disorder Society-sponsored revision of the Unified Parkinson's Disease Rating Scale (MDS-UPDRS): Scale presentation and clinimetric testing results. *Mov. Disord.* **2008**, *23*, 2129–2170. [CrossRef] [PubMed]
33. Nasreddine, Z.S.; Phillips, N.A.; Bédirian, V.; Charbonneau, S.; Whitehead, V.; Collin, I.; Cummings, J.L.; Chertkow, H. The Montreal Cognitive Assessment, MoCA: A brief screening tool for mild cognitive impairment. *J. Am. Geriatr. Soc.* **2005**, *53*, 695–699. [CrossRef] [PubMed]
34. Saltagi, A.K.; Saltagi, M.Z.; Nag, A.K.; Wu, A.W.; Higgins, T.S.; Knisely, A.; Ting, J.Y.; Illing, E.A. Diagnosis of Anosmia and Hyposmia: A Systematic Review. *Allergy Rhinol.* **2021**, *12*, 21526567211026568. [CrossRef]
35. Sixel-Doring, F.; Trautmann, E.; Mollenhauer, B.; Trenkwalder, C. Associated factors for REM sleep behavior disorder in Parkinson disease. *Neurology* **2011**, *77*, 1048–1054. [CrossRef]
36. Comella, C.L.; Nardine, T.M.; Diederich, N.J.; Stebbins, G.T. Sleep-related violence, injury, and REM sleep behavior disorder in Parkinson's disease. *Neurology* **1998**, *51*, 526–529. [CrossRef] [PubMed]
37. Sobreira-Neto, M.A.; Pena-Pereira, M.A.; Sobreira, E.S.T.; Chagas, M.H.N.; Fernandes, R.M.F.; Tumas, V.; Eckeli, A.L. High frequency of sleep disorders in Parkinson's disease and its relationship with quality of life. *Eur. Neurol.* **2017**, *78*, 330–337. [CrossRef] [PubMed]
38. García-Lorenzo, D.; Longo-Dos Santos, C.; Ewenczyk, C.; Leu-Semenescu, S.; Gallea, C.; Quattrocchi, G.; Pita Lobo, P.; Poupon, C.; Benali, H.; Arnulf, I.; et al. The coeruleus/subcoeruleus complex in rapid eye movement sleep behaviour disorders in Parkinson's disease. *Brain* **2013**, *136*, 2120–2129. [CrossRef] [PubMed]
39. Slow, E.J.; Postuma, R.B.; Lang, A.E. Implications of nocturnal symptoms towards the early diagnosis of Parkinson's disease. *J. Neural Transm.* **2014**, *121* (Suppl. 1), S49–S57. [CrossRef]
40. Boeve, B.F.; Silber, M.H.; Saper, C.B.; Ferman, T.J.; Dickson, D.W.; Parisi, J.E.; Benarroch, E.E.; Ahlskog, J.E.; Smith, G.E.; Caselli, R.C.; et al. Pathophysiology of REM sleep behaviour disorder and relevance to neurodegenerative disease. *Brain* **2007**, *130*, 2770–2788. [CrossRef]
41. St Louis, E.K.; Boeve, A.R.; Boeve, B.F. REM Sleep Behavior Disorder in Parkinson's Disease and Other Synucleinopathies. *Mov. Disord.* **2017**, *32*, 645–658. [CrossRef]
42. Doty, R.L. Olfactory dysfunction in neurodegenerative diseases: Is there a common pathological substrate? *Lancet Neurol.* **2017**, *16*, 478–488. [CrossRef] [PubMed]

43. Stiasny-Kolster, K.; Doerr, Y.; Möller, J.C.; Höffken, H.; Behr, T.M.; Oertel, W.H.; Mayer, G. Combination of 'idiopathic' REM sleep behaviour disorder and olfactory dysfunction as possible indicator for alpha-synucleinopathy demonstrated by dopamine transporter FP-CIT-SPECT. *Brain* **2005**, *128*, 126–137. [CrossRef] [PubMed]
44. Postuma, R.B.; Lang, A.E.; Massicotte-Marquez, J.; Montplaisir, J. Potential early markers of Parkinson disease in idiopathic REM sleep behavior disorder. *Neurology* **2006**, *66*, 845–851. [CrossRef] [PubMed]
45. Wong, J.C.; Li, J.; Pavlova, M.; Chen, S.; Wu, A.; Wu, S.; Gao, X. Risk factors for probable REM sleep behavior disorder: A community-based study. *Neurology* **2016**, *86*, 1306–1312. [CrossRef] [PubMed]
46. Kang, S.H.; Yoon, I.Y.; Lee, S.D.; Han, J.W.; Kim, T.H.; Kim, K.W. REM sleep behavior disorder in the Korean elderly population: Prevalence and clinical characteristics. *Sleep* **2013**, *36*, 1147–1152. [CrossRef]
47. Haba-Rubio, J.; Frauscher, B.; Marques-Vidal, P.; Toriel, J.; Tobback, N.; Andries, D.; Preisig, M.; Vollenweider, P.; Postuma, R.; Heinzer, R. Prevalence and determinants of rapid eye movement sleep behavior disorder in the general population. *Sleep* **2018**, *41*, zsx197. [CrossRef]
48. Solla, P.; Cannas, A.; Ibba, F.C.; Loi, F.; Corona, M.; Orofino, G.; Marrosu, M.G.; Marrosu, F. Gender differences in motor and non-motor symptoms among Sardinian patients with Parkinson's disease. *J. Neurol. Sci.* **2012**, *323*, 33–39. [CrossRef]
49. Martinez-Martin, P.; Falup Pecurariu, C.; Odin, P.; van Hilten, J.J.; Antonini, A.; Rojo-Abuin, J.M.; Borges, V.; Trenkwalder, C.; Aarsland, D.; Brooks, D.J.; et al. Gender-related differences in the burden of non-motor symptoms in Parkinson's disease. *J. Neurol.* **2012**, *259*, 1639–1647. [CrossRef]
50. Solla, P.; Masala, C.; Liscia, A.; Piras, R.; Ercoli, T.; Fadda, L.; Hummel, T.; Haenher, A.; Defazio, G. Sex-related differences in olfactory function and evaluation of possible confounding factors among patients with Parkinson's disease. *J. Neurol.* **2020**, *267*, 57–63. [CrossRef]
51. Russillo, M.C.; Andreozzi, V.; Erro, R.; Picillo, M.; Amboni, M.; Cuoco, S.; Barone, P.; Pellecchia, M.T. Sex Differences in Parkinson's Disease: From Bench to Bedside. *Brain Sci.* **2022**, *12*, 917. [CrossRef]

Disclaimer/Publisher's Note: The statements, opinions and data contained in all publications are solely those of the individual author(s) and contributor(s) and not of MDPI and/or the editor(s). MDPI and/or the editor(s) disclaim responsibility for any injury to people or property resulting from any ideas, methods, instructions or products referred to in the content.

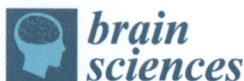 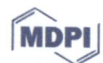

Brief Report

GABA$_A$ Receptor Benzodiazepine Binding Sites and Motor Impairments in Parkinson's Disease

Nicolaas I. Bohnen [1,2,3,4,*], Jaimie Barr [1,4], Robert Vangel [1], Stiven Roytman [1], Rebecca Paalanen [2,3], Kirk A. Frey [1,2], Peter J. H. Scott [1] and Prabesh Kanel [1,3]

[1] Department of Radiology, University of Michigan, Ann Arbor, MI 48109, USA; jaimieba@umich.edu (J.B.); rvangel@umich.edu (R.V.); stivenr@umich.edu (S.R.); kfrey@umich.edu (K.A.F.); pjhscott@umich.edu (P.J.H.S.); prabeshk@umich.edu (P.K.)
[2] Department of Neurology, University of Michigan, Ann Arbor, MI 48109, USA; rebecca.paalanen@gmail.com
[3] Morris K. Udall Center of Excellence for Parkinson's Disease Research, University of Michigan, Ann Arbor, MI 48109, USA
[4] Neurology Service and GRECC, VA Ann Arbor Healthcare System, Ann Arbor, MI 48105, USA
* Correspondence: nbohnen@umich.edu; Tel.: +1-734-936-1168

Abstract: Flumazenil is an allosteric modulator of the γ-aminobutyric acid-A receptor (GABA$_A$R) benzodiazepine binding site that could normalize neuronal signaling and improve motor impairments in Parkinson's disease (PD). Little is known about how regional GABA$_A$R availability affects motor symptoms. We investigated the relationship between regional availability of GABA$_A$R benzodiazepine binding sites and motor impairments in PD. Methods: A total of 11 Patients with PD (males; mean age 69.0 ± 4.6 years; Hoehn and Yahr stages 2–3) underwent [^{11}C]flumazenil GABA$_A$R benzodiazepine binding site and [^{11}C]dihydrotetrabenazine vesicular monoamine transporter type-2 (VMAT2) PET imaging and clinical assessment. Stepwise regression analysis was used to predict regional cerebral correlates of the four cardinal UPDRS motor scores using cortical, striatal, thalamic, and cerebellar flumazenil binding estimates. Thalamic GABA$_A$R availability was selectively associated with axial motor scores (R^2 = 0.55, F = 11.0, β = −6.4, p = 0.0009). Multi-ligand analysis demonstrated significant axial motor predictor effects by both thalamic GABA$_A$R availability (R^2 = 0.47, β = −5.2, F = 7.2, p = 0.028) and striatal VMAT2 binding (R^2 = 0.30, β = −3.9, F = 9.1, p = 0.019; total model: R^2 = 0.77, F = 11.9, p = 0.0056). Post hoc analysis demonstrated that thalamic [^{11}C]methyl-4-piperidinyl propionate cholinesterase PET and K_1 flow delivery findings were not significant confounders. Findings suggest that reduced thalamic GABA$_A$R availability correlates with worsened axial motor impairments in PD, independent of nigrostriatal degeneration. These findings may augur novel non-dopaminergic approaches to treating axial motor impairments in PD.

Keywords: axial motor impairment; benzodiazepine binding site; dopamine; GABA$_A$ receptor; Parkinson's disease; PET

1. Introduction

Axial motor impairments represent a significant cause of disability in Parkinson's disease (PD). Dopaminergic medications are often not efficacious in treating these symptoms [1]. Cholinergic system dysfunction has been implicated in some components of postural instability and gait difficulties in PD, in particular falls and sensory processing during postural control, but not with overall severity of axial motor impairments when accounting for nigrostriatal nerve terminal losses [2–4]. Postural control and gait functions are mediated by widespread neural networks that cannot be captured by a simplistic model of single neurotransmitter system changes. There is increasing interest in the dysfunction of co-localized neurotransmitter functions to better understand the complexity of the multisystem nature of the neurodegeneration in PD.

γ-aminobutyric acid (GABA) is the major inhibitory neurotransmitter in the central nervous system. GABA binds to and mediates its effects via post-synaptic ionotropic $GABA_A$ receptors ($GABA_AR$) and pre- and post-synaptic metabotropic $GABA_B$ receptors [5]. The role of GABA neurotransmission has been little studied in PD, despite the fact that the two major outflows of the basal ganglia, principal neurons of the globus pallidus internus, and of the substantia nigra pars reticulata largely employ inhibitory GABA to connect to areas outside the basal ganglia and that increased GABA activity from these nuclei has been demonstrated previously by both electrophysiologic and mRNA analyses in parkinsonian animal models [6–8]. Regional imbalance of the major inhibitory central nervous system transmitter activity may have propagating effects on the neuronal network activity underlying motor impairments in PD [9,10].

Benzodiazepine binding sites are present in a significant subset of cerebral $GABA_A$ receptors [11]. Flumazenil is a short-acting intravenously administered silent allosteric modulator of the $GABA_AR$ benzodiazepine binding site, which rapidly improves motor impairments in PD, including postural instability and gait difficulties [12,13]. Based on current basal ganglia functional models of PD, flumazenil could affect neuronal signaling at several brain regions; there is, however, a knowledge gap about the relationship between availability of regional cerebral $GABA_AR$ benzodiazepine binding sites and specific motor impairments in human PD. There are relatively few in vivo imaging reports regarding the impairment of $GABA_AR$ benzodiazepine binding sites in the brain in PD. An in vivo imaging report by Japanese researchers found a correlation between reduced cerebral $GABA_AR$ benzodiazepine binding sites in the cortex as determined by [^{123}I]iomazenil single-photon computed emission tomography and greater motor disability in PD but did not report on regions other than the cortex or striatal dopaminergic loss [14,15]. To address in more detail the role of $GABA_AR$ benzodiazepine binding sites, we investigated the relationship between in vivo regional cerebral availability of $GABA_AR$ benzodiazepine binding sites with [^{11}C]flumazenil PET and motor impairments while accounting for nigrostriatal nerve terminal losses and cholinergic activity in subjects with PD.

2. Materials and Methods

2.1. Subjects and Clinical Test Battery

This cross-sectional study involved the analysis of 11 PD subjects (males, mean age 69.0 ± 4.6 years (SD; range 63–76); mean Mini-Mental State Examination score of 28.4 ± 2.4 (range 22–30); and mean duration of motor disease of 10.5 ± 4.1 years (range 5–15)). Subjects met the United Kingdom Parkinson's Disease Society Brain Bank clinical diagnostic criteria [16]. Abnormal striatal [^{11}C]dihydrotetrabenazine PET findings were consistent with the diagnosis of PD in all subjects. No subjects had a history of a large artery stroke or other significant intracranial disease. Mean modified Hoehn and Yahr stage was 2.6 ± 0.3 (range 2–3) with 1 subject in stage 2, 5 in stage 2.5 and 5 in stage 3 [17]. No subjects were taking benzodiazepine, (anti)cholinergic or neuroleptic drugs. Nine subjects were taking a combination of dopamine agonist and carbidopa–levodopa medications and two were using carbidopa–levodopa alone. All subjects completed the Unified Parkinson's Disease Rating Scale (UPDRS) [18]. Subjects were examined and underwent [^{11}C]dihydrotetrabenazine PET imaging in the morning after withholding dopaminergic drugs overnight. Mean motor UPDRS score was 28.3 ± 11.6 (range 10–48). UPDRS motor scores were divided into cardinal motor sub-scores for tremor (items 20 and 21), rigidity (item 22), distal appendicular bradykinesia (items 23–26 and 31), and axial symptoms (items 27–30).

This study was approved by the Institutional Review Boards of Ann Arbor Department of Veterans Affairs Medical Center and the University of Michigan. Written informed consent was obtained from all subjects prior to any research procedures.

2.2. Imaging Techniques

All subjects underwent brain MRI, $GABA_AR$ benzodiazepine binding site imaging using [^{11}C]flumazenil PET, and [^{11}C]dihydrotetrabenazine vesicular monoamine transporter type-2 (VMAT2) PET imaging. Acetylcholinesterase PET imaging using the [^{11}C]methyl-4-piperidinyl propionate (PMP) ligand was available in 10 subjects for additional analysis. [^{11}C]flumazenil, [^{11}C]dihydrotetrabenazine and [^{11}C]PMP were prepared as described previously [19–21]. A bolus/infusion protocol was used for [^{11}C]flumazenil dynamic PET imaging with intravenous bolus injection containing 40% of the total administered 10 mCi [^{11}C]flumazenil dosage over 15 s, followed by continuous infusion of the remaining tracer at a constant rate for 62 min [19]. A bolus infusion was also used for [^{11}C]dihydrotetrabenazine vesicular monoamine transporter type 2 (VMAT2) dynamic PET imaging with bolus injection of 55% of a 15 mCi dose, while the remaining 45% of the dose was continuously infused over the next 60 min [22]. Dynamic acetylcholinesterase PET scanning was performed for 70 min following an intravenous bolus of 15 mCi [^{11}C]PMP. VMAT2 (used to quantify the degree of nigrostriatal striatal dopaminergic denervation) and acetylcholinesterase PET (used to quantify cholinergic thalamic binding) denervation were used for our post-analysis. The three PET scans were performed as part of a single study with two PET scans on the same day and the third one within days.

MRI was performed on a 3 Tesla Philips Achieva system (Philips, Best, The Netherlands) and PET imaging was performed in 3D imaging mode with an ECAT EXACT HR+ tomograph (Siemens Molecular Imaging, Inc., Knoxville, TN, USA) as previously reported [2].

2.3. Imaging Analysis

All image frames were spatially coregistered within subjects with a rigid-body transformation to reduce the effects of subject motion during the imaging session [23]. Interactive Data Language (IDL version 8.7) image analysis software (Research systems, Inc., Boulder, CO, USA) was used to manually trace volumes of interest on the MRI scan. Traced volumes of interest included the bilateral striatum (putamen and caudate nucleus), thalamus, pons, cerebellum, and neocortex. Neocortical volume of interest definition used semi-automated threshold delineation of the neocortical grey matter signal on the MRI images [24].

[^{11}C]flumazenil distribution volume ratios were estimated using the Logan plot graphical analysis method [25]. The input kinetics for the reference tissue were derived from the pons, where the [^{11}C]flumazenil binding is predominantly accounted for by free and nonspecifically bound radiotracer [26,27]. [^{11}C]dihydrotetrabenazine distribution volume ratios were estimated also using the Logan plot graphical analysis method [25] with the striatal time activity curves as the input function and the total neocortex as reference tissue, a reference region overall low in VMAT2 binding sites, with the assumption that the nondisplaceable distribution is uniform across the brain at equilibrium to allow accurate and stable assessment of VMAT2 binding when using the distribution volume ratio [22]. Acetylcholinesterase [^{11}C]PMP hydrolysis rates (k_3) were estimated using the striatal volume as the input tissue region [28].

2.4. Statistical Analysis

Stepwise regression analyses were used to predict cortical, striatal, thalamic and cerebellar flumazenil binding estimates from the four cardinal motor UPDRS scores as defined in Section 2.1. Analyses were performed using SAS version 9.3, (SAS institute, Cary, NC, USA). We also performed post hoc confounder analysis for the dopaminergic and cholinergic PET ligands. Post hoc confounder analysis was also performed using the K_1 proxy flow images extracted from the flumazenil PET kinetic model. A model was considered significant if its *p*-value fell below our Bonferroni-adjusted α of 0.0125 (0.05/4 models).

3. Results

3.1. Availability of Regional Cerebral GABA$_A$R Benzodiazepine Binding Sites and UPDRS Motor Scores

Significant findings were present for the thalamic region with axial motor scores as the only significant variable in the model ($R^2 = 0.55$, $F = 11.0$, $\beta = -6.4$, $p = 0.0009$, significant after correction for multiple testing). Tremor was the only variable that entered the model for the cortex ($R^2 = 0.42$, $F = 6.6$, $\beta = -4.9$, $p = 0.03$), which was no longer significant after correction for the effects of multiple testing. No cardinal UPDRS motor scores entered the regression models for the striatum or cerebellum.

3.2. Post Hoc Analysis of Thalamic GABA$_A$R Benzodiazepine Binding Site Availability, Acetylcholinesterase Hydrolysis Rate, and VMAT2 and Axial UPDRS Motor Scores

A subgroup of 10 subjects completed all three PET ligand studies. Stepwise regression analysis was used to best predict axial UPDRS motor scores from thalamic GABA$_A$R benzodiazepine binding site availability, thalamic acetylcholinesterase hydrolysis rate, striatal VMAT2 activity, age, and duration of motor disease. The overall model was significant ($R^2 = 0.77$, $F = 11.9$, $p = 0.0056$) with significant contributions from both the thalamic GABA$_A$R benzodiazepine binding site availability ($R^2 = 0.47$, $\beta = -5.2$, $F = 7.2$, $p = 0.028$), and striatal VMAT2 binding ($R^2 = 0.30$, $\beta = -3.9$, $F = 9.1$, $p = 0.019$). Thalamic acetylcholinesterase hydrolysis rates, age, and duration of disease did not meet the entry criteria for the model.

3.3. Post Hoc Analysis of Thalamic [^{11}C]Flumazenil K_1 Flow Effects and Axial UPDRS Motor Scores

Although the above findings show that other neurotransmitters, such as dopamine or acetylcholine were not confounders for our GABA$_A$R findings, we used the K_1 proxy flow images from the flumazenil PET kinetic model as an additional step to confirm that neural processes other than the two non-GABAergic neurotransmitters (dopamine and acetylcholine) may not play a significant role. This is because reduced gray matter flow is a marker of the global neurodegenerative process (or global neural integrity) and may be associated with glutamatergic activity (the most common neurotransmitter in the brain). For this purpose, we computed thalamic K_1 flow derived from the [^{11}C]flumazenil kinetic model. Results showed no significant effect of thalamic K_1 flow measures in the prediction of axial motor UPDRS scores ($F = 2.92$, $\beta = -2.6$, $p = 0.13$). Furthermore, entering the thalamic K_1 flow measure together with the thalamic [^{11}C]flumazenil receptor binding measure not only failed to show a significant effect for the thalamic K_1 flow measure but actually further strengthened the effect of the [^{11}C]flumazenil receptor binding measure in the prediction of axial motor scores ($F = 20.3$, $\beta = -6.7$, $p = 0.0028$; total model $F = 8.9$, $p = 0.009$, Figure 1).

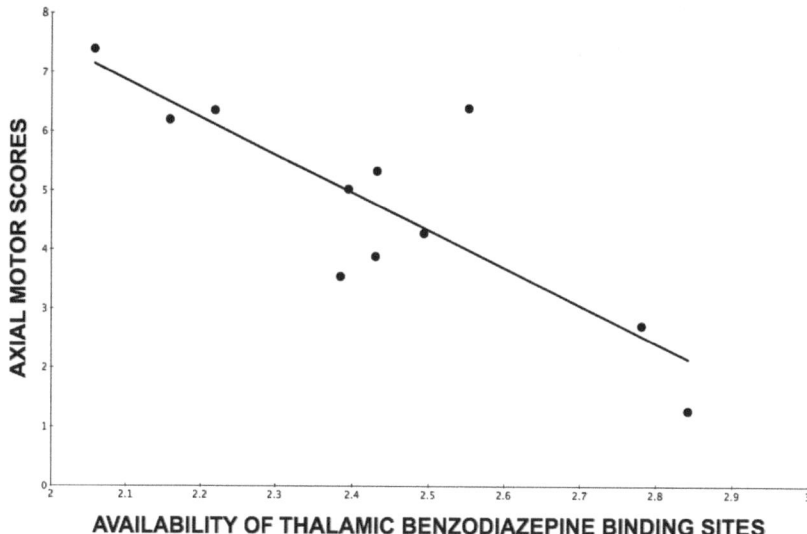

Figure 1. Line of best fit through a scatterplot of axial motor impairment scores over availability of thalamic benzodiazepine binding sites as assessed by [^{11}C]flumazenil PET distribution volume ratios.

4. Discussion

The thalamus is a key structure involved in motor control. The thalamus receives inhibitory inputs from the basal ganglia and excitatory signals from the cerebellum and cortex. Additional modulation in the form of monoaminergic and cholinergic signaling acts on the thalamus. Together, inputs to the thalamus act to modulate information received from the cortical regions resulting in motor control [29]. Our findings indicate that decreased availability of thalamic GABA$_A$R benzodiazepine binding sites, reflecting increased GABAergic activity, is correlated with increased axial motor impairments in PD, independent of the degree of nigrostriatal degeneration. This may be compatible with the postulated basal ganglia model that the dopamine-denervated striatal nuclei provide inhibitory control over the globus pallidus internus and the substantia nigra pars reticulata [30], effectively "releasing" the tonic GABAergic inhibition mediated by the output structures of the basal ganglia [31]. As such, any dopaminergic hypoactivity within the striatum would therefore lead to a relative increase in inhibitory outflow from the basal ganglia [32]. Consequently, the subthalamic nucleus sends strong excitatory efferent signals to the globus pallidus internus and the substantia nigra pars reticulata, meaning that any increase in the firing rate of subthalamic nucleus neurons leads directly to an increased firing rate within globus pallidus internus and the substantia nigra pars reticulata neurons, in turn inhibiting the thalamic and brainstem structures resulting in mobility disturbances in PD [33]. In short, the dopaminergic hypoactivity in the striatum results in a comparative abundance of GABAergic inhibitory outputs from the basal ganglia to the thalamic region that ultimately leads to increased axial impairment in PD.

Indeed, recent research supports this model; one study demonstrated a correlation between increased GABA in the basal ganglia and axial motor impairment in PD [34], and another study demonstrated that GABA$_A$R antagonism restored dopaminergic firing in the striatum and improved motor symptoms in mouse models [35]. There is also evidence that direct thalamic pathology may contribute to the pathophysiology of motor impairments in PD. For example, a post-mortem study demonstrated a 30–50% loss of cells in the center-median/parafascicular complex, which normally provides important glutaminergic feedback from the thalamus to the putamen [29]. [^{11}C]flumazenil binding site densities may serve as an indicator of synaptic neuropil integrity or may be an indicator of a disease-specific disturbance at the $GABA_A$ receptor level. The former rationale is derived from the fact that GABA receptors are expressed on virtually all cortical and subcortical synaptic terminals. We performed a post hoc analysis to test the possibility that thalamic [^{11}C]flumazenil $GABA_AR$ benzodiazepine binding site availability findings may be confounded by loss of neuronal integrity. For this purpose, we computed thalamic K_1 flow measures derived from the [^{11}C]flumazenil kinetic model but did not find a significant effect. Similar findings have been reported for the [^{123}I]iomazenil single-photon computed emission tomography studies in PD where the authors also found an association between reduced cerebral $GABA_AR$ benzodiazepine binding site availability and increased motor disability in PD, which could not be explained by flow or perfusion data, suggesting a specific alteration of $GABA_A$ receptors rather than of generalized synaptic or neuronal integrity [15].

These findings support our previous reports on in vivo imaging studies that demonstrated correlations between cholinergic innervation changes and posture, falls, and sensory processing during postural changes [3,24,36,37]. These findings agree with pharmacological studies, showing a benefit of cholinesterase drug treatment and a reduction in falls in subjects with PD with no significant changes in parkinsonian motor rating scores [38,39].

Our results also showed an independent effect for the integrity of nigrostriatal dopaminergic nerve terminals and axial motor impairments in PD. Although axial motor impairments are relatively refractory to dopaminergic treatments, a subset of these impairments are or remain responsive to these drugs [40]. Furthermore, there is emerging evidence for GABA and dopamine co-releasing neurotransmission from substantia nigra pars compacta (SNpc) and ventral tegmental area dopaminergic neurons [41,42]. Animal models of PD suggest that dopaminergic activity in the SNpc may be inhibited due to aberrant tonic inhibition, thought to be the result of excessive astrocytic GABA, leading to further imbalance between dopamine and GABA [43]. These observations illustrate the intricate interplay between these two major neurotransmitter changes and how it may be derailed by nigrostriatal denervation [8].

Our findings of an association between motor impairments and altered $GABA_AR$ availability may not be limited to Lewy body parkinsonism but may potentially also apply to other types of parkinsonian disorders. For example, a [^{11}C]flumazenil $GABA_AR$ benzodiazepine binding site PET study in patients with vascular parkinsonism with and without gait disturbances found that striatal [^{11}C]flumazenil uptake was inversely correlated with the motor UPDRS scores and [^{11}C]flumazenil binding reductions were associated with the presence of gait disturbance [44]. However, comparisons of these findings and our present results are limited as—at least pure—vascular parkinsonism would not manifest with nigrostriatal degeneration [45], which, inherent to its dysfunction, would lead to a relative increase in inhibitory outflow from the basal ganglia [32].

As previously stated, axial symptoms of PD are often resistant to treatment with dopaminergic replacement therapy [1]. Additionally, treatment with deep brain stimulation (DBS), which commonly targets the subthalamic nucleus and globus pallidus internus, fails to alleviate axial symptoms and may worsen axial disability. Subthalamic nucleus DBS, specifically, has been correlated with greater axial impairment post-surgery [46]. This is in line with our findings as increased firing of excitatory efferents from the subthalamic nucleus may lead to increased inhibition of the thalamic and brainstem regions. Alternative treatments to address the relative hyper GABAergic activity in these regions may lead to breakthroughs in the treatment of axial impairment.

Our findings augur $GABA_AR$ benzodiazepine binding site allosteric modulator drug treatment approaches to manage axial motor impairments in PD. Flumazenil is a fused imidazobenzodiazepine, which serves therapeutically as a $GABA_AR$ benzodiazepine binding site blocker [47]. Ondo and Hunter reported findings of single-dose (0.5 mg) intravenous flumazenil administration in eight PD patients and found significant improvements in total UPDRS motor scores, where the axial motor UPDRS sub-score tended to account for most of this improvement [12]. These flumazenil treatment data are compatible with the more selective association of reduced GABA$_A$R benzodiazepine binding site availability and axial motor scores in our study.

Limitations of this study include the size and homogeneity of our sample. Because the patients were recruited from a veteran's hospital, all the participants were male. This, in combination with the limited sample size, could influence the generalizability of the present findings with specific axial motor impairments, such as falls or freezing of gait. In addition, research into specific subtypes of axial impairments, such as patients with falls or freezing of gait, may lead to symptom-specific findings of GABA$_A$R benzodiazepine binding site availability. Another limitation is the lack of a normal control or active disease control group to allow for the investigation of differential effects from normal aging or disease-specific effects of PD. Further studies based on a larger, more diverse study population, preferably with longitudinal follow up, are needed to more thoroughly investigate the role of GABA$_A$R benzodiazepine binding site availability in the neural network underlying motor impairments in PD.

We conclude that thalamic GABA$_A$R benzodiazepine binding site availability is inversely correlated with axial motor impairments in PD, independent from the degree of nigrostriatal degeneration. These findings may augur novel non-dopaminergic approaches to treating axial motor impairments in PD.

Author Contributions: Conceptualization, N.I.B.; methodology, N.I.B., K.A.F. and P.J.H.S.; software, P.K.; validation, N.I.B.; formal analysis, N.I.B. and P.K.; investigation, N.I.B.; resources, N.I.B.; data curation, P.K.; writing—original draft preparation, N.I.B., J.B. and R.V.; writing—review and editing, N.I.B., P.K., J.B., R.P., S.R. and R.V.; visualization, N.I.B.; supervision, N.I.B.; project administration, N.I.B.; funding acquisition, N.I.B. All authors have read and agreed to the published version of the manuscript.

Funding: This research was supported by the Michael J. Fox Foundation, Department of Veterans Affairs (grant number I01 RX000317), and the National Institutes of Health (grant numbers P01 NS015655 and RO1 NS070856).

Institutional Review Board Statement: This study was conducted in accordance with the Declaration of Helsinki, and approved by the Institutional Review Boards of the Ann Arbor Department of Veterans Affairs Medical Center and the University of Michigan (HUM00130361, 14 September 2017).

Informed Consent Statement: Informed consent was obtained from all subjects involved in this study.

Data Availability Statement: The data that support the findings of this study are available on reasonable request from the corresponding author. The data are not publicly available due to their containing information that could compromise the privacy of research participants.

Acknowledgments: The authors thank all patients for their time commitment, and research assistants, PET technologists, cyclotron operators, and chemists, for their assistance with this study.

Conflicts of Interest: N.I.B. receives research support from the National Institutes of Health, Michael J. Fox Foundation, and Ann Arbor Department of Veterans Affairs. K.A.F. receives research support from the National Institutes of Health, GE Healthcare, and AVID Radiopharmaceuticals. K.A.F. is a consultant for AVID Radiopharmaceuticals, MIMVista, Bayer-Schering, and GE healthcare, and holds equity (common stock) in GE, Bristol-Myers, Merck, and Novo-Nordisk. The funders had no role in the design of this study; in the collection, analyses, or interpretation of data; in the writing of the manuscript; or in the decision to publish the results.

References

1. Bloem, B.R.; Steijns, J.A.; Smits-Engelsman, B.C. An update on falls. *Curr. Opin. Neurol.* **2003**, *16*, 15–26. [CrossRef] [PubMed]
2. Bohnen, N.I.; Muller, M.L.; Kotagal, V.; Koeppe, R.A.; Kilbourn, M.R.; Gilman, S.; Albin, R.L.; Frey, K.A. Heterogeneity of cholinergic denervation in Parkinson's disease without dementia. *J. Cereb. Blood Flow Metab.* **2012**, *32*, 1609–1617. [CrossRef] [PubMed]
3. Muller, M.L.; Albin, R.L.; Kotagal, V.; Koeppe, R.A.; Scott, P.J.; Frey, K.A.; Bohnen, N.I. Thalamic cholinergic innervation and postural sensory integration function in Parkinson's disease. *Brain* **2013**, *136*, 3282–3289. [CrossRef] [PubMed]

4. Roytman, S.; Paalanen, R.; Griggs, A.; David, S.; Pongmala, C.; Koeppe, R.A.; Scott, P.J.H.; Marusic, U.; Kanel, P.; Bohnen, N.I. Cholinergic system correlates of postural control changes in Parkinson's disease freezers. *Brain* **2023**, *146*, 3243–3257. [CrossRef] [PubMed]
5. Bowery, N.G.; Bettler, B.; Froestl, W.; Gallagher, J.P.; Marshall, F.; Raiteri, M.; Bonner, T.I.; Enna, S.J. International Union of Pharmacology. XXXIII. Mammalian gamma-aminobutyric acid$_{(B)}$ receptors: Structure and function. *Pharmacol. Rev.* **2002**, *54*, 247–264. [CrossRef] [PubMed]
6. Filion, M.; Tremblay, L. Abnormal spontaneous activity of globus pallidus neurons in monkeys with MPTP-induced parkinsonism. *Brain Res.* **1991**, *547*, 142–151. [CrossRef] [PubMed]
7. Vila, M.; Levy, R.; Herrero, M.T.; Ruberg, M.; Faucheux, B.; Obeso, J.A.; Agid, Y.; Hirsch, E.C. Consequences of nigrostriatal denervation on the functioning of the basal ganglia in human and nonhuman primates: An in situ hybridization study of cytochrome oxidase subunit I mRNA. *J. Neurosci.* **1997**, *17*, 765–773. [CrossRef]
8. Borgkvist, A.; Avegno, E.M.; Wong, M.Y.; Kheirbek, M.A.; Sonders, M.S.; Hen, R.; Sulzer, D. Loss of Striatonigral GABAergic Presynaptic Inhibition Enables Motor Sensitization in Parkinsonian Mice. *Neuron* **2015**, *87*, 976–988. [CrossRef]
9. Boecker, H. Imaging the role of GABA in movement disorders. *Curr. Neurol. Neurosci. Rep.* **2013**, *13*, 385. [CrossRef]
10. Boccalaro, I.L.; Schwerdel, C.; Cristia-Lara, L.; Fritschy, J.M.; Rubi, L. Dopamine depletion induces neuron-specific alterations of GABAergic transmission in the mouse striatum. *Eur. J. Neurosci.* **2020**, *52*, 3353–3374. [CrossRef]
11. Sieghart, W.; Sperk, G. Subunit composition, distribution and function of GABA(A) receptor subtypes. *Curr. Top Med. Chem.* **2002**, *2*, 795–816. [CrossRef]
12. Ondo, W.G.; Hunter, C. Flumazenil, a GABA antagonist, may improve features of Parkinson's disease. *Mov. Disord.* **2003**, *18*, 683–685. [CrossRef] [PubMed]
13. Ondo, W.G.; Silay, Y.S. Intravenous flumazenil for Parkinson's disease: A single dose, double blind, placebo controlled, cross-over trial. *Mov. Disord.* **2006**, *21*, 1614–1617. [CrossRef] [PubMed]
14. Kawabata, K.; Tachibana, H.; Sugita, M.; Fukuchi, M. Impairment of benzodiazepine receptor in Parkinson's disease evaluated by 123I-iomazenil SPECT. *Kaku Igaku* **1996**, *33*, 391–397. [PubMed]
15. Kawabata, K.; Tachibana, H. Evaluation of benzodiazepine receptor in the cerebral cortex of Parkinson's disease using 123I-iomazenil SPECT. *Nihon Rinsho* **1997**, *55*, 244–248. [PubMed]
16. Hughes, A.J.; Daniel, S.E.; Kilford, L.; Lees, A.J. Accuracy of clinical diagnosis of idiopathic Parkinson's disease: A clinico-pathological study of 100 cases. *J. Neurol. Neurosurg. Psychiatry* **1992**, *55*, 181–184. [CrossRef]
17. Goetz, C.G.; Poewe, W.; Rascol, O.; Sampaio, C.; Stebbins, G.T.; Counsell, C.; Giladi, N.; Holloway, R.G.; Moore, C.G.; Wenning, G.K.; et al. Movement Disorder Society Task Force report on the Hoehn and Yahr staging scale: Status and recommendations. *Mov. Disord.* **2004**, *19*, 1020–1028. [CrossRef]
18. Fahn, S. Unified Parkinson's disease rating scale. *Recent Dev. Park. Dis.* **1987**, *0*, 153–163.
19. Frey, K.A.; Holthoff, V.A.; Koeppe, R.A.; Jewett, D.M.; Kilbourn, M.R.; Kuhl, D.E. Parametric in vivo imaging of benzodiazepine receptor distribution in human brain. *Ann. Neurol.* **1991**, *30*, 663–672. [CrossRef]
20. Jewett, D.M.; Kilbourn, M.R.; Lee, L.C. A simple synthesis of [11C]dihydrotetrabenazine (DTBZ). *Nucl. Med. Biol.* **1997**, *24*, 197–199. [CrossRef]
21. Shao, X.; Hoareau, R.; Runkle, A.C.; Tluczek, L.J.M.; Hockley, B.G.; Henderson, B.D.; Scott, P.J.H. Highlighting the versatility of the Tracerlab synthesis modules. Part 2: Fully automated production of [11C]-labeled radiopharmaceuticals using a Tracerlab FXC-Pro. *J. Label. Compd. Radiopharm.* **2011**, *54*, 819–838. [CrossRef]
22. Koeppe, R.A.; Frey, K.A.; Kuhl, D.E.; Kilbourn, M.R. Assessment of extrastriatal vesicular monoamine transporter binding site density using stereoisomers of [11C]dihydrotetrabenazine. *J. Cereb. Blood Flow Metab.* **1999**, *19*, 1376–1384. [CrossRef]
23. Minoshima, S.; Koeppe, R.A.; Fessler, J.A.; Mintun, M.A.; Berger, K.L.; Taylor, S.F.; Kuhl, D.E. Integrated and Automated Data-Analysis Method for Neuronal Activation Studies Using O-15-Water Pet. *Int. Congr. Ser.* **1993**, *1030*, 409–417.
24. Bohnen, N.I.; Frey, K.A.; Studenski, S.; Kotagal, V.; Koeppe, R.A.; Constantine, G.M.; Scott, P.J.; Albin, R.L.; Muller, M.L. Extra-nigral pathological conditions are common in Parkinson's disease with freezing of gait: An in vivo positron emission tomography study. *Mov. Disord.* **2014**, *29*, 1118–1124. [CrossRef] [PubMed]
25. Logan, J.; Fowler, J.S.; Volkow, N.D.; Wang, G.J.; Ding, Y.S.; Alexoff, D.L. Distribution volume ratios without blood sampling from graphical analysis of PET data. *J. Cereb. Blood Flow Metab.* **1996**, *16*, 834–840. [CrossRef]
26. Millet, P.; Graf, C.; Buck, A.; Walder, B.; Ibanez, V. Evaluation of the reference tissue models for PET and SPECT benzodiazepine binding parameters. *Neuroimage* **2002**, *17*, 928–942. [CrossRef] [PubMed]
27. Odano, I.; Halldin, C.; Karlsson, P.; Varrone, A.; Airaksinen, A.J.; Krasikova, R.N.; Farde, L. [18F]flumazenil binding to central benzodiazepine receptor studies by PET—Quantitative analysis and comparisons with [11C]flumazenil. *Neuroimage* **2009**, *45*, 891–902. [CrossRef] [PubMed]
28. Nagatsuka Si, S.; Fukushi, K.; Shinotoh, H.; Namba, H.; Iyo, M.; Tanaka, N.; Aotsuka, A.; Ota, T.; Tanada, S.; Irie, T. Kinetic analysis of [(11)C]MP4A using a high-radioactivity brain region that represents an integrated input function for measurement of cerebral acetylcholinesterase activity without arterial blood sampling. *J. Cereb. Blood Flow Metab.* **2001**, *21*, 1354–1366. [CrossRef]
29. Halliday, G.M. Thalamic changes in Parkinson's disease. *Park. Relat. Disord.* **2009**, *15* (Suppl. S3), S152–S155. [CrossRef]
30. Nambu, A. A new dynamic model of the cortico-basal ganglia loop. *Prog. Brain Res.* **2004**, *143*, 461–466. [CrossRef]

31. Takakusaki, K.; Habaguchi, T.; Ohtinata-Sugimoto, J.; Saitoh, K.; Sakamoto, T. Basal ganglia efferents to the brainstem centers controlling postural muscle tone and locomotion: A new concept for understanding motor disorders in basal ganglia dysfunction. *Neuroscience* **2003**, *119*, 293–308. [CrossRef] [PubMed]
32. Lewis, S.J.; Barker, R.A. A pathophysiological model of freezing of gait in Parkinson's disease. *Park. Relat. Disord.* **2009**, *15*, 333–338. [CrossRef]
33. Lewis, S.J.; Shine, J.M. The Next Step: A Common Neural Mechanism for Freezing of Gait. *Neuroscientist* **2016**, *22*, 72–82. [CrossRef]
34. O'Gorman Tuura, R.L.; Baumann, C.R.; Baumann-Vogel, H. Beyond Dopamine: GABA, Glutamate, and the Axial Symptoms of Parkinson Disease. *Front. Neurol.* **2018**, *9*, 806. [CrossRef]
35. Emmanouilidou, E.; Minakaki, G.; Keramioti, M.V.; Xylaki, M.; Balafas, E.; Chrysanthou-Piterou, M.; Kloukina, I.; Vekrellis, K. GABA transmission via ATP-dependent K+ channels regulates alpha-synuclein secretion in mouse striatum. *Brain* **2016**, *139*, 871–890. [CrossRef] [PubMed]
36. Bohnen, N.I.; Kanel, P.; Zhou, Z.; Koeppe, R.A.; Frey, K.A.; Dauer, W.T.; Albin, R.L.; Müller, M.L. Cholinergic system changes of falls and freezing of gait in Parkinson's disease. *Ann. Neurol.* **2019**, *85*, 538–549. [CrossRef] [PubMed]
37. Bohnen, N.I.; Muller, M.L.; Koeppe, R.A.; Studenski, S.A.; Kilbourn, M.A.; Frey, K.A.; Albin, R.L. History of falls in Parkinson disease is associated with reduced cholinergic activity. *Neurology* **2009**, *73*, 1670–1676. [CrossRef]
38. Chung, K.A.; Lobb, B.M.; Nutt, J.G.; Horak, F.B. Effects of a central cholinesterase inhibitor on reducing falls in Parkinson disease. *Neurology* **2010**, *75*, 1263–1269. [CrossRef]
39. Henderson, E.J.; Lord, S.R.; Brodie, M.A.; Gaunt, D.M.; Lawrence, A.D.; Close, J.C.; Whone, A.L.; Ben-Shlomo, Y. Rivastigmine for gait stability in patients with Parkinson's disease (ReSPonD): A randomised, double-blind, placebo-controlled, phase 2 trial. *Lancet Neurol.* **2016**, *15*, 249–258. [CrossRef]
40. Bohnen, N.I.; Cham, R. Postural control, gait, and dopamine functions in parkinsonian movement disorders. *Clin. Geriatr. Med.* **2006**, *22*, 797–812. [CrossRef]
41. Tritsch, N.X.; Ding, J.B.; Sabatini, B.L. Dopaminergic neurons inhibit striatal output through non-canonical release of GABA. *Nature* **2012**, *490*, 262–266. [CrossRef] [PubMed]
42. Tritsch, N.X.; Oh, W.J.; Gu, C.; Sabatini, B.L. Midbrain dopamine neurons sustain inhibitory transmission using plasma membrane uptake of GABA, not synthesis. *Elife* **2014**, *3*, e01936. [CrossRef] [PubMed]
43. Heo, J.Y.; Nam, M.H.; Yoon, H.H.; Kim, J.; Hwang, Y.J.; Won, W.; Woo, D.H.; Lee, J.A.; Park, H.J.; Jo, S.; et al. Aberrant Tonic Inhibition of Dopaminergic Neuronal Activity Causes Motor Symptoms in Animal Models of Parkinson's Disease. *Curr. Biol.* **2020**, *30*, 276–291.e279. [CrossRef] [PubMed]
44. Ihara, M.; Tomimoto, H.; Ishizu, K.; Yoshida, H.; Sawamoto, N.; Hashikawa, K.; Fukuyama, H. Association of vascular parkinsonism with impaired neuronal integrity in the striatum. *J. Neural Transm.* **2007**, *114*, 577–584. [CrossRef]
45. Gerschlager, W.; Bencsits, G.; Pirker, W.; Bloem, B.R.; Asenbaum, S.; Prayer, D.; Zijlmans, J.C.; Hoffmann, M.; Brucke, T. [123I]beta-CIT SPECT distinguishes vascular parkinsonism from Parkinson's disease. *Mov. Disord.* **2002**, *17*, 518–523. [CrossRef]
46. Zampogna, A.; Cavallieri, F.; Bove, F.; Suppa, A.; Castrioto, A.; Meoni, S.; Pélissier, P.; Schmitt, E.; Bichon, A.; Lhommée, E.; et al. Axial impairment and falls in Parkinson's disease: 15 years of subthalamic deep brain stimulation. *NPJ Park. Dis.* **2022**, *8*, 121. [CrossRef]
47. Haefely, W.; Hunkeler, W. The story of flumazenil. *Eur. J. Anaesthesiol. Suppl.* **1988**, *2*, 3–13.

Disclaimer/Publisher's Note: The statements, opinions and data contained in all publications are solely those of the individual author(s) and contributor(s) and not of MDPI and/or the editor(s). MDPI and/or the editor(s) disclaim responsibility for any injury to people or property resulting from any ideas, methods, instructions or products referred to in the content.

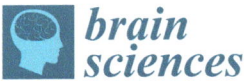

Review

Advances on Cellular Clonotypic Immunity in Amyotrophic Lateral Sclerosis

Giuseppe Schirò [1,†], Vincenzo Di Stefano [1], Salvatore Iacono [1], Antonino Lupica [1], Filippo Brighina [1], Roberto Monastero [1] and Carmela Rita Balistreri [2,*,†]

[1] Section of Neurology, Department of Biomedicine, Neurosciences and Advanced Diagnostics (BiND), University of Palermo, 90127 Palermo, Italy
[2] Cellular and Molecular Laboratory, Department of Biomedicine, Neurosciences and Advanced Diagnostics (BiND), University of Palermo, 90134 Palermo, Italy
* Correspondence: carmelarita.balistreri@unipa.it
† These authors contributed equally to this work.

Abstract: Amyotrophic lateral sclerosis (ALS) is a fatal neuromuscular disease, characterized by the progressive degeneration of the upper and lower motor neurons in the cortex and spinal cord. Although the pathogenesis of ALS remains unclear, evidence concerning the role of the clonotypic immune system is growing. Adaptive immunity cells often appear changed in number, or in terms of their activation profiles, both peripherally and centrally; however, their role in ALS appears conflictive. Data from human and animal model studies, which are currently reported in the literature, show that each subset of lymphocytes and their mediators may mediate a protective or toxic mechanism in ALS, affecting both its progression and risk of death. In the present review, an attempt is made to shed light on the actual role of cellular clonotypic immunity in ALS by integrating recent clinical studies and experimental observations.

Keywords: Amyotrophic lateral sclerosis (ALS); neurodegeneration; neuroinflammation; neuromuscular disease; autoimmunity; the clonotypic immune system

1. Introduction

Amyotrophic lateral sclerosis (ALS) is a neurological disease characterized by the irreversible and progressive loss of motor neurons located both at the cortical level—the so-called *first motor neurons*—in the gray matter of the spinal cord, and in the nuclei of the cranial nerves—the so-called *second motor neurons* [1]. Sporadic ALS accounts for about 90% of cases of the disease, whereas about 10% of ALS cases are hereditary due to genetic variants in numerous genes, including: the chromosome 9 open reading frame 72 (C9ORF72), Cu/Zn superoxide dismutase (SOD1), TAR DNA-binding protein 43 (TDP-43), and fused-in sarcoma/translocated liposarcoma (FUS/TLS) genes. These variations usually occur with autosomal dominant transmission (see Figure 1) [2]. The pathogenesis of both sporadic and familial forms is complex, partially clear, and certainly not restricted to a single factor (i.e., genetic factors may account for part of the pathogenesis, but they are also strictly related to several triggering and driving factors). The strong involvement of the immune system has been also documented. It is well recognized that the innate immunity plays a pivotal role in the central nervous system (CNS) and homeostasis, but also contributes to the onset of ALS. Accordingly, under physiological CNS conditions, innate immunity induces neuroinflammation to contain infections and eliminate pathogens, cell debris, and aggregated or misfolded proteins. With ALS, neuroinflammation is continuous and harmful for CNS cells; this constitutes the typical hallmark of the disease [3,4]. Moreover, in recent years, adaptive (or clonotypic) immunity [5] has emerged in studies concerning CNS health and disease; indeed, it is a fundamental component with a double function. First, it mediates immune-surveillance and defends against neurotropic viruses [6,7], as well as maintaining CNS homeostasis and integrity. It also promotes neurogenesis and improves cognitive function. With CNS degenerative diseases (i.e., ALS), clonotypic immunity commonly shows dysregulated and abnormal immune responses [4]. Accordingly, clonotypic immune cells often appear to be peripherally and centrally changed in several activation profiles. Data from human and animal model studies are currently reported in the literature. They provide the evidence on the capacity of each subset of lymphocytes, and their mediators, of caning mediate a protective or toxic mechanism in ALS, affecting both its progression and risk of death. In the present review, an attempt is made to shed light on the actual role of cellular clonotypic immunity in ALS by integrating recent clinical studies and experimental observations.

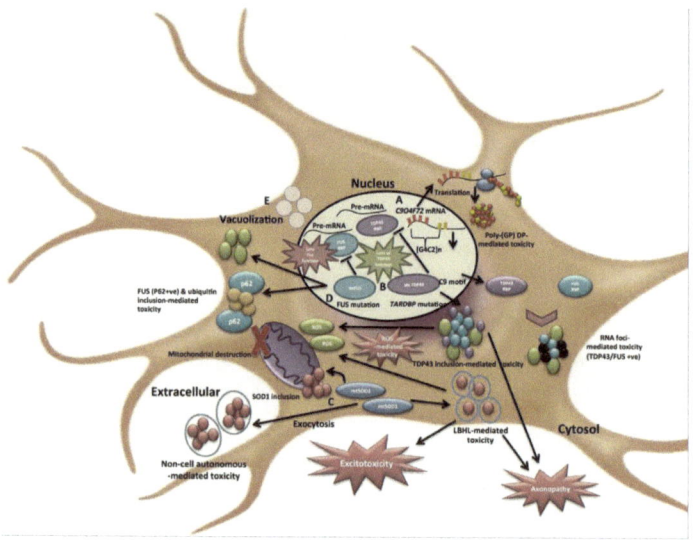

Figure 1. Pathophysiological effects induced by *C9OR72, TARDBP, SOD1, and FUS* gene mutations that are associated with the onset of ALS. A: The C9ORF72 mutation induces a gain-of-function (GOF) mechanism. More precisely, GGGGCC (G4C2), when translocated to its cytosol form, aggregates poly-(GP) dipeptide-repeat proteins (DPR), or misfolded proteins, to produce aggregates of ubiquitinated (U) RNA foci that are associated with TDP43 or FUS proteins, which are both mediating neuronal toxins. B: The transactive response of the DNA-binding protein (TARDBP) mutation triggers both the loss of function (LOF) and GOF mechanisms. C: The superoxide dismutase 1 (SOD1) mutation provokes a GOF mechanism. Mutant SOD1 dimers in the cytosol collect as SOD1 inclusions within mitochondria, and Lewy-body-like hyaline (LBLH) inclusions in the cytosol, where they can trigger mitochondrial reactive oxygen species (ROS) a generation later, thus causing mitochondrial destruction. D: The fused-in sarcoma (FUS) mutation mediates both LOF and GOF mechanisms. Mutant FUS proteins cause LOF by preventing normal FUS from binding to pre-mRNA. E: Cytosol vacuolization is caused by all the above-mentioned mutations. **By Biorender software.**

2. Recent Evidence on Clonotypic Immunity in ALS

The interplay between the clonotypic immune system and ALS emerges from the results of several clinical and experimental studies. For example, ALS patients are more often affected by autoimmune diseases [8], and the presence or absence of cognitive impairment in ALS patients has been associated with different peripheral immune profiles, with lower total lymphocytes, CD4+, B cell counts, and CD8+ lymphocytes in patients with cognitive decline than in those without objective cognitive impairment [9]. Current evidence on the biological effects, mediated by mutations in the abovementioned genes, additionally underlines a close relationship between the onset and progression of ALS and clonotypic responses of the immune system. Among them, mutations in the C9orf72 gene, which are particularly expressed in B cells and characterized by an expansion of the GGGGCC sequence within an intronic region [10], represent the most frequent cause of inherited ALS, and they indirectly reveal the close relationship between the disease and the active participation of the clonotypic immune system. Interestingly, C9orf72 knockout (KO) mouse models, with mild motor deficits, exhibit a dysregulated immune response, which is characterized by T-cell activation, overproduction of autoantibodies and cytokines, and signs of massive leukocyte infiltration, such as lymphadenopathy and splenomegaly, thus causing the development of a systemic lupus erythematosus-like disease [11]. C9orf72 KO mice also show the absence of mitochondrial degradation with Stimulator of Interferon Genes (STING) signaling, thus leading to the maintenance of interferon production and the activation of adaptive immunity [12]. Furthermore, mice harboring loss-of-function mutations in the ortholog of C9ORF72 develop splenomegaly, neutrophilia, thrombocytopenia, increased expression of inflammatory cytokines, and severe autoimmunity, ultimately leading to a high mortality rate [13]. Moreover, mice with full C9orf72 ablations show a typical induction of ALS pathological hallmarks, including motor neuron degeneration, gliosis, and increased ubiquitination, which is associated with a massive infiltration (detected by postmortem histopathological analyses) of histiocytes/macrophages and lymphocytes (particularly B220/CD45R-positive B-lymphocytes) in the CNS, as well as in the spleen, bone marrow, liver, kidneys, and lungs [14]. In addition, ALS patients with the C9orf72 mutation have higher levels of Interferon-α (INF-α) in their cerebrospinal fluid (CSF), when compared with ALS patients having other mutations [15] (see Figure 1). Interesting data on the relevant role of chronic inflammation in ALS also come from studies examining familial forms of the disease. These forms are evoked by FUS mutations, whose evidence suggests that the FUS protein may be a common component of clonotypic immune inclusions in non-SOD1 ALS [16]. Significant evidence concerning the role of clonotypic immunity and inflammation in ALS pathogeneses also emerges from the causative and susceptibility genes associated with the TDP-43 pathology, which are highly expressed in innate immune cells and increasingly implicated in key immune and inflammatory pathways, such as GRN and TBK1 [17].

In addition, it has been also reported that different subsets with different functions are involved, depending on the stage of the disease. T cells have been shown to enhance the survival of motoneuron cells (MNs) in Superoxide dismutase (SOD)1 mutant mice through protective neuroinflammation, which is likely to occur via Interleukin-4 (IL-4), and they infiltrate the spinal cord and brain in abundance during ALS progression [18]. Motor impairment has also been shown to be accompanied by a decline in the functions of regulatory T cells, which inhibits microglia activation in SOD1 mutant mice [19]. These data might suggest that neuroprotective functions of the immune system may prevail at an early stage of the disease, although other studies are needed to confirm this (see Figure 2). The progression of the disease is, however, accompanied by several changes in the immune system, such as: the acquisition of an inflammatory phenotype via microglia cells [20], thymic involution [21], increased levels of pro-inflammatory cytokines [22], and leucocyte infiltration into the central nervous system (CNS) [18]. In ALS, the infiltration of lymphocytes into the CNS has different consequences depending on the cell type. Accordingly, CD4+ CD25+ regulatory T cells (Tregs) and CD4+ T helper (Th)2 cells tend to mediate a neuroprotective effect, whereas the presence of CD4+ Th1, CD4+ Th17, cytotoxic CD8+, and Natural killer (NK) cells, and effector T lymphocytes (Teffs), is associated with a more rapid progression of ALS and an increased risk of death [22,23]. Few data are available on the role of B lymphocytes, plasma cells, and antibodies in the pathogenesis of ALS. Cases of paraneoplastic ALS with specific anti-neuronal antibodies deserve particular attention, because these are extremely rare forms of the disease; thus, definitively diagnosing these forms is difficult. However, the description of some of these forms in a recent review [24] suggests that there may be an interaction between cancer and neurodegeneration in ALS which is mediated by the immune system.

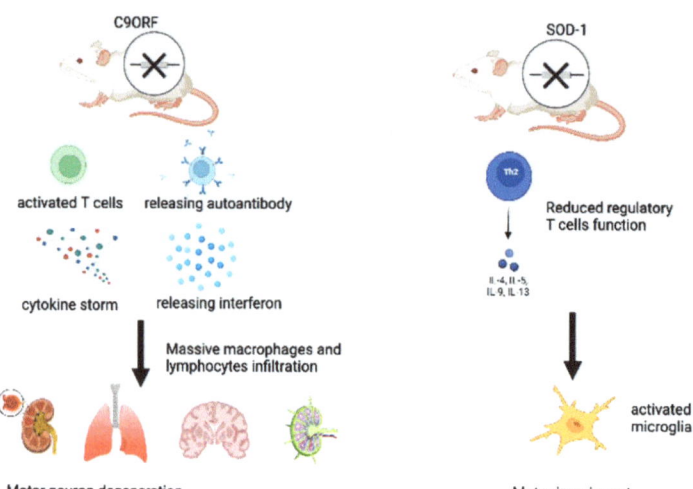

Figure 2. *C9ORF* and *SOD1* mouse models which are mainly used for providing evidence concerning the involvement of the clonotypic immune system in the pathogenesis of ALS. **By Biorender software**.

The evidence available in the literature for each of these cell types is described and discussed in this review.

3. T Helper 17 Cells (Th17)

Changes in the clonotypic cellular composition of the immune system have been found in ALS patients. A peripheral increase in the number of Th17 T cells has been found to be positively correlated with ALS symptom severity and disease progression [25]. In addition, patients with ALS have been shown to have increased levels of Interleukin-17 (IL-17), in both the serum and CSF [26]. Furthermore, higher levels of IL-17 have been quantified in ALS patients when compared with patients with primary progressive multiple sclerosis (PPMS) [27]. Among the Th17-related cytokines, only IL-17A has been shown to have a clear pathogenetic role in ALS models. Indeed, MNs of patients with ALS, derived from the differentiation of induced pluripotent stem cells, were found to express the receptor for IL-17A (IL-17AR), and they were vulnerable to its neurotoxic action in a dose-dependent manner; however, they were not damaged by exposure to IL-17F. Furthermore, targeting IL-17A has been shown to protect MNs from death [25]. Similarly, Th17 and IL-17A were shown to impair MNs survival in a FUS-related ALS mutant model [28]. IL-17 secreting cells, CD8+ T cells, and mast cells, have been observed to infiltrate the gray matter of the spinal cord in ALS patients. In these subjects, increased peripheral levels of IL-17A have been reported to mirror the decreased serum levels of IL-10, which has anti-inflammatory effects. This could help explain the increased susceptibility to the effects of IL-17A [29].

4. CD8+ T Cells

CD8 + cells have been shown to be activated both peripherally and intrathecally in ALS patients, compared with healthy controls, dementia patients, and PPMS [30]. A high percentage of CD8+ lymphocytes has been found to be negatively associated with ALS prognosis, and its increase has been correlated with the risk of death [31]. Although it was initially reported that the infiltration, of the spinal cord by CD8+ lymphocytes, occurs in the later stages of the disease, in a mouse model, a recent work has also revealed their presence in the early stages of the disease [32]. CD8+ lymphocytes infiltrating the spinal cord of a SOD1^{G93A} mouse model of ALS have been shown to interact with MNs through the major histocompatibility complex class I (MHC-I), and they induce killing by involving Fas and granzyme mechanisms [33]; however, the role of CD8+ lymphocytes in ALS, mediated by their interaction with MHC-I, has proven to be rather complex and still unclear. Although CD8+ lymphocytes have been shown to be toxic for spinal cord MNs in ALS models, some protective effects have been observed at a more peripheral level. More specifically, using a SOD1^{G93A} mouse model, the absence of the interaction between the sciatic nerve, MHC-I on the surface of the motor axon, and CD8+ lymphocytes appears to accelerate atrophy and the denervation of hindlimb muscles, thus indicating the onset of disease symptoms; however, it has been shown that the lack of interaction between CD8+ lymphocytes and microglia in the spinal cord protects cervical MNs from death and it delays disease onset [34].

5. Natural Killer (NK) Cells

The presence of NK cells, which contribute to innate and adaptive immunity, was observed in the spinal cord, and the motor cortex of postmortem tissues, of sporadic ALS (sALS) patients, whereas the presence of these cells was not found in the tissues that were used as controls. In contrast, NK cell levels were shown to be reduced in the peripheral blood of sALS patients compared with controls [35,36]. Similarly, postmortem data in humans and SOD1^{G93A} mice have reported that NK cells infiltrate the motor cortex and the spinal cord with a peak concentration occurring during the early phase of the disease, and a decreased number during motor decline. In addition, it has been observed that such mice express high levels of activation markers on their cell surfaces. In SOD1^{G93A} and TDP43^{A315T} mice, early treatment with anti-NK cell antibodies has been shown to increase survival and delay the onset of the disease [36]; however, NK cell depletion has been shown to prolong survival in female, but not male, SOD1 mice, thus suggesting that NK cells are related to ALS in a sex-specific manner [37]. In addition, it is also important to consider the subtype of NK cells rather than their total number. Indeed, although some authors noted no change in the total number of NK cells in the CSF of their study patients compared with controls, cell characterization in the slow-progression ALS group showed an increase in the number of regulatory, rather than cytotoxic, NK cells [25]. In general, the immune aspects of NK cells in ALS are poorly explored, and further investigations are needed given the complexity of the topic, as shown by a possible paraneoplastic case of MNs in the disease, with a rapid progression that is associated with NK cell leukemia [38].

6. Regulatory T (Treg) Cells

It has been reported that the CD4+ CD25+ Treg levels correlate with the rate of disease progression in ALS patients and mice models. Using the Appel ALS score (AALS), 54 patients with ALS were clinically evaluated, and they were divided into two groups according to disease progression. The 28 patients with a slowly progressing version of the disease (AALS points per month <1.5) had a percentage of Treg lymphocytes that did not vary from the controls. In contrast, the 26 patients with a rapidly progressing version of ALS (AALS points per month $\geq$1.5) showed a percentage of Treg cells that were reduced by about one-third compared with controls and patients with a less aggressive version of the disease [39]. In another study from Sheean and colleagues, the levels of Treg lymphocytes in 24 male and 9 female ALS patients were found to be inversely correlated with the rate of progression, although no clear difference was found between the Treg cell levels of ALS patients and those of the control group [40].

In Cu^{2+}/Zn^{2+} SOD1 mutant (mSOD1) ALS mice, an increase in the number of Treg lymphocytes was found in the early stages of the slowly progressing version of the disease. This has been shown to improve the course of the disease as the expression of IL-4 is increased and the protective role of M2 microglia is enhanced. In addition, the transfer of CD4+ T lymphocytes from SOD1 mutated mice, with an increased number of Tregs, to SOD1$^{-/-}$ mice, has been shown to reduce disease progression when compared with the transfer of wild-type CD4+ T lymphocytes [41].

Thus, the course of ALS appears to be characterized by an initial phase in which the neuroprotective role of the immune system dominates, and a second phase that is characterized by the development of neurotoxicity via microglia and proinflammatory

Teffs [22]. Furthermore, it has been observed that Treg cells support the neuroprotective phase of the disease by inhibiting microglia through the production of IL-4, and Teffs through the production of IL-4, IL-10, and Transforming Growth Factor-β [19].

7. B-Cells and Immunoglobulins

Although some authors initially suggested that that B-cell, and even anti-retroviral immune responses, may be present in ALS [42], few data are available on the involvement of B cells in ALS, and in any case, their role appears to be very limited. B cells isolated from SOD1 mouse models of ALS before, during, and after the onset of disease showed a phenotype and responsiveness that was like those of the wild-type mice. In addition, the SOD1 mice that were lacking mature B cells, because they were blocked at the pro-B cell stage, were shown to develop the disease with clinical features that were identical to those of the control SOD1 mice [43]. It has been shown that possible signs of B cell involvement in some mechanisms of the disease arose mostly from indirect signals. Indeed, autoantibodies against neurofilaments, actin, and desmin have been found in the spinal cord of ALS patients, and these antibodies have been shown to positively correlate with disease severity [44]. In contrast, the presence of anti-SOD1 antibodies has shown a positive association with survival in sALS patients [45]; however, it should be noted that although T helper lymphocytes and cytotoxic T lymphocytes infiltrate the areas affected by degeneration, no infiltration by B lymphocytes has been found in the tissues of ALS patients [46], although the expression of the IgG subclass in ALS has been found to be altered [47], which suggests some dysfunction in the B lymphocytes.

Two animal models of autoimmunity, developed for ALS study, were used to explore the role of IgG reactivity in ALS. The first involves experimental autoimmune motor neuron disease that was induced via the inoculation of purified MNs and characterized by the loss of lower MNs. The second involves experimental autoimmune gray matter disease (EAGMD), which was induced via the inoculation of homogenate from the ventral horn of the spinal cord, thus leading to the death of the upper and lower MNs. Both models mimic ALS with respect to the depletion of MNs in terms of their neurophysiological findings [48]. The passage of serum immunoglobulins, which were isolated from both models and transferred to control mice, appears to passively reproduce some alterations in the animal-derived models, such as increased calcium levels within MNs and the increased release of acetylcholine from the axons of spinal MNs; the latter alteration suggests a possible role of an antibody-mediated response in ALS, with respect to interactions concerning the neuromuscular junction [48,49]. In ALS, the IgG accumulation in MNs has been described as inducing altered calcium homeostasis, and the inoculation of anti-MNs antibodies induces similar alterations in mice [50]. Similarly, Polgár and colleagues observed that serum transfers from ALS patients with the C9orf72 mutation into ventral spinal cord mice causes increased calcium levels in MNs, thus resulting in neurodegeneration [51]; similar data were provided by Obál and colleagues through the long-term intraperitoneal injection of sera from ALS patients [52].

8. Immunotherapy in ALS: Promising Data

Promising results have been reported in the literature concerning the potential role of the clonotypic immune system in negatively influencing the course of ALS. This has led to the development of substances which use immunomodulators, and which produce biological effects of particular interest. Accordingly, some authors have shown that Treg cell dysfunction is transient, and their expansion, under different environmental conditions, can lead to a recovery of their functions. Subsequent autologous transplantations of these cells have also been shown to slow the progression of sALS in a phase I clinical trial [53]; therefore, such approaches seem promising. In Table 1 below, the main immuno-modulatory agents and treatment options, that have been examined in ALS patients and animal models thus far, are shown. They show interesting results and may also encourage further studies on larger cohorts to validate their effects and find any possible adverse reactions. They may also elucidate the actual role of clonotypic cells in ALS. This could enable the development of more appropriate treatments for preclinical and clinical stages of ALS which could delay or halt its onset and progression. In addition, works based on omics technologies that are used to characterize and detect the clonotypic subsets in ALS, as well as its onset and progression stages, could enable the development of personalized therapies. Overall, if confirmed, these research hypotheses will play an important role in terms of ALS treatment and prognosis, with significant economic implications for national health care systems.

Table 1. Main immune-modulating agents and treatment options that have been evaluated in ALS patients and in animal models.

Treatment	Dose and Administration	Number of Cases or Types of Animal Model	Laboratory and/or Clinical Outcomes	References
Aldesleukin	Intravenous Low dose of Interleukin-2 for five days at week 1, 5, and 9.	Twenty-four patients	Increase in Treg response; no significant change in terms of a reduction in circulating lymphocytes in ALS patients when compared with the placebo group.	[54]
Dimethyl fumarate	Oral administration of 480 mg daily for 36 weeks.	Seventy-two patients	No significant effects in terms of a reduction in circulating lymphocytes in ALS patients compared with the placebo group.	[55]
RNS60	Weekly intravenous infusion and daily nebulization.	Thirteen patients	No changes in biomarkers (i.e., FOXP3 mRNA and IL-17 levels).	[56]
RNS60	300 µL/mouse intraperitoneally every other day.	C57BL/6-SOD1G93A	Increase in CD4+/Foxp3+ T regulatory cells and neuroprotection.	[57]
RNS60	Three hundred and seventy-five mL intravenously administered for 24 weeks, once a week, and 4 mL/day administered via nebulization on the other days.	Seventy-two patients	Slower decline of forced vital capacity and bulbar dysfunctions in the patients treated with RNS60 compared with the placebo group.	[58]
Infusions of autologous Treg in ALS	Intravenous Tregs 106 cells/kg, initially four doses over 2 months, and in later stages, four doses over 4 months of the disease (n. 8 total infusions).	Three patients with sALS	Increase in Treg function and a slower disease progression, measured in accordance with the Appel ALS scale for each patient.	[53]
Fingolimod	Oral administration, dose of 0.5 mg/day for 4 weeks.	Eighteen patients with ALS	Reduction of circulating lymphocytes in ALS patients. No effects on ALSFRS-R.	[59]
Glatiramer acetate	Subcutaneous injection of 40 mg/day.	Three hundred and sixty-six patients with ALS enrolled in a phase II clinical trial	No effects on ALSFRS-R.	[60]
Tocilizumab	Treatment of PMBCs overnight with 2 µg/mL apo-G37R + 10 µg/mL tocilizumab.	Four patients with ALS	Reduction of the secretion of cytokynes and chemiokynes from the PMBCs of patients.	[61]

9. Conclusions

Recent data suggest that ALS, the classic neurodegenerative disease, usually having a rapid progression, is characterized by inflammation, which may also involve cells of clonotypic immunity, in addition to glial activation, and consequently, the induction of innate immunity [62]. At present, the early pathogenetic role of such cells cannot be hypothesized, even if it has been shown in an animal model of SOD1-ALS T-lymphocytes, that such cells infiltrate the CNS before the onset of symptoms [63]; however, the balance between CD4+ and CD8+, and between Treg and Teffs cells, has been reported to influence the prognosis of the disease (see Figure 3). In addition, there is no clear association between the dysfunctions of the immune system, particularly those regarding the clonotypic immunity, and the different clinical forms of ALS. The higher incidence of autoimmune diseases, such as myasthenia gravis, polymyositis, dermatomyositis, and type I diabetes mellitus [8] in ALS patients, suggests an increased reactivity of the immune system. We speculate that the progressive neurodegeneration causes the release of autoantigens and triggers the antibody-mediated response. In contrast, other authors have hypothesized that the formation of aggregates by SOD1 and TDP-43, which is triggered by CD4+ cells, may elicit an immune response in the CNS towards certain antigens [62]. Certainly, other studies are needed for clearing such relevant aspect, by facilitating the development of related treatments.

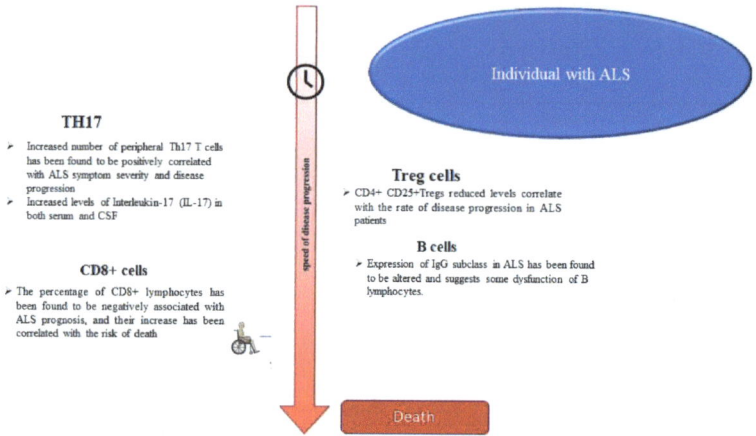

Figure 3. Correlation between the number and levels of clonotypic cells and related cytokines in terms of disease progression and outcomes. **By Biorender software**.

Author Contributions: Conceptualization G.S. and C.R.B.; literature research G.S.; S.I., A.L. and V.D.S.; data curation, G.S., S.I., V.D.S.; figure preparation, S.I. and C.R.B.; writing—original draft preparation, G.S. and C.R.B.; writing—review and editing C.R.B., F.B., V.D.S. and R.M.; visualization, C.R.B.; supervision, C.R.B. All authors have read and agreed to the published version of the manuscript.

Funding: This research received no external funding.

Institutional Review Board Statement: Not applicable.

Informed Consent Statement: Not applicable.

Data Availability Statement: Not applicable.

Conflicts of Interest: These authors declare no conflict of interest.

References

1. Hulisz, D. Amyotrophic Lateral Sclerosis: Disease State Overview. *Am. J. Manag. Care* **2018**, *24*, S320–S326. [PubMed]
2. Chia, R.; Chiò, A.; Traynor, B.J. Novel genes associated with amyotrophic lateral sclerosis: Diagnostic and clinical implications. *Lancet Neurol.* **2018**, *17*, 94–102. [CrossRef]
3. Liu, E.; Karpf, L.; Bohl, D. Neuroinflammation in Amyotrophic Lateral Sclerosis and Frontotemporal Dementia and the Interest of Induced Pluripotent Stem Cells to Study Immune Cells Interactions With Neurons. *Front. Mol. Neurosci.* **2021**, *14*, 767041. [CrossRef] [PubMed]
4. Mayne, K.; White, J.A.; Mcmurran, C.E.; Rivera, F.J.; De La Fuente, A.G. Aging and Neurodegenerative Disease: Is the Adaptive Immune System a Friend or Foe? *Front. Aging Neurosci.* **2020**, *12*, 572090. [CrossRef]
5. Chaplin, D.D. Overview of the immune response. *J. Allergy Clin. Immunol.* **2010**, *125*, S3–S23. [CrossRef]
6. Ellwardt, E.; Walsh, J.T.; Kipnis, J.; Zipp, F. Understanding the Role of T Cells in CNS Homeostasis. *Trends Immunol.* **2016**, *37*, 154–165. [CrossRef]

7. Radjavi, A.; Smirnov, I.; Kipnis, J. Brain antigen-reactive CD4+ T cells are sufficient to support learning behavior in mice with limited T cell repertoire. *Brain Behav. Immun.* **2014**, *35*, 58–63. [CrossRef]
8. Longinetti, E.; Sveinsson, O.; Press, R.; Ye, W.; Ingre, C.; Piehl, F.; Fang, F. ALS patients with concurrent neuroinflammatory disorders; a nationwide clinical records study. *Amyotroph. Lateral Scler. Front. Degener.* **2022**, *23*, 209–219. [CrossRef]
9. Yang, Y.; Pan, D.; Gong, Z.; Tang, J.; Li, Z.; Ding, F.; Liu, M.; Zhang, M. Decreased blood CD4+ T lymphocyte helps predict cognitive impairment in patients with amyotrophic lateral sclerosis. *BMC Neurol.* **2021**, *21*, 157. [CrossRef]
10. Mori, K.; Weng, S.-M.; Arzberger, T.; May, S.; Rentzsch, K.; Kremmer, E.; Schmid, B.; Kretzschmar, H.A.; Cruts, M.; Van Broeckhoven, C.; et al. The *C9orf72* GGGGCC Repeat Is Translated into Aggregating Dipeptide-Repeat Proteins in FTLD/ALS. *Science* **2013**, *339*, 1335–1338. [CrossRef]
11. Atanasio, A.; Decman, V.; White, D.; Ramos, M.; Ikiz, B.; Lee, H.-C.; Siao, C.-J.; Brydges, S.; LaRosa, E.; Bai, Y.; et al. C9orf72 ablation causes immune dysregulation characterized by leukocyte expansion, autoantibody production and glomerulonephropathy in mice. *Sci. Rep.* **2016**, *6*, 23204. [CrossRef] [PubMed]
12. McCauley, M.E.; O'Rourke, J.G.; Yáñez, A.; Markman, J.L.; Ho, R.; Wang, X.; Chen, S.; Lall, D.; Jin, M.; Muhammad, A.K.M.G.; et al. C9orf72 in myeloid cells suppresses STING-induced inflammation. *Nature* **2020**, *585*, 96–101. [CrossRef] [PubMed]
13. Burberry, A.; Suzuki, N.; Wang, J.-Y.; Moccia, R.; Mordes, D.A.; Stewart, M.H.; Suzuki-Uematsu, S.; Ghosh, S.; Singh, A.; Merkle, F.T.; et al. Loss-of-function mutations in the *C9ORF72* mouse ortholog cause fatal autoimmune disease. *Sci. Transl. Med.* **2016**, *8*, 347ra93. [CrossRef] [PubMed]
14. Sudria-Lopez, E.; Koppers, M.; De Wit, M.; Van Der Meer, C.; Westeneng, H.-J.; Zundel, C.A.C.; Youssef, S.A.; Harkema, L.; De Bruin, A.; Veldink, J.H.; et al. Full ablation of C9orf72 in mice causes immune system-related pathology and neoplastic events but no motor neuron defects. *Acta Neuropathol.* **2016**, *132*, 145–147. [CrossRef] [PubMed]
15. Chiu, I.M.; Chen, A.; Zheng, Y.; Kosaras, B.; Tsiftsoglou, S.A.; Vartanian, T.K.; Brown, R.H.; Carroll, M.C. T lymphocytes potentiate endogenous neuroprotective inflammation in a mouse model of ALS. *Proc. Natl. Acad. Sci. USA* **2008**, *105*, 17913–17918. [CrossRef] [PubMed]
16. Deng, H.-X.; Zhai, H.; Bigio, E.H.; Yan, J.; Fecto, F.; Ajroud, K.; Mishra, M.; Ajroud-Driss, S.; Heller, S.; Sufit, R.; et al. FUS-immunoreactive inclusions are a common feature in sporadic and non-SOD1 familial amyotrophic lateral sclerosis. *Ann. Neurol.* **2010**, *67*, 739–748. [CrossRef]
17. Bright, F.; Chan, G.; van Hummel, A.; Ittner, L.; Ke, Y. TDP-43 and Inflammation: Implications for Amyotrophic Lateral Sclerosis and Frontotemporal Dementia. *Int. J. Mol. Sci.* **2021**, *22*, 7781. [CrossRef]
18. Zhao, W.; Beers, D.R.; Liao, B.; Henkel, J.S.; Appel, S.H. Regulatory T lymphocytes from ALS mice suppress microglia and effector T lymphocytes through different cytokine-mediated mechanisms. *Neurobiol. Dis.* **2012**, *48*, 418–428. [CrossRef]
19. Boillée, S.; Yamanaka, K.; Lobsiger, C.S.; Copeland, N.G.; Jenkins, N.A.; Kassiotis, G.; Kollias, G.; Cleveland, D.W. Onset and Progression in Inherited ALS Determined by Motor Neurons and Microglia. *Science* **2006**, *312*, 1389–1392. [CrossRef]
20. Hooten, K.G.; Beers, D.R.; Zhao, W.; Appel, S.H. Protective and Toxic Neuroinflammation in Amyotrophic Lateral Sclerosis. *Neurotherapeutics* **2015**, *12*, 364–375. [CrossRef]
21. Seksenyan, A.; Ron-Harel, N.; Azoulay, D.; Cahalon, L.; Cardon, M.; Rogeri, P.; Ko, M.K.; Weil, M.; Bulvik, S.; Rechavi, G.; et al. Thymic involution, a co-morbidity factor in amyotrophic lateral sclerosis. *J. Cell. Mol. Med.* **2009**, *14*, 2470–2482. [CrossRef] [PubMed]
22. Ehrhart, J.; Smith, A.J.; Kuzmin-Nichols, N.; Zesiewicz, T.A.; Jahan, I.; Shytle, R.D.; Kim, S.-H.; Sanberg, C.D.; Vu, T.H.; Gooch, C.L.; et al. Humoral factors in ALS patients during disease progression. *J. Neuroinflamm.* **2015**, *12*, 127. [CrossRef] [PubMed]
23. De Marchi, F.; Munitic, I.; Amedei, A.; Berry, J.D.; Feldman, E.L.; Aronica, E.; Nardo, G.; Van Weehaeghe, D.; Niccolai, E.; Prtenjaca, N.; et al. Interplay between immunity and amyotrophic lateral sclerosis: Clinical impact. *Neurosci. Biobehav. Rev.* **2021**, *127*, 958–978. [CrossRef] [PubMed]
24. Yang, Z.; He, L.; Ren, M.; Lu, Y.; Meng, H.; Yin, D.; Chen, S.; Zhou, Q. Paraneoplastic Amyotrophic Lateral Sclerosis: Case Series and Literature Review. *Brain Sci.* **2022**, *12*, 1053. [CrossRef]
25. Jin, M.; Günther, R.; Akgün, K.; Hermann, A.; Ziemssen, T. Peripheral proinflammatory Th1/Th17 immune cell shift is linked to disease severity in amyotrophic lateral sclerosis. *Sci. Rep.* **2020**, *10*, 5941. [CrossRef]
26. Jin, M.; Akgün, K.; Ziemssen, T.; Kipp, M.; Günther, R.; Hermann, A. Interleukin-17 and Th17 Lymphocytes Directly Impair Motoneuron Survival of Wildtype and FUS-ALS Mutant Human iPSCs. *Int. J. Mol. Sci.* **2021**, *22*, 8042. [CrossRef]
27. Rentzos, M.; Rombos, A.; Nikolaou, C.; Zoga, M.; Zouvelou, V.; Dimitrakopoulos, A.; Alexakis, T.; Tsoutsou, A.; Samakovli, A.; Michalopoulou, M.; et al. Interleukin-17 and interleukin-23 are elevated in serum and cerebrospinal fluid of patients with ALS: A reflection of Th17 cells activation? *Acta Neurol. Scand.* **2010**, *122*, 425–429. [CrossRef]
28. Saresella, M.; Piancone, F.; Tortorella, P.; Marventano, I.; Gatti, A.; Caputo, D.; Lunetta, C.; Corbo, M.; Rovaris, M.; Clerici, M. T helper-17 activation dominates the immunologic milieu of both amyotrophic lateral sclerosis and progressive multiple sclerosis. *Clin. Immunol.* **2013**, *148*, 79–88. [CrossRef]
29. Fiala, M.; Chattopadhay, M.; La Cava, A.; Tse, E.; Liu, G.; Lourenco, E.; Eskin, A.; Liu, P.T.; Magpantay, L.; Tse, S.; et al. IL-17A is increased in the serum and in spinal cord CD8 and mast cells of ALS patients. *J. Neuroinflamm.* **2010**, *7*, 76. [CrossRef]
30. Rolfes, L.; Schulte-Mecklenbeck, A.; Schreiber, S.; Vielhaber, S.; Herty, M.; Marten, A.; Pfeuffer, S.; Ruck, T.; Wiendl, H.; Gross, C.C.; et al. Amyotrophic lateral sclerosis patients show increased peripheral and intrathecal T-cell activation. *Brain Commun.* **2021**, *3*, fcab157. [CrossRef]

31. Cui, C.; Ingre, C.; Yin, L.; Li, X.; Andersson, J.; Seitz, C.; Ruffin, N.; Pawitan, Y.; Piehl, F.; Fang, F. Correlation between leukocyte phenotypes and prognosis of amyotrophic lateral sclerosis. *eLife* **2022**, *11*, e74065. [CrossRef] [PubMed]
32. Chiot, A.; Lobsiger, C.S.; Boillée, S. New insights on the disease contribution of neuroinflammation in amyotrophic lateral sclerosis. *Curr. Opin. Neurol.* **2019**, *32*, 764–770. [CrossRef] [PubMed]
33. Coque, E.; Salsac, C.; Espinosa-Carrasco, G.; Varga, B.; Degauque, N.; Cadoux, M.; Crabé, R.; Virenque, A.; Soulard, C.; Fierle, J.K.; et al. Cytotoxic CD8 $^+$ T lymphocytes expressing ALS-causing SOD1 mutant selectively trigger death of spinal motoneurons. *Proc. Natl. Acad. Sci. USA* **2019**, *116*, 2312–2317. [CrossRef]
34. Nardo, G.; Trolese, M.C.; Verderio, M.; Mariani, A.; De Paola, M.; Riva, N.; Dina, G.; Panini, N.; Erba, E.; Quattrini, A.; et al. Counteracting roles of MHCI and CD8+ T cells in the peripheral and central nervous system of ALS SOD1G93A mice. *Mol. Neurodegener.* **2018**, *13*, 42. [CrossRef] [PubMed]
35. Murdock, B.J.; Zhou, T.; Kashlan, S.R.; Little, R.J.; Goutman, S.; Feldman, E.L. Correlation of Peripheral Immunity With Rapid Amyotrophic Lateral Sclerosis Progression. *JAMA Neurol.* **2017**, *74*, 1446–1454. [CrossRef] [PubMed]
36. Garofalo, S.; Cocozza, G.; Porzia, A.; Inghilleri, M.; Raspa, M.; Scavizzi, F.; Aronica, E.; Bernardini, G.; Peng, L.; Ransohoff, R.M.; et al. Natural killer cells modulate motor neuron-immune cell cross talk in models of Amyotrophic Lateral Sclerosis. *Nat. Commun.* **2020**, *11*, 1773. [CrossRef]
37. Murdock, B.J.; Famie, J.P.; Piecuch, C.E.; Raue, K.D.; Mendelson, F.E.; Pieroni, C.H.; Iniguez, S.D.; Zhao, L.; Goutman, S.A.; Feldman, E.L. Natural killer cells associate with amyotrophic lateral sclerosis in a sex- and age-dependent manner. *JCI Insight* **2021**, *6*, e147129. [CrossRef] [PubMed]
38. La Bella, V.; Iannitto, E.; Cuffaro, L.; Spataro, R. A rapidly progressive motor neuron disease associated to a natural killer cells leukaemia. *J. Neurol. Sci.* **2019**, *398*, 117–118. [CrossRef]
39. Henkel, J.S.; Beers, D.R.; Wen, S.; Rivera, A.L.; Toennis, K.M.; Appel, J.E.; Zhao, W.; Moore, D.H.; Powell, S.Z.; Appel, S.H. Regulatory T-lymphocytes mediate amyotrophic lateral sclerosis progression and survival. *EMBO Mol. Med.* **2013**, *5*, 64–79. [CrossRef]
40. Sheean, R.K.; McKay, F.C.; Cretney, E.; Bye, C.; Perera, N.D.; Tomas, D.; Weston, R.A.; Scheller, K.J.; Djouma, E.; Menon, P.; et al. Association of Regulatory T-Cell Expansion With Progression of Amyotrophic Lateral Sclerosis. *JAMA Neurol.* **2018**, *75*, 681–689. [CrossRef]
41. Beers, D.R.; Zhao, W.; Wang, J.; Zhang, X.; Wen, S.; Neal, D.; Thonhoff, J.R.; Alsuliman, A.S.; Shpall, E.J.; Rezvani, K.; et al. ALS patients' regulatory T lymphocytes are dysfunctional, and correlate with disease progression rate and severity. *JCI Insight* **2017**, *2*, e89530. [CrossRef] [PubMed]
42. Westarp, M.E.; Fuchs, D.; Bartmann, P.; Hoff-Jörgensen, R.; Clausen, J.; Wachter, H.; Kornhuber, H.H. Amyotrophic lateral sclerosis an enigmatic disease with B-cellular and anti-retroviral immune responses. *Eur. J. Med.* **1993**, *2*, 327–332. [PubMed]
43. Naor, S.; Keren, Z.; Bronshtein, T.; Goren, E.; Machluf, M.; Melamed, D. Development of ALS-like disease in SOD-1 mice deficient of B lymphocytes. *J. Neurol.* **2009**, *256*, 1228–1235. [CrossRef] [PubMed]
44. Niebroj-Dobosz, I.; Dziewulska, D.; Janik, P. Auto-antibodies against proteins of spinal cord cells in cerebrospinal fluid of patients with amyotrophic lateral sclerosis (ALS). *Folia Neuropathol.* **2006**, *44*, 191–196. [PubMed]
45. van Blitterswijk, M.; Gulati, S.; Smoot, E.; Jaffa, M.; Maher, N.; Hyman, B.T.; Ivinson, A.J.; Scherzer, C.; Schoenfeld, D.A.; Cudkowicz, M.E.; et al. Anti-superoxide dismutase antibodies are associated with survival in patients with sporadic amyotrophic lateral sclerosis. *Amyotroph. Lateral Scler.* **2011**, *12*, 430–438. [CrossRef] [PubMed]
46. Engelhardt, J.I.; Tajti, J.; Appel, S.H. Lymphocytic infiltrates in the spinal cord in amyotrophic lateral sclerosis. *Arch Neurol.* **1993**, *50*, 30–36. [CrossRef] [PubMed]
47. Ostermeyer-Shoaib, B.; Patten, B.M. IgG subclass deficiency in amyotrophic lateral sclerosis. *Acta Neurol. Scand.* **2009**, *87*, 192–194. [CrossRef]
48. Appel, S.H.; Engelhardt, J.I.; García, J.; Stefani, E. Autoimmunity and ALS: A Comparison of Animal Models of Immune-Mediated Motor Neuron Destruction and Human ALS. *Adv. Neurol.* **1991**, *56*, 405–412.
49. Engelhardt, J.I.; Siklós, L.; Appel, S.H. Altered Calcium Homeostasis and Ultrastructure in Motoneurons of Mice Caused by Passively Transferred Anti-motoneuronal IgG. *J. Neuropathol. Exp. Neurol.* **1997**, *56*, 21–39. [CrossRef]
50. Engelhardt, J.I.; Siklós, L.; Kőműves, L.; Smith, R.G.; Appel, S.H. Antibodies to calcium channels from ALS patients passively transferred to mice selectively increase intracellular calcium and induce ultrastructural changes in motoneurons. *Synapse* **1995**, *20*, 185–199. [CrossRef]
51. Polgár, T.F.; Meszlényi, V.; Nógrádi, B.; Körmöczy, L.; Spisák, K.; Tripolszki, K.; Széll, M.; Obál, I.; Engelhardt, J.I.; Siklós, L.; et al. Passive Transfer of Blood Sera from ALS Patients with Identified Mutations Results in Elevated Motoneuronal Calcium Level and Loss of Motor Neurons in the Spinal Cord of Mice. *Int. J. Mol. Sci.* **2021**, *22*, 9994. [CrossRef] [PubMed]
52. Obál, I.; Nógrádi, B.; Meszlényi, V.; Patai, R.; Ricken, G.; Kovacs, G.G.; Tripolszki, K.; Széll, M.; Siklós, L.; Engelhardt, J.I. Experimental Motor Neuron Disease Induced in Mice with Long-Term Repeated Intraperitoneal Injections of Serum from ALS Patients. *Int. J. Mol. Sci.* **2019**, *20*, 2573. [CrossRef] [PubMed]
53. Thonhoff, J.R.; Beers, D.R.; Zhao, W.; Pleitez, M.; Simpson, E.P.; Berry, J.D.; Cudkowicz, M.E.; Appel, S.H. Expanded autologous regulatory T-lymphocyte infusions in ALS. *Neurol. Neuroimmunol. Neuroinflamm.* **2018**, *5*, e465. [CrossRef] [PubMed]

54. Camu, W.; Mickunas, M.; Veyrune, J.-L.; Payan, C.; Garlanda, C.; Locati, M.; Juntas-Morales, R.; Pageot, N.; Malaspina, A.; Andreasson, U.; et al. Repeated 5-day cycles of low dose aldesleukin in amyotrophic lateral sclerosis (IMODALS): A phase 2a randomised, double-blind, placebo-controlled trial. *eBioMedicine* **2020**, *59*, 102844. [CrossRef]
55. Vucic, S.; Henderson, R.D.; Mathers, S.; Needham, M.; Schultz, D.; Kiernan, M.C. The TEALS study group Safety and efficacy of dimethyl fumarate in ALS: Randomised controlled study. *Ann. Clin. Transl. Neurol.* **2021**, *8*, 1991–1999. [CrossRef]
56. Vallarola, A.; Sironi, F.; Tortarolo, M.; Gatto, N.; De Gioia, R.; Pasetto, L.; De Paola, M.; Mariani, A.; Ghosh, S.; Watson, R.; et al. RNS60 exerts therapeutic effects in the SOD1 ALS mouse model through protective glia and peripheral nerve rescue. *J. Neuroinflamm.* **2018**, *15*, 65. [CrossRef]
57. Paganoni, S.; Alshikho, M.J.; Luppino, S.; Chan, J.; Ba, L.P.; Schoenfeld, D.; Dpt, P.L.A.; Babu, S.; Zürcher, N.R.; Loggia, M.L.; et al. A pilot trial of RNS60 in amyotrophic lateral sclerosis. *Muscle Nerve* **2018**, *59*, 303–308. [CrossRef]
58. Beghi, E.; Pupillo, E.; Bianchi, E.; Bonetto, V.; Luotti, S.; Pasetto, L.; Bendotti, C.; Tortarolo, M.; Sironi, F.; Camporeale, L.; et al. Effect of RNS60 in amyotrophic lateral sclerosis: A phase II multicentre, randomized, double-blind, placebo-controlled trial. *Eur. J. Neurol.* **2022**; *online ahead of print*. [CrossRef]
59. Berry, J.D.; Paganoni, S.; Atassi, N.; Macklin, E.A.; Goyal, N.; Rivner, M.; Simpson, E.; Appel, S.; Grasso, D.L.; Mejia, N.I.; et al. Phase IIa trial of fingolimod for amyotrophic lateral sclerosis demonstrates acceptable acute safety and tolerability. *Muscle Nerve* **2017**, *56*, 1077–1084. [CrossRef]
60. Meininger, V.; Drory, V.E.; Leigh, P.N.; Ludolph, A.; Robberecht, W.; Silani, V. Glatiramer acetate has no impact on disease progression in ALS at 40 mg/day: A double-blind, randomized, multicentre, placebo-controlled trial. *Amyotroph. Lateral Scler.* **2009**, *10*, 378–383. [CrossRef]
61. Mizwicki, M.T.; Milan, F.; Magpantay, L.; Aziz, N.; Sayre, J.; Liu, G.; Siani, A.; Chan, D.; Martinez-Maza, O.; Chattopadhyay, M.; et al. Tocili-zumab Attenuates Inflammation in ALS Patients through Inhibition of IL6 Receptor Signaling. *Am. J. Neurodegener. Dis.* **2012**, *1*, 305.
62. Lima-Junior, J.R.; Sulzer, D.; Arlehamn, C.S.L.; Sette, A. The role of immune-mediated alterations and disorders in ALS disease. *Hum. Immunol.* **2021**, *82*, 155–161. [CrossRef] [PubMed]
63. Alexianu, M.E.; Kozovska, M.; Appel, S.H. Immune reactivity in a mouse model of familial ALS correlates with disease progression. *Neurology* **2001**, *57*, 1282–1289. [CrossRef] [PubMed]

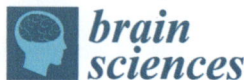

Article

The Role of Superoxide Dismutase 1 in Amyotrophic Lateral Sclerosis: Identification of Signaling Pathways, Regulators, Molecular Interaction Networks, and Biological Functions through Bioinformatics

Sharad Kumar Suthar [1] and Sang-Yoon Lee [1,2,*]

[1] Neuroscience Research Institute, Gachon University, Incheon 21565, Republic of Korea
[2] Department of Neuroscience, College of Medicine, Gachon University, Incheon 21936, Republic of Korea
* Correspondence: rchemist@gachon.ac.kr

Abstract: Mutations in superoxide dismutase 1 (SOD1) result in misfolding and aggregation of the protein, causing neurodegenerative amyotrophic lateral sclerosis (ALS). In recent years, several new SOD1 variants that trigger ALS have been identified, making it increasingly crucial to understand the SOD1 toxicity pathway in ALS. Here we used an integrated bioinformatics approach, including the Ingenuity Pathway Analysis (IPA) tool to analyze signaling pathways, regulators, functions, and network molecules of SOD1 with an emphasis on ALS. IPA toxicity analysis of SOD1 identified superoxide radicals' degradation, apelin adipocyte, ALS, NRF2-mediated oxidative stress response, and sirtuin signaling as the key signaling pathways, while the toxicity of SOD1 is exerted via mitochondrial swelling and oxidative stress. IPA listed CNR1, APLN, BTG2, MAPK, DRAP1, NFE2L2, SNCA, and CG as the upstream regulators of SOD1. IPA further revealed that mutation in SOD1 results in hereditary disorders, including ALS. The exploration of the relationship between SOD1 and ALS using IPA unveiled SOD1-ALS pathway molecules. The gene ontology (GO) analysis of SOD1-ALS pathway molecules with ShinyGO reaffirmed that SOD1 toxicity results in ALS and neurodegeneration. The GO analysis further identified enriched biological processes, molecular functions, and cellular components for SOD1-ALS pathway molecules. The construction of a protein–protein interaction network of SOD1-ALS pathway molecules using STRING and further analysis of that network with Cytoscape identified ACTB followed by TP53, IL6, CASP3, SOD1, IL1B, APP, APOE, and VEGFA as the major network hubs. Taken together, our study provides insight into the molecular underpinning of SOD1's toxicity in ALS.

Keywords: superoxide dismutase 1; antioxidant; amyotrophic lateral sclerosis; canonical pathways; regulators; molecular interaction network; biological functions; toxicity

1. Introduction

Copper/zinc-binding superoxide dismutase 1 (SOD1) is primarily an antioxidant enzyme present in the cytosol, outer-mitochondrial membrane, and intermembrane space of the mitochondria (Figure 1) [1–3]. It detoxifies superoxide radicals ($O_2^{\bullet-}$) expelled by mitochondria and generated by other redox reactions into molecular oxygen (O_2) and hydrogen peroxide (H_2O_2) [4,5]. As well as acting as an antioxidant, SOD1 via localization from the cytosol to the nucleus combats oxidative stress by regulating the transcription of antioxidant genes involved in cellular defense [6].

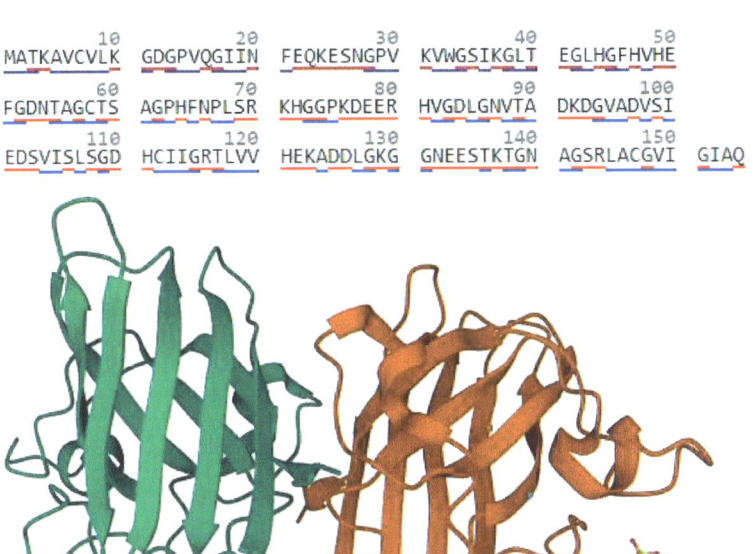

Figure 1. Amino acid sequence and three-dimensional structure of SOD1 (PDB ID: 1PU0). SOD1 is a 32 kDa homodimer protein of 154 amino acids. The red underline of amino acid letters indicates polar residues, while the blue underline indicates hydrophobic residues.

Around three decades ago, the identification of the first SOD1 mutation in a group of familial amyotrophic lateral sclerosis (ALS) patients changed the perception of SOD1 being a protective antioxidant to the culprit in ALS [7]. ALS is a neurodegenerative disease characterized by the progressive loss of motor neurons in the spinal cord, leading to spasticity, generalized weakness, muscle atrophy, and paralysis [8,9]. More than 200 different SOD1 mutations have been reported to cause familial ALS [10], accounting for approximately 20% of familial and 2.3% of sporadic ALS [11].

Although wild-type SOD1 is a stable homodimeric protein [12–15], the mutation in SOD1 decreases the net repulsive charge in the structure, undermining the protein architecture [16]. The destabilized SOD1 mutant in ALS triggers misfolding and aggregation via abnormal disulfide cross-linking, forming toxic inclusions in the mitochondria of neuronal cells [16,17]. The exact mechanism by which SOD1 induces toxicity in ALS remains unknown [18,19].

The number of SOD1 variants in ALS has steadily increased over the last decade (Table S1) [10], while the molecules conveying SOD1 toxicity in ALS remain far from being deciphered, prompting us to investigate SOD1 toxicity in ALS. In this study, we used a set of computational tools, including Ingenuity Pathway Analysis (IPA), STRING, and Cytoscape to analyze the canonical pathways, regulators, functions, and molecular interaction network of SOD1, with an emphasis on SOD1 toxicity in ALS. Our study provides a list of molecules that serve as a bridge between SOD1 and ALS and potentially convey SOD1-imparted toxicity in ALS. The wet-lab researchers can build upon our findings to elucidate the mechanism and pathway of SOD1 toxicity in ALS.

2. Materials and Methods

2.1. IPA Toxicity Analysis of SOD1

The SOD1 gene (gene ID 6647) obtained as a text file from the National Center for Biotechnology Information (NCBI) [20] database was imported onto the IPA server for new core analysis [21]. The gene identification (GI) number of SOD1 was defined. The "Tox Analysis" function was selected for the new core analysis. The Ingenuity Knowledge Base was used as a reference source. Both direct and indirect relationships with reference to the gene were considered for the predictions. For interaction network generation, 35 molecules per network and 25 networks per analysis were chosen. Along with the interaction network, casual networks were also considered for the predictions. All node types (such as chemicals, complexes, cytokines, diseases, enzymes, functions, etc.) and all data sources were selected for the predictions. For miRNA confidence, only experimentally observed values were considered. Only the human species was considered for predictions. Furthermore, tissues and primary cells, and all types of mutations were selected for the predictions. Right-tailed Fisher's exact test was used to rank the predictions, where the smaller p-value indicates the higher significance of the results. Wherever required the data obtained from IPA were plotted in the Figure formats using GraphPad Prism [22,23].

2.2. IPA Exploration of the Pathway/Pathway Molecules between SOD1 and ALS

IPA "genes and chemicals" search of "SOD1" provided the SOD1 gene, which was added to the new pathway to be created between SOD1 and ALS [21]. Similarly, IPA "diseases and functions" search of "amyotrophic lateral sclerosis" provided the list of ALS and associated 631 molecules, which were also added to the pathway to be built between SOD1 and ALS (These 631 molecules were associated with ALS, and not all molecules were associated with SOD1) [21]. To build the path between SOD1 and ALS (predicting molecules connecting SOD1 and ALS), molecules displaying both direct and indirect relationships with SOD1 and ALS were chosen with a direction of relationship from SOD1 to ALS. Ingenuity Knowledge Base was used as a source of molecules and relationships among them. Upon following these steps, IPA identified 87 molecules as nodes between SOD1 and ALS. These node molecules were added to the SOD1-ALS pathway, which resulted in the final SOD1-ALS pathway. The created path was further organized with IPA path designer feature to create the figure for publication. Additionally, the molecule activity predictor (MAP) feature of IPA predicted the effect of increased activity of SOD1 on pathway molecules.

2.3. Gene Ontology Analysis of SOD1-ALS Pathway Genes

The ShinyGO v0.76.3 online tool was used for the gene ontology (GO) enrichment analysis of IPA-predicted SOD1-ALS pathway molecules (Table S2; http://bioinformatics.sdstate.edu/go/) [24]. For this, the list of SOD1-ALS pathway molecules identified by IPA was imported on the ShinyGO server and submitted for analysis. ShinyGO first converts all query genes to ENSEMBL gene IDs or STRING-db protein IDs for analysis. Only the human species were selected for analysis. The false discovery rate (FDR) cutoff was set at 0.05 for the predictions. ShinyGO calculates FDR based on the nominal p-value from the hypergeometric test.

2.4. Construction of Molecular Interaction Network of SOD1-ALS Pathway Molecules

The protein–protein interaction (PPI) network of SOD1-ALS pathway molecules (Table S2) was constructed with STRING v11.5, a tool developed by a consortium of academic organizations (https://string-db.org/cgi/input) [25]. For this, the list of IPA-predicted SOD1-ALS pathway molecules (Table S2) was imported onto the STRING server. For PPI network construction, the "multiple proteins" feature of STRING was used. *Homo sapiens* was selected as the organism for the network construction.

The STRING-constructed PPI network was exported to Cytoscape v3.9.1, an open-source software platform, for further analysis using the STRING option "send network to Cytoscape" (https://cytoscape.org/) [26]. The Cytoscape option "analyze network", available in the tools category, was used for the analysis of the STRING constructed network. After subjecting the network to analysis in Cytoscape we deselected STRING features of the network such as the glass ball effect, STRING style labels, and STRING style colors. This enabled the network to be designed according to Cytoscape's features. For the mapping of the PPI network we used the Cytoscape option "style-node-size" followed by column as degree and mapping type as continuous mapping to display the node size corresponding to the degree of the node's network, while we used the Cytoscape option "style-node-fill color" followed by column as degree and mapping type as continuous mapping to indicate the node color according to the degree of the node's network.

3. Results

3.1. Identification of Canonical Pathways, Regulatory Molecules, Biological Functions and Toxicity Outcome of SOD1

IPA toxicity analysis of SOD1 identified superoxide radicals' degradation as the leading signaling pathway followed by apelin adipocyte signaling, amyotrophic lateral sclerosis signaling, NRF2-mediated oxidative stress response, and sirtuin signaling pathways (Figure 2A). IPA toxicity analysis also revealed upstream regulators of SOD1. Cannabinoid receptor 1 (CNR1) was predicted to be the most important upstream regulator of SOD1. Additionally, IPA identified apelin (APLN), B-cell translocation gene 2 or BTG anti-proliferation factor 2 (BTG2), mitogen-activated protein kinase (MAPK), Dr1 associated protein 1 (DRAP1), nuclear factor erythroid 2-related factor 2 (NFE2L2), α-synuclein (SNCA), and cathepsin G (CG) as the upstream regulators of SOD1 (Figure 2B). In contrast to its protective antioxidant function, mutations in SOD1 result in brain diseases. According to the IPA analysis, hereditary disorders such as familial ALS are the leading outcome of SOD1-associated anomalous functions. Anomalies in SOD1 can also result in neurological diseases, ophthalmic diseases, organismal injuries and abnormalities, and psychological disorders. (Figure 2C). In accordance with SOD1's involvement in a variety of diseases and disorders, our study found that SOD1 toxicity and response to it is manifested through mitochondrial swelling, renal injury associated with superoxide radicals, oxidative stress, NRF2-mediated oxidative stress response, and liver necrosis (Figure 2D). SOD1 performs a variety of molecular and cellular functions. Our study discovered that SOD1 plays a key role in cell death and survival, cellular assembly and organization, post-translation modification, cellular compromise, and free radical scavenging (Figure 2E). Additionally, SOD1 is involved in physiological system development and processes. IPA identified the role of SOD1 in behavior, embryonic development, hematological system development and functions, nervous system development and functions, and reproductive system development and functions (Figure 2F).

3.2. Identification of SOD1-ALS Pathway Molecules

Mutation in SOD1 leads to the development of ALS. We used IPA to identify the molecules which are altered in response to SOD1 mutant-induced toxicity in ALS. IPA mapped 87 molecules which orchestrate a direct or indirect network between SOD1 and ALS (Figure 3). IPA identified PARK7 (Parkinson protein 7) as one of the key SOD1-ALS pathway molecules. PARK7 displayed a direct relationship with SOD1. Given the role of PARK7 as a sensor of oxidative stress, its critical relationship with SOD1 was not surprising. In addition to PARK7, IPA revealed several molecules that are central to protein aggregopathy as a part of the SOD1-ALS pathway, such as ALS2, FUS (ALS6; fusion gene), PFN1 (ALS18; profilin-1), APP (AD1; Aβ precursor protein), OPTN (ALS12; optineurin), and CLU (clusterin). The presence of these molecules in the SOD1–ALS pathway suggests that SOD1 inclusions precipitate the aggregation of other similar proteins, intensifying ALS symptoms.

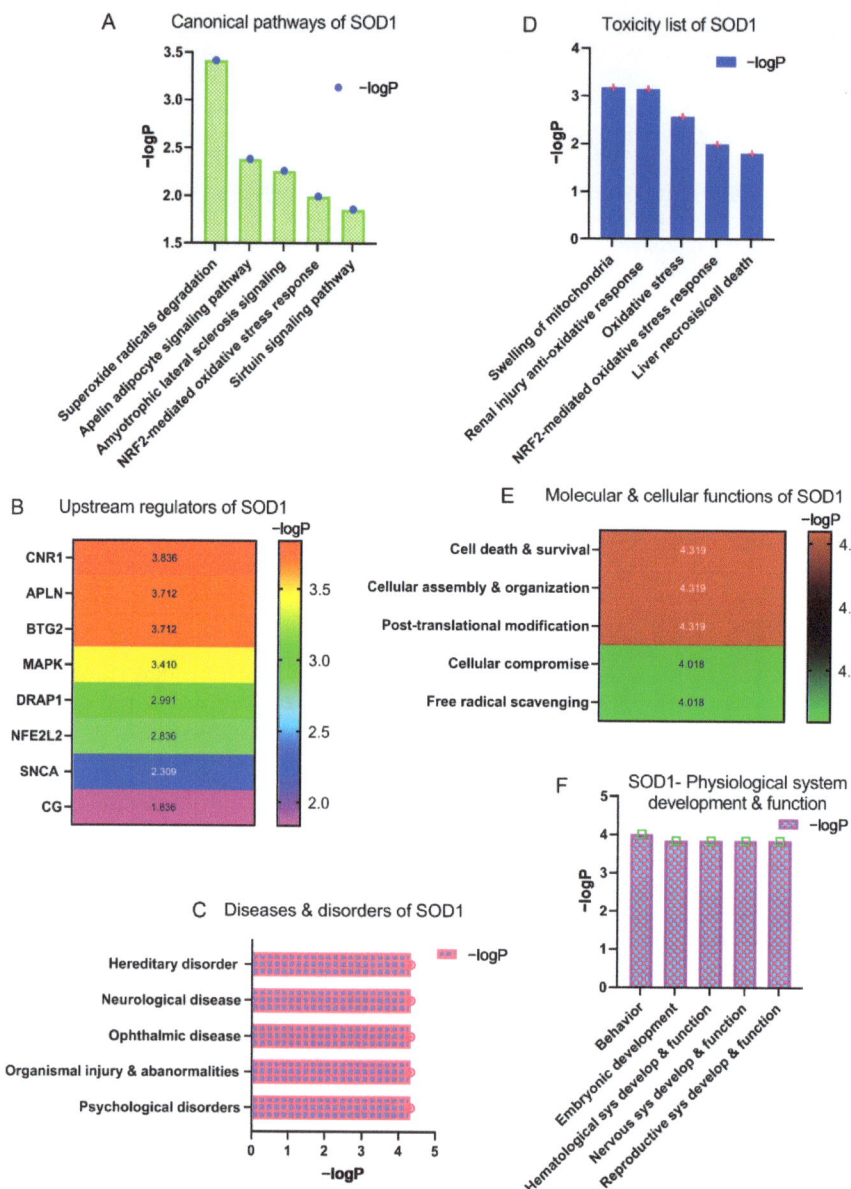

Figure 2. Canonical pathways, regulators, biological functions, role, and toxicity of SOD1. (**A**) Canonical signaling pathways of SOD1. (**B**) The upstream regulators of SOD1. (**C**) Diseases and disorders caused by abnormal expression of SOD1. (**D**) The list of toxicities caused by abnormal expression of SOD1. (**E**) Molecular and cellular functions of SOD1. (**F**) The role of SOD1 in physiological system development and its functions in organ systems. −logP indicates −log$_{10}$(*p*-value), sys—system, develop—development.

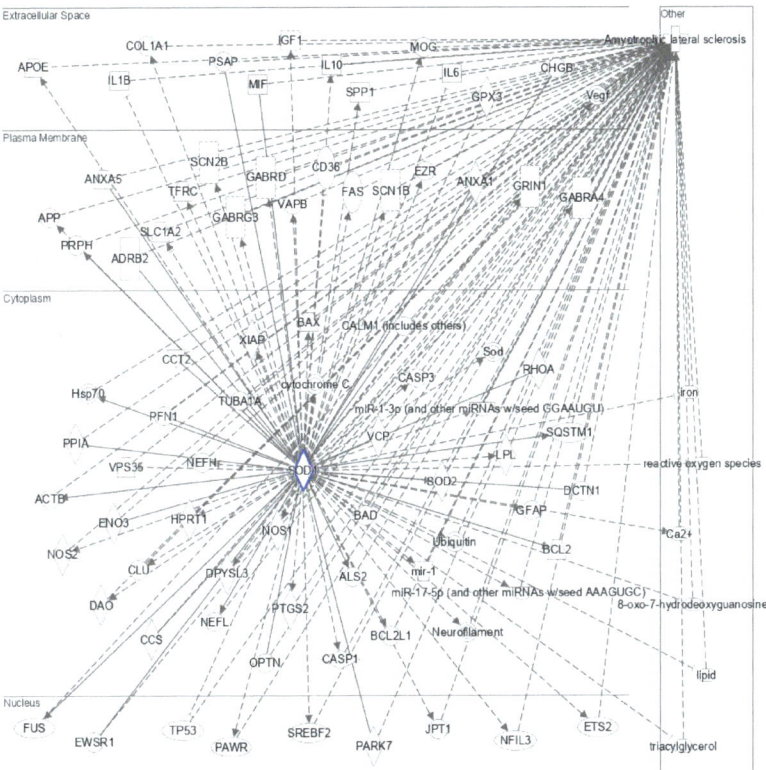

Figure 3. SOD1-ALS pathway molecules that are altered in response to SOD1 mutation and play a role in the development of amyotrophic lateral sclerosis, identified by IPA. Solid lines represent direct interaction, while dotted lines represent indirect interaction.

IPA highlighted that impaired lipid homeostasis and metabolism plays a crucial role in the development of SOD1-triggered ALS. This was evident by the presence of several molecules related to lipid regulation and catabolism in the SOD1-ALS pathway, such as SREBF2 (sterol regulatory element binding transcription factor 2), APOE (apolipoprotein E), PSAP (prosaposin), and LPL (lipoprotein lipase).

SOD1-induced toxicity in ALS also alters neurotransmission in the brain. Various transport proteins and neurotransmitters, specifically those present in the plasma membrane such as SLC1A2 (solute carrier family 1 member 2), GABRG3 (gamma-aminobutyric acid type A receptor subunit gamma3), GABRD (gamma-aminobutyric acid type A receptor subunit delta), GRIN1 (glutamate receptor ionotropic, NMDA 1), GABRA4 (gamma-aminobutyric acid type A receptor subunit alpha4), SCN1B (sodium voltage-gated channel beta subunit 1), SCN2B (sodium voltage-gated channel beta subunit 2), VAPB (VAMP-associated protein B/C), and ANXA5 (annexin A5) appeared as members of the SOD1-ALS pathway.

SOD1 is abundantly present in the cytoplasm, where the SOD1 aggregates are bound to interact with molecules concerning cytoskeleton dynamics. IPA identified cytoplasm molecules regulating neuronal architecture, namely RHOA (Ras homolog family member A), DPYSL3 (dihydropyrimidinase-like 3), TUBA1A (tubulin alpha 1A), ACTB (B-actin), and NEFL (neurofilament light chain) as a part of SOD1-ALS pathway molecules. In addition to dysregulating cytoskeleton architectural constituents, SOD1 aggregates impair the function of traffic proteins. IPA showed that DCTN1 (dynactin 1) and VPS35 (vacuolar protein sorting ortholog 35), which are involved in the retrograde transport of proteins, are altered in response to SOD1 toxicity.

The overwhelming presence of inflammation and immune response factors, such as TP53 (tumor protein 53; nucleus), PAWR (pro-apoptotic WT1 regulator), BAX (BCL2 associated X protein), BAD (BCL2 associated agonist of cell death), BCL2 (B-cell lymphoma-2), CASP1 (caspase 1), CASP3 (caspase 3), PTGS2 (prostaglandin-endoperoxide synthase 2/COX2), NOS (nitric oxide synthase), XIAP (X-linked inhibitors of apoptosis), CD36 (cluster of differentiation 36), FAS (Fas cell surface death receptor/TNFRSF6), IL1B, IL6, IGF1 (insulin-like growth factor 1), VEGF (vascular endothelial growth factor A), GPX3 (glutathione peroxidase 3), SQSTM (sequestosome 1), SPP1 (secreted phosphoprotein 1), ANXA1 (annexin A1), and PPIA (peptidylprolyl isomerase A) in ALS-SOD1 pathway indicates that SOD1-induced ALS development is markedly associated with inflammation and immune response. Many of these inflammatory and immune response markers are known to activate ERK/MAPK signaling pathway.

3.3. GO Analysis of SOD1-ALS Pathway Genes

IPA identified 87 molecules, including 75 genes associated with SOD1 toxicity, leading to the development of ALS (Figure 3; Table S2). These genes were further subjected to GO analysis to shed a light on the relationship between SOD1 and ALS and decipher the role of these molecules (genes) in the SOD1-ALS pathway. The GO analysis of SOD1-ALS network molecules unraveled that ALS and neurodegeneration pathways were significantly higher enriched than other pathways (Figures 4 and S1–S3). The SOD1-ALS pathway molecules such as BAD, ALS2, NOS2, BAX, NOS1, FUS, OPTN, VAPB, PRPH, SOD1, CASP3, VCP (valosin-containing protein), TUBA1A, BCL2L1, BCL2, GRIN1, DCTN1, GPX3, and NEFL play a critical role in the development of SOD1-induced ALS (Figure S2) and neurodegeneration (Figure S3). Additionally, SOD1-ALS pathway molecules, such as ACTB, PFN1, SLC1A2, CASP1, and TP53 also play a part in the development of SOD1-provoked ALS (Figure S2), while FAS, PTGS2, PARK7, IL1B, IL6, APP, and CALM1 (calmodulin 1) engage in SOD1-triggered neurodegeneration in ALS (Figure S3).

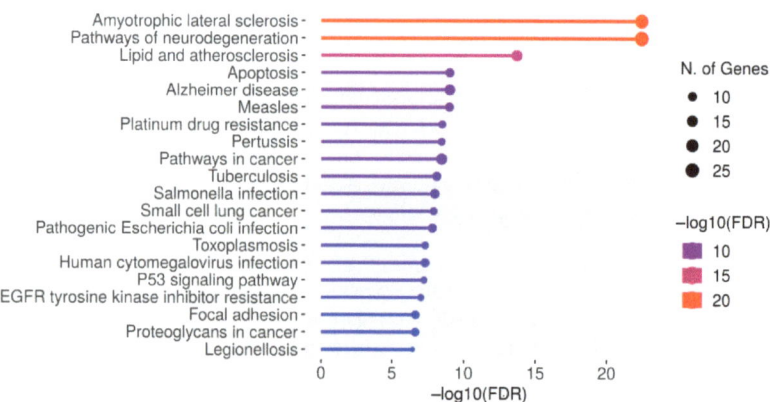

Figure 4. The GO analysis of IPA-predicted SOD1-ALS pathway molecules by ShinyGO. The GO analysis identified amyotrophic lateral sclerosis and neurodegeneration signaling as the key pathways.

The GO analysis also identified enriched biological processes (BP), molecular functions (MF), and cellular components (CC) of SOD1-ALS pathway molecules (Table 1). The GO analysis revealed response to chemical, regulation of biological quality, response to organic substance, positive regulation of transport, and signaling as the top-enriched biological processes of SOD1-ALS network molecules. The highest-enriched molecular functions associated with SOD1-ALS network molecules were identical protein binding, protein binding, protein domain specific binding, enzyme binding, and signaling receptor binding. The GO analysis identified vesicle, extracellular space, extracellular region, cell junction, and synapse as the most enriched cellular components of SOD1-ALS pathway molecules.

Table 1. The GO enrichment analysis of SOD1-ALS pathway molecules, highlighting top-enriched biological processes, molecular functions, and cellular components.

	Description (Term)	Gene Counts	p-Value
BP	Response to chemical (GO:0042221)	55	7.84×10^{-23}
	Regulation of biological quality (GO:0065008)	53	3.34×10^{-22}
	Response to organic substance (GO:0010033)	47	8.62×10^{-22}
	Positive regulation of transport (GO:0051050)	29	4.89×10^{-20}
	Signaling (GO:0023052)	56	1.02×10^{-19}
MF	Identical protein binding (GO:0042802)	38	2.88×10^{-20}
	Protein binding (GO:0005515)	62	4.54×10^{-19}
	Protein domain specific binding (GO:0019904)	18	8.00×10^{-11}
	Enzyme binding (GO:0019899)	29	2.83×10^{-10}
	Signaling receptor binding (GO:0005102)	23	4.65×10^{-09}
CC	Vesicle (GO:0031982)	43	7.79×10^{-14}
	Extracellular space (GO:0005615)	37	5.07×10^{-12}
	Extracellular region (GO:0005576)	41	2.86×10^{-11}
	Cell junction (GO:0030054)	28	2.63×10^{-10}
	Synapse (GO:0045202)	23	2.30×10^{-10}

3.4. Construction and Analysis of Interaction Network of SOD1-ALS Pathway Molecules

IPA-predicted SOD1-ALS pathway molecules (75 genes) were imported on the STRING server for the construction of a molecular interaction network (PPI network). The STRING-constructed interaction network displayed 75 nodes, 510 edges, 13.6 average node degree, 0.624 average local clustering coefficient, 174 expected number of edges, and PPI enrichment *p*-value of <1.0×10^{-16}. The PPI network constructed on STRING was imported to Cytoscape for analysis. The Cytoscape network analysis revealed ACTB as the major network hub followed by TP53, IL6, CASP3, SOD1, IL1B, APP, APOE, VEGFA, IL10, PTGS2, ANXA5, RHOA, and SQSTM1 (Figure 5). The observance of ACTB as a prominent network hub was not surprising since SOD1 is mainly located in the cytoplasm and ACTB is a major component of the cytoskeleton. APP is a major neurodegenerative amyloid protein that likely contributes to the development and progression of ALS upon mutation in SOD1. APOE, besides being co-expressed with APP, mediates the clearance of lipoproteins. The dysregulation of APOE alters the lipid profile in the body, which may contribute to SOD1-induced ALS. The finding of inflammatory and immune response mediators as major network hubs is consistent with the marked presence of inflammatory and immune response mediators in the SOD1-ALS pathway identified by IPA.

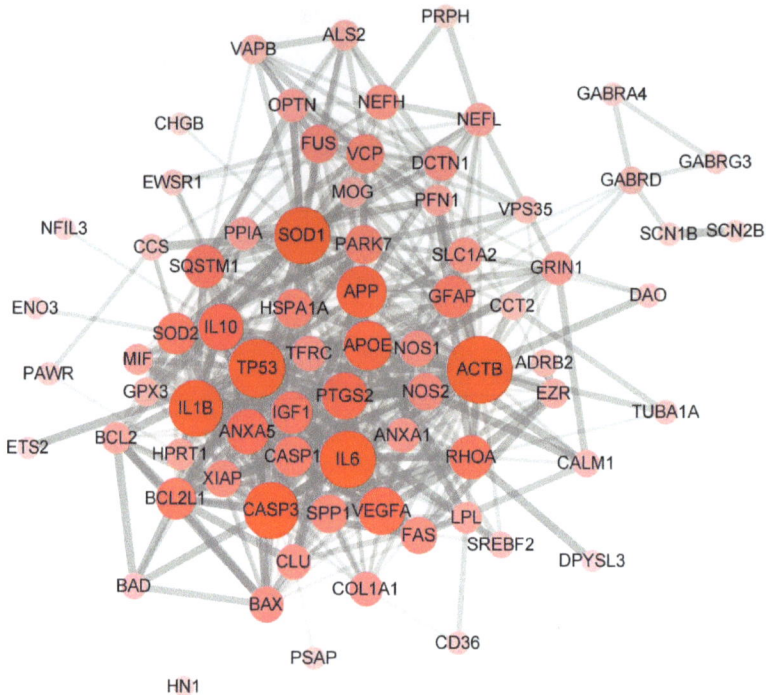

Figure 5. The molecular interaction network (PPI network) of IPA-identified SOD1-ALS pathway molecules. The PPI network was constructed using STRING and analyzed with Cytoscape. The Cytoscape network analysis predicted ACTB followed by TP53, IL6, CASP3, SOD1, IL1B, APP, APOE, and VEGFA as the major network hubs. The nodes' size and color intensity correspond to the size of the network hub.

4. Discussion

IPA QIAGEN is one of the leading tools for the analysis and interpretation of data acquired from omics experiments [21]. With IPA one can predict the expression, toxicity, metabolomics, and a variant effect analysis of molecule(s). SOD1 is an antioxidant enzyme, but mutations in SOD1 result in cellular stress and the progressive development of ALS. The number of SOD1 variants that trigger ALS continues to rise. This piqued our interest to extract more information about the role and toxicity of SOD1, with an emphasis on its toxicity in ALS. SOD1 detoxifies superoxide radicals into oxygen and hydrogen peroxide (Figure S4). Hydrogen peroxide is further broken down by catalase into water and oxygen. Apelin (APLN) is an adipocytokine. Under hypoxic conditions, hypoxia-inducible factor 1 subunit alpha (HIF1A) activates APLN, which in turn increases the activity of SOD1 via MAPK-ERK1/2 and AMPK axes (Figure S5). The mutated SOD1 is susceptible to misfolding, resulting in the formation of aggregate species in ALS (Figure S2). The misfolded SOD1 conformers have been implicated in the degeneration of spinal cord motor neurons (Figure S3). In addition, the misfolded SOD1 species not only impair normal SOD1 functions but also exhibit unusual interactions with other proteins, thus contributing to SOD1 toxicity via both loss and gain of functions [18]. NRF2, also known as nuclear factor erythroid 2-related factor 2, is a transcription factor, encoded by the NFE2L2 gene. Reactive oxygen species under oxidative stress activate NFE2L2 via RAS, MAP3K1/5/7, and PKC signaling. Following activation, NFE2L2 in the nucleus transcripts several genes, including SOD1 (Figure S6). However, under oxidative stress conditions, SOD1 oxidation leads to impaired dimer formation and misfolded proteins, resulting in the oligomerization and aggregate formation of SOD1. Sirtuin (SIRT5)-SOD1 interaction takes place in mitochondria, where under normal physiological conditions SIRT5 activates SOD1, leading to the detoxification of reactive oxygen species.

CNR1 was identified as the foremost regulator of SOD1 (Figure 2B). In the case of mutant SOD1-induced ALS, the expression of CNR1 increases while endocannabinoids accumulate in the spinal cord. This suggests that endocannabinoids play a protective role against neurodegeneration, and CNR1 might be a potential therapeutic target for ALS. The role of SOD1 regulator APLN was discussed earlier in the apelin adipocyte signaling pathway. Another regulator, BTG2, activates the antioxidant transcription factor NFE2L2, which in turn elevates the level of SOD1. Similar to BTG, MAPK also regulates SOD1 via the activation of NFE2L2. DRAP1 is a transcription repressor gene that is elevated in hypoxic conditions and likely governs SOD1 activity in conjunction with HIF1. SNCA, like SOD1, is an aggregate-forming protein, which potentiates SOD1 toxicity by accelerating SOD1 oligomerization. Similar to other upstream regulators, CG (CTSG) may also play a crucial role in oxidative stress.

Mutation in SOD1 compromises its functions, resulting in hereditary and neurological diseases including ALS (Figure 2C). SOD1 mutants tend to form aggregates that cause mitochondrial dysfunction, leading to neuronal cell death (Figure 2D). At the same time, oxidative stress promotes and potentiates SOD1 aggregation, resulting in exacerbated cell death. Furthermore, SOD1 regulates molecular and cellular functions such as cell death and survival via BCL2-BAX molecules, while it maintains cellular architecture via ACTN (Figure 2E). The post-translational modification of SOD1 causes misfolding of SOD1 in the cytoplasm and mitochondria. The misfolded protein in the mitochondria oligomerizes to form aggregates. The aggregated SOD1 loses its capacity to neutralize reactive oxygen species, impairing the electron transport chain (ETC). The cascade of events further leads to the release of mitochondrial cytochrome C through the formation of the BAX-BAK channel, which destroys mitochondrial homeostasis and results in caspase-mediated cell death (Figure S2) [18].

Since ALS was predicted to be the major outcome of SOD1 toxicity, we explored the pathway molecules between SOD1 toxicity and ALS. Our study discovered a network of molecules transmitting SOD1 toxicity, resulting in the development of ALS (Figure 3). Based on the IPA-identified SOD1-ALS pathway molecules, it can be assumed that SOD1-induced toxicity in ALS is accompanied by aggregation of other misfolded proteins, lipid dysregulation, impaired neurotransmission, compromised vesicular transport, and perturbed cytoskeleton dynamics. In addition to this, the plethora of immune and inflammatory mediators are altered during the course of SOD1-triggered ALS development. However, whether IPA-identified SOD1-ALS pathway molecules are altered due to explicit SOD1 toxicity or they are altered as a result of secondary non-specific or host stress response to SOD1 toxicity, remains to be discerned. The comparison of the molecular interaction network of wild-type SOD1 and mutant SOD1 could shed a light on this issue. Furthermore, SOD1 toxicity network molecules can be compared with the toxicity network of other amyloid proteins like APP, MAPT (tau), SNCA, and HTT (Huntingtin) to conclude which IPA-identified SOD1-ALS pathway molecules are exclusive to SOD1 toxicity only. We further subjected IPA-identified molecules to GO analysis, which ascertained the IPA finding that SOD1-ALS network molecules are most significantly associated with ALS and neurodegeneration signaling pathways (Figures 4 and S1–S3). The GO-enriched biological processes, such as response to chemical and response to organic substance, indicate the cellular response of SOD1-ALS network molecules against SOD1 toxicity, whereas regulation of biological quality highlights the up- or down-regulation of network molecules as a result of SOD1 toxicity (Table 1). The GO-enriched molecular functions, such as identical protein binding and protein binding, suggest the interaction of SOD1 homodimer with network molecules and the binding of network molecules with the interacting proteins, respectively (Table 1). The GO-enriched top-ranked cellular component vesicle points to the association of network molecules with apoptotic bodies and cytoplasmic vesicles (Table 1).

To analyze the interactions among IPA-predicted SOD1-ALS pathway molecules, we constructed a PPI network using STRING, which was analyzed with Cytoscape (Figure 5). The appearance of cytoplasmic ACTB as the largest network hub is understandable since it regulates neuronal cell growth and motility and preserves cellular architecture. SOD1, APP, and APOE drive amyloid pathology in the brain and spinal cord, while amyloidosis-resulted neuroinflammation and cell death are mediated by TP53, IL6, CASP3, IL1B, and VEGFA.

5. Conclusions

In light of the growing number of SOD1 variants causing ALS, researchers are still struggling to understand the complex SOD1 interaction network at work in ALS and neurodegeneration. In this study we used an integrated bioinformatics approach to analyze the role and function of SOD1, with an emphasis on uncovering SOD1 network molecules in ALS. Our study identified signaling pathways, regulators, and molecular interaction network of SOD1 that dominates ALS. Researchers in the wet lab can build upon our findings to elucidate the mechanism by which SOD1 mutants cause amyloid pathology.

Supplementary Materials: The following supporting information can be downloaded at: https://www.mdpi.com/article/10.3390/brainsci13010151/s1, Figure S1: Interactive pathway plot for SOD1-ALS network molecules predicted by ShinyGO analysis, Figure S2: Amyotrophic lateral sclerosis pathway, Figure S3: Neurodegeneration pathway, Figure S4: Superoxide radicals' degradation by SOD1, Figure S5: The role of SOD1 in the apelin adipocyte signaling pathway, Figure S6: (**A**) NRF2-mediated oxidative stress response signaling pathway in the extracellular space and cytoplasm. (**B**) The role of SOD1 in the NRF2-mediated oxidative stress response signaling pathway in the nucleus; Table S1: SOD1 variants causing amyotrophic lateral sclerosis, Table S2: The list of SOD1-ALS pathway molecules identified by IPA, genes used for ShinyGO analysis, and construction of a molecular interaction network on STRING.

Author Contributions: S.K.S. conceived the idea, performed the analysis, and wrote and reviewed the manuscript. S.-Y.L. conceived the idea, provided suggestions, and reviewed the manuscript. All authors have read and agreed to the published version of the manuscript.

Funding: This work was supported by Korea Health Technology R & D project through the Korea Health Industry Development Institute (KHIDI), funded by the Ministry for Health and Welfare, Korea research grant No. HI14C1135 and Gachon University research grant No. GCU-2019-0724.

Institutional Review Board Statement: Not applicable.

Informed Consent Statement: Not applicable.

Data Availability Statement: Not applicable.

Acknowledgments: S.K.S. received a Brain Pool Fellowship (No. 2021H1D3A2A02044867) from the National Research Foundation (NRF) of Korea. The authors would like to thank Bharath Kumar Eriboina, QIAGEN for providing the IPA trial version license.

Conflicts of Interest: The authors declare no conflict of interest.

References

1. McCord, J.M.; Fridovich, I. Superoxide Dismutase. An Enzymic Function for Erythrocuprein (Hemocuprein). *J. Biol. Chem.* **1969**, *244*, 6049–6055. [CrossRef] [PubMed]
2. Sturtz, L.A.; Diekert, K.; Jensen, L.T.; Lill, R.; Culotta, V.C. A Fraction of Yeast Cu,Zn-Superoxide Dismutase and its Metallochaperone, CCS, Localize to the Intermembrane Space of Mitochondria. A Physiological Role for SOD1 in Guarding Against Mitochondrial Oxidative Damage. *J. Biol. Chem.* **2001**, *276*, 38084–38089. [CrossRef]
3. Mesecke, N.; Terziyska, N.; Kozany, C.; Baumann, F.; Neupert, W.; Hell, K.; Herrmann, J.M. A Disulfide Relay System in the Intermembrane Space of Mitochondria that Mediates Protein Import. *Cell* **2005**, *121*, 1059–1069. [CrossRef] [PubMed]
4. Field, L.S.; Furukawa, Y.; O'Halloran, T.V.; Culotta, V.C. Factors Controlling the Uptake of Yeast Copper/Zinc Superoxide Dismutase into Mitochondria. *J. Biol. Chem.* **2003**, *278*, 28052–28059. [CrossRef] [PubMed]

5. Montllor-Albalate, C.; Kim, H.; Thompson, A.E.; Jonke, A.P.; Torres, M.P.; Reddi, A.R. SOD1 Integrates Oxygen Availability to Redox Regulate NADPH Production and the Thiol Redoxome. *Proc. Natl. Acad. Sci. USA* **2022**, *119*, e2023328119. [CrossRef] [PubMed]
6. Tsang, C.K.; Liu, Y.; Thomas, J.; Zhang, Y.; Zheng, X.F.S. Superoxide Dismutase 1 Acts as a Nuclear Transcription Factor to Regulate Oxidative Stress Resistance. *Nat. Commun.* **2014**, *5*, 3446. [CrossRef]
7. Rosen, D.R.; Siddique, T.; Patterson, D.; Figlewicz, D.A.; Sapp, P.; Hentati, A.; Donaldson, D.; Goto, J.; O'Regan, J.P.; Deng, H.X.; et al. Mutations in Cu/Zn Superoxide Dismutase Gene are Associated with Familial Amyotrophic Lateral Sclerosis. *Nature* **1993**, *362*, 59–62. [CrossRef]
8. Mulder, D.W.; Kurland, L.T.; Offord, K.P.; Beard, C.M. Familial Adult Motor Neuron Disease: Amyotrophic Lateral Sclerosis. *Neurology* **1986**, *36*, 511–517. [CrossRef]
9. Bruijn, L.I.; Miller, T.M.; Cleveland, D.W. Unraveling the Mechanisms Involved in Motor Neuron Degeneration in ALS. *Annu. Rev. Neurosci.* **2004**, *27*, 723–749. [CrossRef]
10. ALSoD—Amyotrophic Lateral Sclerosis Online Database. Available online: https://alsod.ac.uk/output/gene.php/SOD1 (accessed on 10 November 2022).
11. Berdyński, M.; Miszta, P.; Safranow, K.; Andersen, P.M.; Morita, M.; Filipek, S.; Żekanowski, C.; Kuźma-Kozakiewicz, M. SOD1 Mutations Associated with Amyotrophic Lateral Sclerosis Analysis of Variant Severity. *Sci. Rep.* **2022**, *12*, 103. [CrossRef]
12. Rodriguez, J.A.; Shaw, B.F.; Durazo, A.; Sohn, S.H.; Doucette, P.A.; Nersissian, A.M.; Faull, K.F.; Eggers, D.K.; Tiwari, A.; Hayward, L.J.; et al. Destabilization of Apoprotein is Insufficient to Explain Cu,Zn-Superoxide Dismutase-linked ALS Pathogenesis. *Proc. Natl. Acad. Sci. USA* **2005**, *102*, 10516–10521. [CrossRef]
13. Banci, L.; Bertini, I.; Boca, M.; Calderone, V.; Cantini, F.; Girotto, S.; Vieru, M. Structural and Dynamic Aspects Related to Oligomerization of Apo SOD1 and its Mutants. *Proc. Natl. Acad. Sci. USA* **2009**, *106*, 6980–6985. [CrossRef] [PubMed]
14. Kumar, V.; Prakash, A.; Pandey, P.; Lynn, A.M.; Hassan, M.I. TFE-induced local unfolding and fibrillation of SOD1: Bridging the experiment and simulation studies. *Biochem. J.* **2018**, *475*, 1701–1719. [CrossRef]
15. Prakash, A.; Kumar, V.; Pandey, P.; Bharti, D.R.; Vishwakarma, P.; Singh, R.; Hassan, M.I.; Lynn, A.M. Solvent sensitivity of protein aggregation in Cu, Zn superoxide dismutase: A molecular dynamics simulation study. *J. Biomol. Struct. Dyn.* **2018**, *36*, 2605–2617. [CrossRef] [PubMed]
16. DiDonato, M.; Craig, L.; Huff, M.E.; Thayer, M.M.; Cardoso, R.M.F.; Kassmann, C.J.; Lo, T.P.; Bruns, C.K.; Powers, E.T.; Kelly, J.W.; et al. ALS Mutants of Human Superoxide Dismutase Form Fibrous Aggregates via Framework Destabilization. *J. Mol. Biol.* **2003**, *332*, 601–615. [CrossRef]
17. Stathopulos, P.B.; Rumfeldt, J.A.O.; Scholz, G.A.; Irani, R.A.; Frey, H.E.; Hallewell, R.A.; Lepock, J.R.; Meiering, E.M. Cu/Zn Superoxide Dismutase Mutants Associated with Amyotrophic Lateral Sclerosis Show Enhanced Formation of Aggregates In Vitro. *Proc. Natl. Acad. Sci. USA* **2003**, *100*, 7021–7026. [CrossRef]
18. Trist, B.G.; Hilton, J.B.; Hare, D.J.; Crouch, P.J.; Double, K.L. Superoxide Dismutase 1 in Health and Disease: How a Frontline Antioxidant Becomes Neurotoxic. *Angew. Chem. Int. Ed. Engl.* **2021**, *60*, 9215–9246. [CrossRef] [PubMed]
19. Peggion, C.; Scalcon, V.; Massimino, M.L.; Nies, K.; Lopreiato, R.; Rigobello, M.P.; Bertoli, A. SOD1 in ALS: Taking Sock in Pathogenic Mechanisms and the Role of Glial and Muscle Cells. *Antioxidants* **2022**, *11*, 614. [CrossRef]
20. NCBI (2022). National Center for Biotechnology (NCBI). Available online: https://www.ncbi.nlm.nih.gov/gene (accessed on 30 September 2022).
21. IPA (2021). Ingenuity Pathway Analysis (IPA), Qiagen. Available online: https://digitalinsights.qiagen.com/products-overview/discovery-insights-portfolio/analysis-and-visualization/qiagen-ipa/ (accessed on 30 September 2022).
22. Suthar, S.K.; Alam, M.M.; Lee, J.; Monga, J.; Joseph, A.; Lee, S.-Y. Bioinformatic Analyses of Canonical Pathways of TSPOAP1 and its Roles in Human Diseases. *Front. Mol. Biosci.* **2021**, *8*, 667947. [CrossRef]
23. Suthar, S.K.; Lee, S.-Y. Ingenuity Pathway Analysis of α-Synuclein Predicts Potential Signaling Pathways, Network Molecules, Biological Functions, and its Role in Neurological Diseases. *Front. Mol. Neurosci.* **2022**, *15*, 1029682. [CrossRef]
24. Ge, S.X.; Jung, D.; Yao, R. ShinyGO: A Graphical Gene-set Enrichment Tool for Animals and Plants. *Bioinformatics* **2020**, *36*, 2628–2629. [CrossRef] [PubMed]
25. Szklarczyk, D.; Franceschini, A.; Wyder, S.; Forslund, K.; Heller, D.; Huerta-Cepas, J.; Simonovic, M.; Roth, A.; Santos, A.; Tsafou, K.P.; et al. STRING v10: Protein-Protein Interaction Networks, Integrated Over the Tree of Life. *Nucleic Acids Res.* **2015**, *43*, D447–D452. [CrossRef] [PubMed]
26. Shannon, P.; Markiel, A.; Ozier, O.; Baliga, N.S.; Wang, J.T.; Ramage, D.; Amin, N.; Schwikowski, B.; Ideker, T. Cytoscape: A Software Environment for Integrated Models of Biomolecular Interaction Networks. *Genome Res.* **2003**, *13*, 2498–2504. [CrossRef] [PubMed]

Disclaimer/Publisher's Note: The statements, opinions and data contained in all publications are solely those of the individual author(s) and contributor(s) and not of MDPI and/or the editor(s). MDPI and/or the editor(s) disclaim responsibility for any injury to people or property resulting from any ideas, methods, instructions or products referred to in the content.

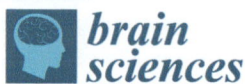 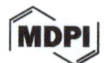

Article

The Spatiotemporal Expression of SOCS3 in the Brainstem and Spinal Cord of Amyotrophic Lateral Sclerosis Mice

Ching-Yi Lin *, Veronica Vanoverbeke, David Trent, Kathryn Willey and Yu-Shang Lee

Department of Neurosciences, Lerner Research Institute, Cleveland Clinic, LRI, NB3-90, 9500 Euclid Ave., Cleveland, OH 44195, USA
* Correspondence: linc@ccf.org

Abstract: Amyotrophic lateral sclerosis (ALS) is characterized by the progressive loss of motor neurons from the brain and spinal cord. The excessive neuroinflammation is thought to be a common determinant of ALS. Suppressor of cytokine signaling-3 (SOCS3) is pathologically upregulated after injury/diseases to negatively regulate a broad range of cytokines/chemokines that mediate inflammation; however, the role that SOCS3 plays in ALS pathogenesis has not been explored. Here, we found that SOCS3 protein levels were significantly increased in the brainstem of the superoxide dismutase 1 (SOD1)-G93A ALS mice, which is negatively related to a progressive decline in motor function from the pre-symptomatic to the early symptomatic stage. Moreover, SOCS3 levels in both cervical and lumbar spinal cords of ALS mice were also significantly upregulated at the pre-symptomatic stage and became exacerbated at the early symptomatic stage. Concomitantly, astrocytes and microglia/macrophages were progressively increased and reactivated over time. In contrast, neurons were simultaneously lost in the brainstem and spinal cord examined over the course of disease progression. Collectively, SOCS3 was first found to be upregulated during ALS progression to directly relate to both increased astrogliosis and increased neuronal loss, indicating that SOCS3 could be explored to be as a potential therapeutic target of ALS.

Keywords: amyotrophic lateral sclerosis (ALS); suppressor of cytokine signaling-3 (SOCS3); pre-Bötzinger Complex (preBötC); neuroinflammation

1. Introduction

Amyotrophic lateral sclerosis (ALS, is often called Lou Gehrig's disease) is a debilitating and devastating neurodegenerative disease characterized by the loss of both upper and lower motor neurons and ultimately paralysis and death, usually resulting from respiratory failure, within 2–5 years of diagnosis [1–4]. The majority of ALS cases are sporadic (sporadic ALS, i.e., sALS) with unknown etiology [5,6], whereas approximately 10% of cases correspond to inherited forms of ALS (familiar ALS, i.e., fALS). Mutations in the gene encoding for the enzyme Cu/Zn superoxide dismutase 1 (SOD1) are observed in approximately 20% of fALS cases [7]. ALS pathogenesis studied in ALS animal models are known to be attributable to oxidative stress, glutamate excitotoxicity, protein misfolding, mitochondrial defects, impaired axonal transport, or inflammation, any of which will eventually lead to motor neuron death. Despite the diverse etiologies of ALS [2,4], increasing evidence shows that progressive injury caused by excessive and extended neuroinflammation is a common determinant. Neuroinflammation is closely linked to the pathogenic mechanisms of acute or chronic neural injury in many diseases, and is regulated by a broad range of cytokines/chemokines [8–11]. A pivotal regulator of a broad range of cytokines/chemokines is Suppressor of cytokine signaling (SOCS). SOCS proteins negatively modulate signaling through the Janus kinase (JAK)/signal transducer and activator of transcription (STAT) pathway [12,13] to regulate neuronal growth and differentiation [14,15]. However, the role of SOCS in the CNS remains unclear.

Suppressors of cytokine signaling-3 (SOCS3), one member of the SOCS family of proteins, binds to gp130 (a common receptor for signal transduction with interleukin-6 (IL-6)), or JAK1 and JAK2, subsequently inhibiting signal transduction [16,17]. Expression of SOCS3 in neurons in particular causes a negative regulatory effect on signal transduction and transcription-3 (STAT3) activation, which consequently contribute to excitotoxic neuronal death and to decrease cell survival and neurite outgrowth in vitro [18–22]. In addition, SOCS3 negative regulation of neuronal survival and axon regeneration has been found both in vivo and in vitro [18,21–24]. SOCS3 is pathologically upregulated after neural injury/diseases to negatively regulate a broad range of cytokines/chemokines that mediate inflammation [13,25,26]; however, the spatiotemporal expression of SOCS3 in ALS has not been investigated previously.

In this study, we observed that SOCS3 levels are significantly upregulated in (a) the pre-Bötzinger Complex (preBötC) of the brainstem and (b) the ventral horn of both cervical and lumbar spinal cord of ALS mice, which are accompanied by increased astrogliosis and decreased neurons, and are related to the neurodegeneration stage of ALS from the pre-symptomatic to early symptomatic stage. Together, these findings demonstrate a potential role for the manipulation of SOCS3 levels to regulate ALS progression, which may uncover a promising and novel potential therapeutic target for balancing an uncontrolled inflammatory response.

2. Methods

2.1. Mice

All mouse experiments were performed in accordance with the protocols approved by the Institutional Animal Care and Use Committee at the Cleveland Clinic. The SOD1-G93A mouse, a transgenic mouse with a glycine (G)-to-alanine (A) conversion at the 93rd codon of the SOD1 gene in high copy number (SOD1-G93A) [27–29], is one of the most commonly used ALS models. SOD1-G93A (B6.Cg-Tg (SOD1*G93A)1Gur/J, Jackson Laboratory, JAX stock number 004435) on a C57BL/6J genetic background were the ALS mice model (ALS mice) used in the entire study. C57BL/6J mice (JAX stock No. 000664) were used as the WT mice for comparison.

All efforts were made to minimize animal suffering as well as the number of animals used. Male mice were used for the experiments throughout this study to exclude the possible impacts of sex difference on disease onset and lifespan [30]. All animals were housed in standard metallic mouse cages (19.5 × 29.5 × 15 cm) with a corncob bedding under standard conditions of constant temperature and controlled lighting (12/12 h light/dark cycle). Humidity was 55%, the temperature was $23 \pm 1\ °C$, and food and water were available ad libitum. The rotarod and grip strength tests were performed during the light period. The animals were euthanized at either 9 weeks (pre-symptomatic stage) or 16 weeks (early symptomatic stage) of age. n = 8/group and then divided to n = 4/time point.

2.2. Rotarod Test

The rotarod test was used to assess motor function in a blinded fashion. Mice were trained on the rotarod twice at one week before recording the data. Beginning at 8 weeks old, all animals (n = 8/group) were weighed and evaluated for signs of a motor deficits using the accelerated rotarod test. For this test, the time for which an animal spent walking on the rotating rod of a rotarod apparatus (BX-ROD-M; Bioseb Instruments US, Pinellas Park, FL, USA) was recorded weekly. Each animal was given three tries. The longest latency (sec) it takes for the mouse to fall off the rod was recorded. The apparatus had an initial speed of 2 rpm, a ramp time of 300 s, and gradually accelerated at a rate of 38/300 rpm/s. The speeds therefore gradually and consistently increased from 2 rpm to 40 rpm over the course of 300 s.

2.3. Grip Strength Test

The Grip strength test was also used to assess the motor function in a blinded fashion. During this test, each mouse was placed on the grip strength meter (BIO-GS4; BX-ROD-M; Bioseb Instruments US, FL, USA), n = 8/group. The tail was pulled gently to impel the mouse to grip the bar with its forelimbs, and then the tail was pulled backwards at a uniform speed until the mouse released its grip. Each animal was given three tries, and the maximal force (g) that the mouse released its grip was recorded as the grip strength.

2.4. Immunohistochemistry (IHC) Analyses

After behavioral tests, ALS and control WT mice were terminated at either 9 or 16 weeks of age for IHC analyses in a blinded fashion. Animals anesthetized using Euthasol were transcardially perfused with ice-cold 0.9% saline followed by 4% paraformaldehyde (PFA). The brains and spinal cords were collected and post-fixed in 4% PFA for 1 day and were then transferred to 30% sucrose solution for 3 days. Frozen cryostat sections (30 μm thick each, 6~8 sections per animal) were incubated with phosphate-buffered saline (PBS) containing 0.3% Triton X-100 for 30 min at room temperature (RT), and then were incubated with the blocking solution (PBS containing 1% normal donkey serum (NDS, Vector Laboratories, Newark, CA), 3% bovine serum albumin (BSA, Sigma-Aldrich, St. Louis, MO, USA), and 0.5% Triton X-100 (Sigma-Aldrich, St. Louis, MO, USA)) for 60 min at RT and, subsequently, double-staining with SOCS3 antibody (rabbit, ab16030, 1:300; Abcam, Waltham, MA, USA) and either NeuN (mouse, MAB377, 1:500; EMD Millipore, Burlington, MA, USA), glial fibrillary acidic protein (GFAP) (mouse, MAB3402, 1:3000; EMD Millipore, Burlington, MA, USA), or ionized calcium-binding adaptor molecule 1 (Iba1) antibody (mouse, MA5-38265, 1:200; ThermoFisher Scientific, Waltham, MA, USA) at RT overnight. After washing in PBS containing 0.3% Triton X-100 three times, secondary donkey anti-rabbit IgG conjugated Alexa 555 (ab150074, 1:1200; Abcam, Waltham, MA, USA) and donkey anti-mouse IgG conjugated Alexa 488 (A-21202, 1:1200; ThermoFisher Scientific) were applied at RT for 2 h. After washing in PBS containing 0.3% Triton X-100 twice and then in PBS once, sections were covered with mounting medium containing Hoechst to stain nuclei (Vector Laboratories, Newark, CA, USA) and analyzed using a Zeiss confocal laser-scanning microscope. Steps were taken to minimize the potential for background staining by (1) application of both NDS and BSA during the incubation with blocking solution, primary antibodies, and secondary antibodies; and (2) conducting the regular staining procedures but with no addition of individual primary antibody against either SOCS3, NeuN, GFAP, or Iba1 to confirm the specificity of antibodies before IHC analyses.

2.5. Statistical Analyses

Standardized areas for sampling in sections (IHC) from each animal in each group were selected using Photoshop and ImageJ. Light intensity and threshold values were maintained at constant levels for all analyses. The mean number of pixels containing immunoreactive product in the sampled area was measured and multiplied by the average intensity. This value was subtracted from background immunolabeled intensity, as measured in a separate adjacent section. Intensities were shown as mean ± standard error of mean (SEM) in units of the percentage of the maximal intensities from the individual animal, which are presented as 100%. Mean values for each animal were then normalized to obtain a percent intensity value for each group of mice. Statistical significance was evaluated using the two-tailed unpaired Student's *t* tests for comparisons between groups. A one-way analysis of variance (ANOVA) followed by a Tukey test, or a two-way ANOVA followed by a Bonferroni test was used for multiple comparisons for IHC intensity. For behavioral assessments, statistical significance was evaluated using a two-way ANOVA followed by a Bonferroni test to determine whether significant differences existed between ALS and WT mice at different time points. Values of $p < 0.05$ were considered to be statistically significant, as evaluated using Graphpad Prism 8.4.3. The statistical analyses were performed in a double blinded fashion.

3. Results

3.1. Motor Function Is Declined in ALS Mice

The ALS mice we used are SOD1-G93A mice (JAX stock No. 004435, Jackson Laboratories) which are on a C57BL/6J background with high copy number of transgene SOD1^{G93A} [27–29]. This is a well-characterized mouse model of ALS that develops initial signs of ALS around P100 (~ disease onset) [27,31–33] and reaches the end of life around P150 [31,33,34]. Disease onset was determined as the time when mice reached maximum body weight [35]. As shown in Figure 1A, ALS mice reached maximum body weight at 14 weeks old, and then gradually decreased their body weight after 15 weeks of age. Given that motor neurons are continuously lost over disease progression in the spinal cords of ALS mice, we used both rotarod and grip strength tests to assess the motor function of ALS mice as the disease progressed. The behavioral tests started at 9-week-old pre-symptomatic mice and ended at 16 weeks of age (early symptomatic stage). In the rotarod test, ALS mice showed a significant reduction in the time spent walking on the rod at 16 weeks of age compared with age-matched wild type (WT) mice (Figure 1B). The time the ALS mice spent on the rotarod was not significantly different at the pre-symptomatic stage (9 weeks of age), but was deteriorated by significantly decreased 77.6 s at the early symptomatic stage (16 weeks of age), as compared to the age-matched WT mice. In the grip strength test, there was no significant difference between ALS mice and WT mice at 9 weeks of age. However, ALS mice showed a significant reduction in grip strength by significantly decreased 27.2 g at 16 weeks of age when ALS progressed, as compared with age-matched WT mice (Figure 1C). Therefore, these data showed that motor dysfunction of ALS mice was progressively evident from pre-symptomatic to early symptomatic stage. We next investigated the spatiotemporal expression of SOCS3 in the relation to the progressive ALS pathology.

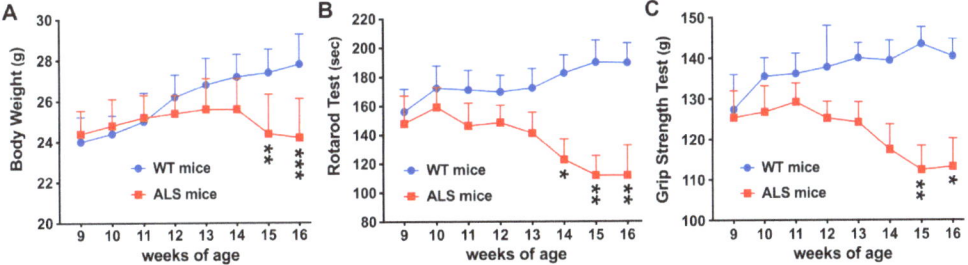

Figure 1. Progression of motor functional deficits in SOD1-G93A mice from 9 to 16 weeks of age. Body weight was measured every week (**A**). Motor function was assessed weekly in mice using the rotarod test (**B**) and Grip strength test (**C**). Data represent mean + SEM. Statistical analysis was performed using a two-way ANOVA followed by a Bonferroni test (* $p < 0.05$, ** $p < 0.01$, and *** $p < 0.001$ vs. age-matched WT mice, n = 8 each group).

3.2. Increased Astrocytes and SOCS3 Upregulation Are Found in the Brainstem of ALS Mice

ALS is noteworthy for upper and lower motor neuron death, which eventually leads to muscle weakness and paralysis. The respiratory dysfunction and eventually respiratory failure especially accounts for a large portion of morbidity and mortality in ALS [36,37]. The brainstem is the structure which modulates breathing, heart function, and more, as well as containing pathways for communication between the brain and the spinal cord. We first used double fluorescent-staining to detect the levels of broad inflammation regulators, SOCS3 and GFAP-positive (GFAP+) astrocytes, in the brainstem of ALS mice. As shown in Figure 2, SOCS3 expression was significantly upregulated in the brainstem of ALS mice, especially in the preBötC of the brainstem (Figure 2D,F,G,I,K,L), compared to WT mice. The preBötC, a portion of the ventrolateral medullary reticular formation is thought to generate the inspiratory breathing rhythm in mammals [38,39]. In the preBötC, ALS-upregulated SOCS3 (Figure 2D,G,K,L) was associated with increased and reactive GFAP+ astrocytes (Figure 2E,H,K,L,N), indicating that the neuroinflammation already started before the disease onset as early as 9 weeks of age as examined, and kept ongoing after disease onset. However, there was no colocalization of SOCS3 and GFAP+ astrocytes (Figure 2F,I,K,L), which indicates that the resource of increased SOCS3 was not from GFAP+ astrocytes in the areas examined.

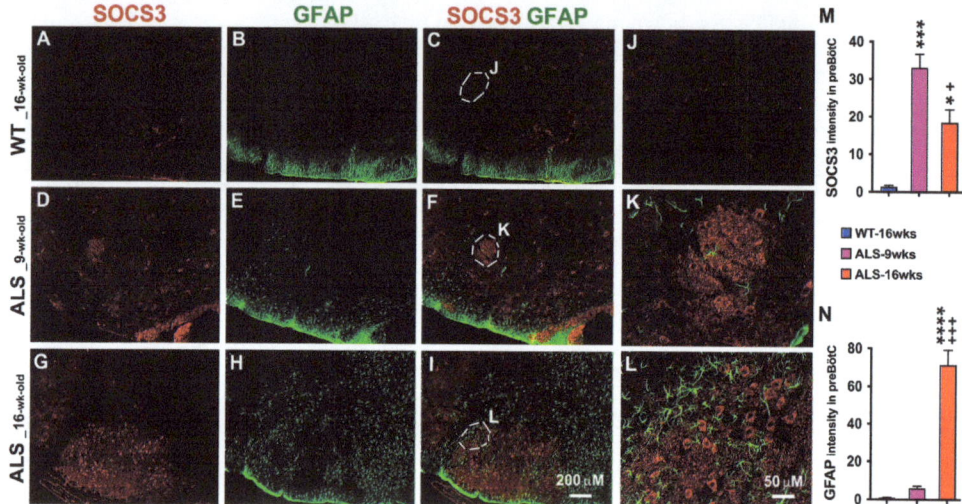

Figure 2. Upregulated SOCS3 in ALS mice is associated with increased astrocytes from the pre-symptomatic to early symptomatic stage in the brainstem. IHC was used to detect SOCS3 and GFAP+ astrocytes. As shown in the representative confocal images (**A–I**), significantly upregulated SOCS3 was observed in ALS mice at both 9 weeks of age (**D,F**) and 16 weeks of age (**G,I**) in the brainstem compared to WT mice (**A,C**). The levels of upregulated SOCS3 (**D,F,G,I**) were directly related with the extent of GFAP expression and astrocyte reactivity (**E,F,H,I,K,L**) over ALS progression. The ALS-induced increases in SOCS3 and GFAP+ astrocytes were especially significant in the preBötC of brainstem, as shown in the higher-magnified images (**K,L**), compared to WT mice (**J**). Graphs represent mean ± SEM of four animals per group per time-point for intensity of SOCS3 (**M**) and GFAP (**N**). * $p < 0.05$, *** $p < 0.001$, and **** $p < 0.0001$ vs. WT mice; + $p < 0.05$, and +++ $p < 0.001$ vs. 9-week-old ALS mice (one-way ANOVA followed by a Tukey test).

3.3. ALS-Upregulated SOCS3 Associates with Increased Neuronal Loss in the Brainstem of ALS Mice

In addition, we used IHC to detect SOCS3 and NeuN+ (a marker for neurons) neurons in the brainstem of ALS mice and found that SOCS3 was significantly increased at the pre-symptomatic stage (9 weeks old, Figure 3D,F,K,M) and became more robust at the early symptomatic stage (16 weeks old, Figure 3G,I,L,M), when compared to WT mice. NeuN+ immunoreactivity was found in gray matter where neuronal cell bodies are located in both WT and ALS mice. Of most importance, the NeuN+ neurons were significantly decreased in the brainstem, especially in the preBötC of the brainstem in ALS mice at the pre-symptomatic stage (Figure 3E,F,K,N), and became even more exacerbated at the early symptomatic phases (Figure 3H,I,L,N), which was negatively related to the upregulated SOCS3 and was associated with neurodegeneration progression in a time-dependent manner. The NeuN+ neurons in the preBötC of the ALS mice were significantly decreased by 30 percent at 9 weeks of age, and were further decreased by 81 percent at 16 weeks of age, as compared to WT mice. Gradual and dramatic neuronal loss in the preBötC of the brainstem may account for the respiratory dysfunction over the ALS progression.

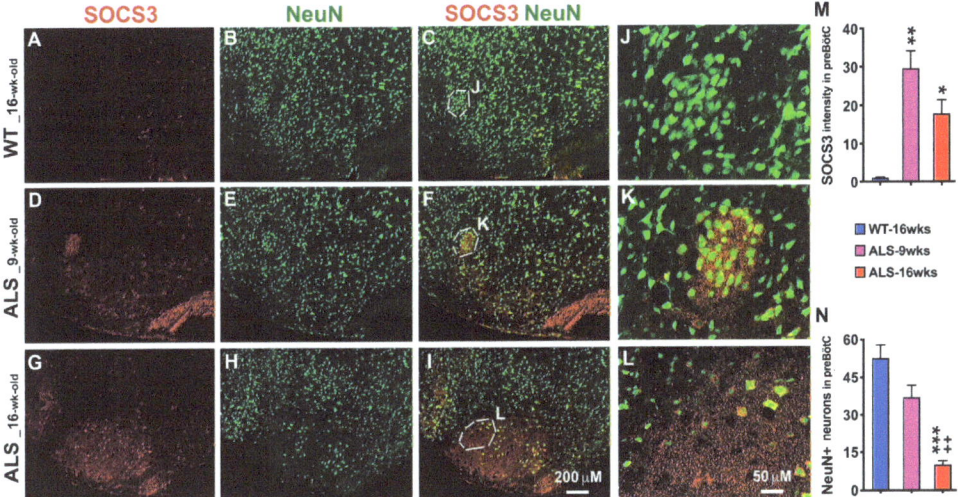

Figure 3. Upregulated SOCS3 in ALS mice during disease progression is directly associated with progressively increased neuronal loss in the brainstem. IHC was used to detect SOCS3 and NeuN+ neurons. As shown in the representative confocal images (**A–L**), significantly upregulated SOCS3 was observed in both 9-week-old (**D,F**) and 16-week-old (**G,I**) ALS mice in the brainstem, compared to WT mice (**A,C**). The levels of upregulated SOCS3 (**D,F,G,I,K,L**) were directly correlated with the extent of neuronal loss (**E,F,H,I,K,L**) over the course of ALS progression. Particularly, the ALS-in-duced increases in SOCS3 and NeuN+ neuronal loss were especially significant in the preBötC of brainstem, as shown in the higher-magnified images (**K,L**) compared to WT mice (**J**). Graphs repre-sent mean ± SEM of four animals per group per time-point for SOCS3 intensity (**M**) and NeuN+ neurons (**N**). * $p < 0.05$, ** $p < 0.01$, and *** $p < 0.001$ vs. WT mice; ++ $p < 0.01$ vs. 9-week-old ALS mice (one-way ANOVA followed by a Tukey test).

3.4. Significant Loss of Neurons When SOCS3 Is Pathologically Upregulated in the Cervical Spinal Cord of ALS Mice

Severe motor neuron loss in the spinal cord is an important feature of ALS mice during disease progression [40]. Accordingly, we next examined the expression levels of SOCS3 in the spinal cords of ALS mice. To determine whether SOCS3 levels are increased in different level of spinal cord before and after the disease onset of ALS, we first examined the expression levels of SOCS3 in the cervical spinal cord at both the pre-symptomatic stage (9 weeks of age) and early symptomatic stage (16 weeks of age) of ALS mice using IHC analyses. As found in the brainstem (Figures 2 and 3), IHC studies showed that the increased SOCS3 was largely located in NeuN+ neurons, especially the large neurons found in the ventral horn where motor neurons are mainly located (arrows in Figure 4F,L). SOCS3 was significantly increased by 12.5 times at 9 weeks of age (Figure 4D,F,M,O), and further increased by 25.3 times at 16 weeks of age (Figure 4J,L,N,O) in the cervical spinal cord of ALS mice, as compared to age-matched WT mice (Figure 4A,G,O). Moreover, not all increased SOCS3 was co-localized with NeuN+ neurons in the ventral horns of the cervical spinal cord; instead, some increased SOCS3 was co-localized with the traced fragment/debris or no signals of NeuN+ immunoreactivity (arrowheads, Figure 4F,L,M,N). These indicate that increased SOCS3 was produced by the dying or lost neurons, or even non-neuronal cells.

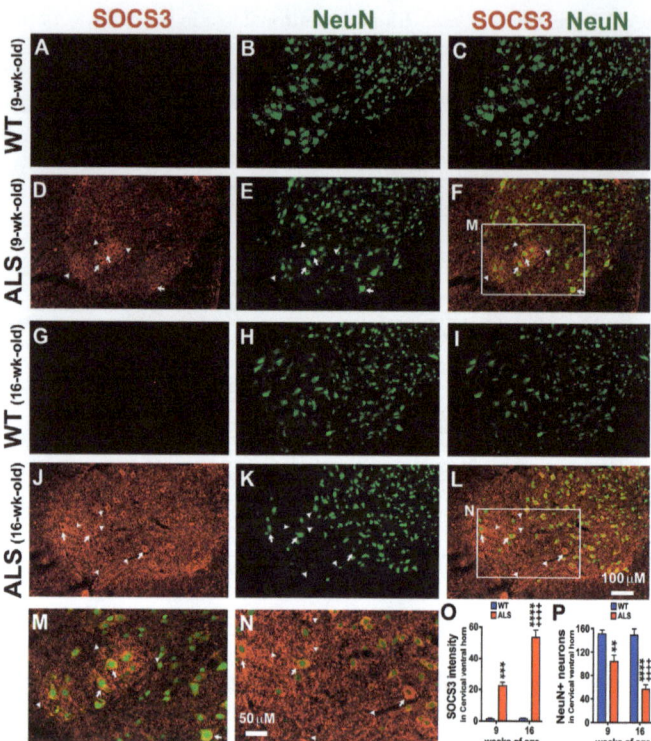

Figure 4. ALS significantly upregulates SOCS3 in the ventral horn of cervical spinal cord where neurons are lost. IHC was used to detect SOCS3 and NeuN+ neurons. Representative confocal im-ages show that SOCS3 levels were significantly upregulated in the ventral horn of the cervical spinal cord in ALS mice at 9 weeks (**D,F**) and 16 weeks (**J,L**) of age, as compared to WT mice at 9 weeks (**A,C**) and 16 weeks (**G,I**) old, respectively. Panels (**M**) and (**N**) are higher magnifications of the boxed areas (the major motor neuron pool in the ventral horn) in panels (**F**) and (**L**), respectively. The NeuN+ neurons were significantly decreased in ALS mice (**E,K,F,L,P**) over disease progression when compared to what found in WT mice (**B,H,C,I,P**). The ALS-increased SOCS3 was either co-localized with NeuN+ neurons (arrows) or not (arrowheads). Graphs represent mean ± SEM of four animals per group per time-point for SOCS3 intensity (**O**) and NeuN+ neurons (**P**). ** $p < 0.01$, *** $p < 0.001$, **** $p < 0.0001$ vs. age-matched WT mice; ++++ $p < 0.0001$ vs. 9-week-old ALS mice (two-way ANOVA followed by a Bonferroni test).

3.5. Significant Neuronal Loss and SOCS3 Upregulation Are Also Found in the Lumbar Spinal Cord of ALS Mice

Given that SOCS3 was highly upregulated in the neurons of the cervical spinal cords of ALS mice at the age of both 9 and 16 weeks (Figure 4), we next examined whether SOCS3 levels are upregulated in the lumbar spinal cords which modulates the hindlimbs function of ALS mice. Similar to what found in the cervical spinal cord (Figure 4), SOCS3 levels were found to be significantly upregulated at the pre-symptomatic stage (9 weeks of age, Figure 5D,F,M,O) and became exacerbated at the early symptomatic stage (16 weeks of age, Figure 5J,L,N,O) of ALS mice in the lumbar spinal cord, particularly in the large NeuN+ neurons found in the ventral horn where motor neurons are mainly located (arrows in Figure 5F,L–N). SOCS3 was significantly increased by 3 times at 9 weeks of age (Figure 5D,F,M,O), and increased by 8.2 times at 16 weeks of age (Figure 5J,L,N,O) in the lumbar spinal cord of ALS mice, as compared to age-matched WT mice (Figure 5A,G,O). The large NeuN+ neurons found in the ventral horn were significantly decreased by

26.5 percent at 9 weeks of age (Figure 5E,F,P) and decreased by 49 percent at 16 weeks of age (Figure 5K,L,P) in the lumbar spinal cord of ALS mice, compared to what we found in age-matched WT mice (Figure 5B,H,P). However, some increased SOCS3 immunoreactivity was not co-localized with NeuN+ neurons (arrowheads, Figure 5F,L–N), indicating that the increased SOCS3 was produced by not only NeuN+ neurons, but also the non-neuronal cells or the previous NeuN+ neurons, but died and were lost.

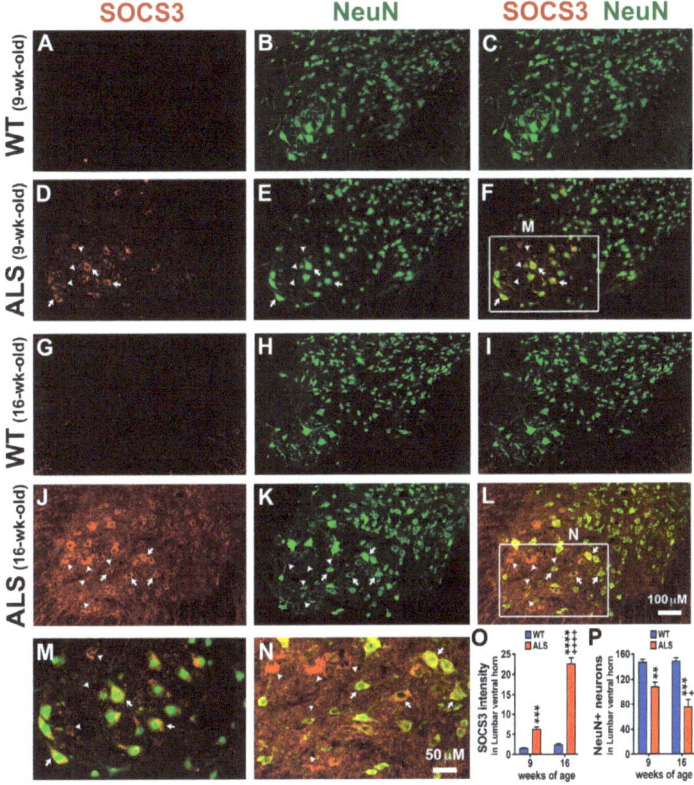

Figure 5. SOCS3 in SOD1-G93A mice is significantly upregulated in the ventral horn of the lumbar spinal cord where neurons are lost. IHC was used to detect SOCS3 and NeuN+ neurons. Representative confocal images showed that SOCS3 was significantly upregulated in the ventral horn of the lumbar spinal cord collected from ALS mice at both 9 (**D,F**) and 16 (**J,L**) weeks of age, as compared to the age-matched WT mice at 9 (**A,C**) and 16 weeks (**G,I**) old, respectively. In contrast, NeuN+ neurons were significantly decreased in ALS mice at both 9 (**E,F**) and 16 (**K,L**) weeks of age, as compared to the age-matched WT mice at 9 (**B,C**) and 16 weeks (**H,I**) old, respectively. Panels (**M**) and (**N**) are higher magnifications of the boxed areas (the major motor neuron pool in the ventral horn) in panels (**F**) and (**L**), respectively. The ALS-increased SOCS3 was either co-localized with NeuN+ neurons (arrows) or not (arrowheads). Graphs represent mean ± SEM of four animals per group per time-point for SOCS3 intensity (**O**) and NeuN+ neurons (**P**). ** $p < 0.01$, *** $p < 0.001$, and **** $p < 0.0001$ vs. age-matched WT mice; + $p < 0.05$ and ++++ $p < 0.0001$ vs. 9-week-old ALS mice (two-way ANOVA followed by a Bon-ferroni test).

3.6. ALS-Upregulated SOCS3 Is Partially Co-Localized with Reactive Microglia/Macrophages in the Lumbar Spinal Cord

During ALS progression, significant microgliosis and astrocytic activation have been found in the spinal cord of ALS mice [41], which contribute to motor neuron degeneration, both in animal models [42,43] and in ALS patients [44]. Since we did not find the increased SOCS3 in astrocytes in the brainstem (Figure 2) and spinal cords. We next examined whether ALS-upregulated SOCS3 was found in microglia/macrophages using IHC analyses of SOCS3 and Iba1. Iba1 is a microglia/macrophage-specific calcium-binding protein [45]. Similar to the increases in SOCS3 levels, the Iba1+ microglia/macrophages were significantly increased by 2.7 times at the pre-symptomatic stage (9 weeks of age) (Figure 6E,F,P), and further increased by 7.3 times at the early symptomatic stage (16 weeks of age) (Figure 6K,L,P) in the lumbar spinal cord of ALS mice, as compared to age-matched WT mice (Figure 6B,H,P). Importantly, the increased SOCS was partially co-localized with Iba1+ microglia/macrophages at 9 weeks of age (arrows in Figure 6F,M), and became more evident at 16 weeks of age (arrows in Figure 6L,N).

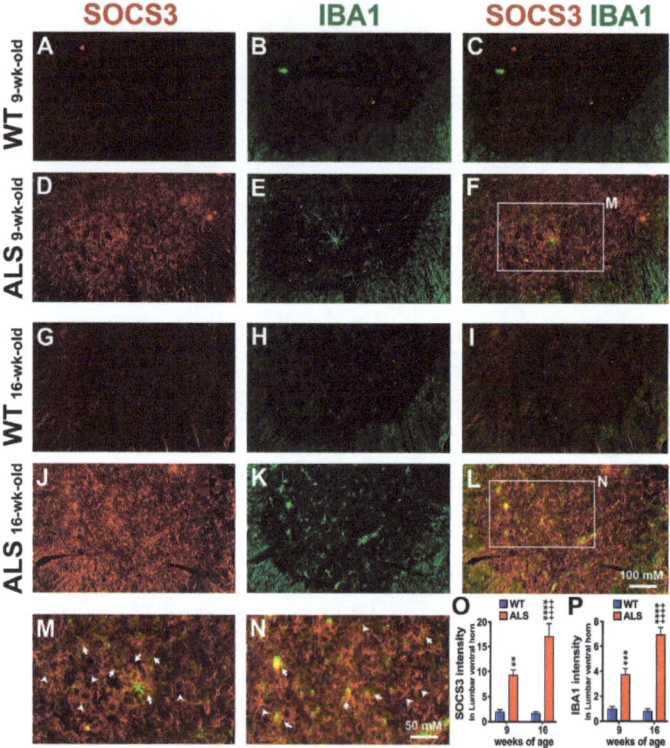

Figure 6. ALS-increased SOCS3 is partially co-localized with increased microglia/macrophages in the ventral horn of the lumbar spinal cord. IHC was used to detect SOCS3 and Iba1+ microglia/macrophages. Representative confocal images showed that SOCS3 was significantly increased in the ventral horn of the lumbar spinal cord collected from ALS mice at both 9 weeks (**D,F**) and 16 weeks (**J,L**) of age when compared to the age-matched WT mice at 9 weeks (**A,C**) and 16 weeks (**G,I**) old, respectively. In addition, Iba1+ microglia/macrophages were significantly increased in ALS mice (**E,K,F,L,P**) when compared to what found in WT mice (**B,H,C,I,P**). Panels (**M**) and (**N**) are higher magnifications of the boxed areas (the major motor neuron pool in the ventral horn) in panels (**F**) and (**L**), respectively. The ALS-increased SOCS3 was either co-localized with Iba1+ microglia/macrophages (arrows) or not (arrowheads). Graphs represent mean ± SEM of four animals per group per time-point for SOCS3 intensity (**O**) and Iba1+ neurons (**P**). ** $p < 0.01$, *** $p < 0.001$, and **** $p < 0.0001$ vs. age-matched WT mice; ++++ $p < 0.0001$ vs. 9-week-old ALS mice (two-way ANOVA followed by a Bonferroni test).

4. Discussion

In this study, we are the first to explore the potential role of SOCS3 in neuroinflammation and neuronal loss in ALS by examining the spatiotemporal expression of SOCS3 in SOD1-G93A ALS mice. IHC analyses showed that SOCS3 protein levels were significantly increased in both the ventral horn of spinal cords and preBötC of the brainstem of ALS mice at the pre-symptomatic stage; such increases were exacerbated at the early symptomatic phase. Concomitantly, SOCS3 levels were significantly upregulated over the course of the disease progression, and were directly related to the increased reactive astrogliosis and significant neuronal loss. Furthermore, SOCS3 levels were significantly upregulated prior to the disease onset, which suggest that SOCS3 may play a role in preceding ALS progression by the regulation of neuroinflammation.

The SOD1-G93A mice we have used are B6.Cg-Tg (SOD1*G93A)1Gur/J which have a high copy number of transgene $SOD1^{G93A}$ to have quicker disease onset and shorter lifespan, as compared to another SOD1-G93A mice with a low copy number of transgene $SOD1^{G93A}$. While there is no universal rule to define the disease onset due to individual variability and disease complication, we have chosen to follow the previous study [35] to determine disease onset as the time when mice reached maximum body weight; it is thus 14 weeks old in this study, as shown in Figure 1. To study if there are dynamic changes in SOCS3 levels as the disease progressed and to avoid the influence of variable disease onset in the SOD1-G93A mice, we have used 9-week-old mice for the pre-symptomatic studies and 16-week-old mice for the early symptomatic studies. The two time points allow us to detect the clear changes in the motor function, SOCS3 levels, astrogliosis, and neuronal loss, which provide critical insights into the dynamic SOCS3 levels as ALS progressed and a reasonable rationale to further investigate the SOCS3 levels in the late symptomatic stage and even the disease endpoint in the future.

An important feature of ALS mice during disease progression is severe motor neuron death that leads to progressive muscle wasting and paralysis [40]. The behavioral performance declined, as shown in Figure 1, and the motor function of ALS mice went into deficit after disease onset. Motor neurons typically have several dendrites and a large cell body which is located in the motor cortex, brainstem, or spinal cord. To study the full neuron profiles involved in the SOCS3 expression, we have chosen an antibody specific to NeuN rather than the motor neuron marker Choline Acetyltransferase (ChAT) for this study. While NeuN is a general neuronal marker, a portion of NeuN+ neurons with increased SOCS3 levels are known to be motor neurons based on their size and location in preBötC of the brainstem and ventral horn of the spinal cord. Importantly, our data show that not only motor neurons, but also another type of neurons are dying or lost with the increases in SOCS3 over ALS progression. Future studies will be needed to use different antibodies, including ChAT, to prove their identity. In addition, the expression of SOCS3 is not found to be different between WT and ALS mice in the cerebral pyramidal cells, which is relatively low, as compared to what we found in the brainstem and spinal cord.

We are interested in investigating SOCS3 expression in the brainstem, as most ALS patients are dying of respiratory complications, while their clinical presentations can be different. We find that SOCS3 levels were significantly increased from the pre-symptomatic to early symptomatic stage in the brainstem, especially in the preBötC. In parallel, we find that the neurons in preBötC of the brainstem were significantly lost over the course of ALS progression, which supports the evidence that dysfunction in the central control of breathing in some ALS patients may be related to preBötC degeneration [36]. Our findings suggest that respiratory neuron pools for breathing control are directly involved in progressive ALS pathology at the very early stage, and challenge the traditional explanation of respiratory failure in ALS, being that it causes motor neuron degeneration resulting in a weakness of the diaphragm and upper airway muscles, compromising the pump and patency of ventilation [46]. While we find that SOCS3 expression is significantly increased in the preBötC of ALS mice based on its unique anatomic location, future studies incorporating specific markers, such as Neurokinin-1 Receptor (NK1R), Somatostatin (SST),

ChAT, and Paired-Like Homeobox 2B (PHOX2B), are needed to more accurately distinguish the preBötC from Nucleus Ambiguus.

Neuroinflammation has been found in both ALS autopsy cases and experimental mouse models, and is a prominent pathological feature that is commonly found at sites of motor neuron injury [47]. Although it is not yet fully understood, an inflammatory process inside the central nervous system (CNS), including pro-inflammatory cytokines, has been considered to contribute to the pathogenesis of ALS [48,49]. It has been postulated that in the earliest stage of ALS, motor neurons release signals to trigger microglia responding in an anti-inflammatory phenotype to release neuroprotective factors in an attempt to repair motor neurons and to protect them from further injury. However, as the disease progress, motor neurons release signals that transform microglia from a protective anti-inflammatory to a cytotoxic pro-inflammatory phenotype, which causes astrocytic dysfunction, astrogliosis, and enhances motor neuron degeneration. While the cause for this phenotypic variability remains unknown; cytokines appear to be likely candidates for such changes [47,49]. Although definitive involvement of the SOCS family of proteins in ALS has not yet been directly explored, SOCS3, a cytokine-inducible protein, has been shown to be required for pro-inflammatory macrophage activation in vivo [50]. Without SOCS3, macrophages develop characteristic anti-inflammatory markers, even when exposed to pro-inflammatory stimuli [50]. These results are consistent with the findings that pro-inflammatory macrophages have been associated with increased SOCS3 [51]. This is also consistent with reports that mice with conditionally deleted SOCS3 expression in nestin-expressing cells have increased STAT3 activation, thereby limiting infiltration of inflammatory cells and subsequent neuron and oligodendrocyte death, which in turn leads to improved functional recovery after spinal cord injury (SCI) [12,52].

It is important to note, however, that although SOCS3 is a member of the SOCS protein family, which was initially characterized by its negative regulatory effects on cytokine signaling, the prevailing and most well-studied function of SOCS3 is to inhibit JAK/STAT signaling. Additional signaling pathways, such as the mitogen-activated protein kinases (MAPK), nuclear factor kappa-light-chain-enhancer of activated B cells (NF-kB) pathways, and insulin signaling are also modulated by SOCS3 [50], as shown in the acute injury models. The situation in a primary neurodegenerative disease may be quite different, and the consensus is that glial (inflammatory) responses drive disease progression in the SOD1-G93A ALS mice [53]. The SOCS3 upregulation found in ALS mice reflects ongoing and chronic neuroinflammation in the nervous system of ALS mice. More experiments will be needed to measure cytokine release and STAT3 activation in order to fully understand the whole picture on how SOCS3 influences the inflammatory responses, which may be the primary driver of ALS. The previous research findings for SOCS3 so far are either supportive or contradictory to each other, which could be due to the complexity of the mechanisms that SOCS3 regulates and the diversity of targets/signaling pathways involved. Additional experiments are therefore required to explore the roles that SOCS3 plays in response to a variety of both physiological and pathological conditions. Therefore, in the case of ALS, it appears evident that it would be extremely useful to investigate the roles of SOCS3, especially in order to develop new therapeutic approaches.

Surprisingly, SOCS3 protein levels were already significantly increased at the pre-symptomatic stage as early as 9 weeks old as examined, indicating that the ongoing neuroinflammation already started during the preclinical phase of the disease and preceded the ALS progression. These preclinical effects may be considered to be critical parameters for the future design of pharmacological trials in ALS. Most importantly, in this study, we are the first to report that increased SOCS3 levels (1) are directly associated with the increases in reactive astrocytes and microglia/macrophages in the ALS mice, and (2) are directly associated with the increases in the neuronal loss over the course of disease progression as early as at the pre-symptomatic stage and become more exaggerated in the early symptomatic stage. These findings support the hypothesis that microglia/macrophages-induced non-cell-autonomous toxicity on neurons is involved in the progressive ALS pathology [35,53,54] and call for further preclinical investigations to determine if SOCS3 plays a role in the pathogenesis of ALS, especially in the relation to the motor neuronal death via the non-cell-autonomous pathway.

5. Conclusions

The studies of the spatiotemporal expression of SOCS3 in ALS not only suggest the involvement of the neuroinflammation-associated non-cell-autonomous pathway in the progressive ALS pathogenesis, but also provide a potential therapeutic target for balancing an uncontrolled neuroinflammatory response through the manipulation of SOCS3 levels to regulate ALS progression.

Author Contributions: C.-Y.L. and Y.-S.L. designed the experiments. K.W. conducted rotarod and grip strength tests. C.-Y.L. and V.V. performed IHC. V.V. and D.T. took the confocal images. K.W. harvested the tissues. D.T. analyzed the data. C.-Y.L. and Y.-S.L. provided support and advice on every experimental step. The manuscript was written by C.-Y.L. and revised by Y.-S.L. All authors have read and agreed to the published version of the manuscript.

Funding: This study was supported by Cleveland Clinic Technology Development Investment Project and Ohio Third Frontier Technology Validation and Start-up Fund: 2022-040.

Institutional Review Board Statement: The animal study protocol was approved by the Institutional Animal Care and Use Committee at the Cleveland Clinic (protocol code Protocol 00003107 and date of approval 4 May 2023).

Informed Consent Statement: Not applicable.

Data Availability Statement: Data are contained within the articles.

Conflicts of Interest: The authors declare no conflicts of interests.

References

1. Wijesekera, L.C.; Leigh, P.N. Amyotrophic lateral sclerosis. *Orphanet J. Rare Dis.* **2009**, *4*, 3. [CrossRef]
2. Palomo, G.M.; Manfredi, G. Exploring new pathways of neurodegeneration in ALS: The role of mitochondria quality control. *Brain Res.* **2015**, *1607*, 36–46. [CrossRef] [PubMed]
3. Cianciulli, A.; Calvello, R.; Porro, C.; Trotta, T.; Panaro, M.A. Understanding the role of SOCS signaling in neurodegenerative diseases: Current and emerging concepts. *Cytokine Growth Factor Rev.* **2017**, *37*, 67–79. [CrossRef] [PubMed]
4. Smith, E.F.; Shaw, P.J.; De Vos, K.J. The role of mitochondria in amyotrophic lateral sclerosis. *Neurosci. Lett.* **2019**, *710*, 132933. [CrossRef]
5. Ferraiuolo, L.; Kirby, J.; Grierson, A.J.; Sendtner, M.; Shaw, P.J. Molecular pathways of motor neuron injury in amyotrophic lateral sclerosis. *Nat. Rev. Neurol.* **2011**, *7*, 616–630. [CrossRef] [PubMed]
6. Abel, O.; Powell, J.F.; Andersen, P.M.; Al-Chalabi, A. ALSoD: A user-friendly online bioinformatics tool for amyotrophic lateral sclerosis genetics. *Hum. Mutat.* **2012**, *33*, 1345–1351. [CrossRef] [PubMed]
7. Rosen, D.R. Mutations in Cu/Zn superoxide dismutase gene are associated with familial amyotrophic lateral sclerosis. *Nature* **1993**, *364*, 362. [CrossRef] [PubMed]
8. Thonhoff, J.R.; Beers, D.R.; Zhao, W.; Pleitez, M.; Simpson, E.P.; Berry, J.D.; Cudkowicz, M.E.; Appel, S.H. Expanded autologous regulatory T-lymphocyte infusions in ALS: A phase I, first-in-human study. *Neurol. Neuroimmunol. Neuroinflamm.* **2018**, *5*, e465. [CrossRef] [PubMed]
9. Lyon, M.S.; Wosiski-Kuhn, M.; Gillespie, R.; Caress, J.; Milligan, C. Inflammation, Immunity, and amyotrophic lateral sclerosis: I. Etiology and pathology. *Muscle Nerve* **2019**, *59*, 10–22. [CrossRef]
10. Wosiski-Kuhn, M.; Lyon, M.S.; Caress, J.; Milligan, C. Inflammation, immunity, and amyotrophic lateral sclerosis: II. immune-modulating therapies. *Muscle Nerve* **2019**, *59*, 23–33. [CrossRef]
11. McCauley, M.E.; Baloh, R.H. Inflammation in ALS/FTD pathogenesis. *Acta Neuropathol.* **2019**, *137*, 715–730. [CrossRef] [PubMed]
12. Baker, B.J.; Akhtar, L.N.; Benveniste, E.N. SOCS1 and SOCS3 in the control of CNS immunity. *Trends Immunol.* **2009**, *30*, 392–400. [CrossRef] [PubMed]
13. Yoshimura, A.; Naka, T.; Kubo, M. SOCS proteins, cytokine signalling and immune regulation. *Nat. Rev. Immunol.* **2007**, *7*, 454–465. [CrossRef] [PubMed]
14. Polizzotto, M.N.; Bartlett, P.F.; Turnley, A.M. Expression of "suppressor of cytokine signalling" (SOCS) genes in the developing and adult mouse nervous system. *J. Comp. Neurol.* **2000**, *423*, 348–358. [CrossRef] [PubMed]
15. Goldshmit, Y.; Greenhalgh, C.J.; Turnley, A.M. Suppressor of cytokine signalling-2 and epidermal growth factor regulate neurite outgrowth of cortical neurons. *Eur. J. Neurosci.* **2004**, *20*, 2260–2266. [CrossRef] [PubMed]

16. Nicholson, S.E.; De Souza, D.; Fabri, L.J.; Corbin, J.; Willson, T.A.; Zhang, J.G.; Silva, A.; Asimakis, M.; Farley, A.; Nash, A.D.; et al. Suppressor of cytokine signaling-3 preferentially binds to the SHP-2-binding site on the shared cytokine receptor subunit gp130. *Proc. Natl. Acad. Sci. USA* **2000**, *97*, 6493–6498. [CrossRef] [PubMed]
17. Schmitz, J.; Weissenbach, M.; Haan, S.; Heinrich, P.C.; Schaper, F. SOCS3 exerts its inhibitory function on interleukin-6 signal transduction through the SHP2 recruitment site of gp130. *J. Biol. Chem.* **2000**, *275*, 12848–12856. [CrossRef]
18. Yadav, A.; Kalita, A.; Dhillon, S.; Banerjee, K. JAK/STAT3 pathway is involved in survival of neurons in response to insulin-like growth factor and negatively regulated by suppressor of cytokine signaling-3. *J. Biol. Chem.* **2005**, *280*, 31830–31840. [CrossRef]
19. Miao, T.; Wu, D.; Zhang, Y.; Bo, X.; Subang, M.C.; Wang, P.; Richardson, P.M. Suppressor of cytokine signaling-3 suppresses the ability of activated signal transducer and activator of transcription-3 to stimulate neurite growth in rat primary sensory neurons. *J. Neurosci.* **2006**, *26*, 9512–9519. [CrossRef]
20. Park, K.W.; Nozell, S.E.; Benveniste, E.N. Protective role of STAT3 in NMDA and glutamate-induced neuronal death: Negative regulatory effect of SOCS3. *PLoS ONE* **2012**, *7*, e50874. [CrossRef]
21. Park, K.W.; Lin, C.Y.; Lee, Y.S. Expression of suppressor of cytokine signaling-3 (SOCS3) and its role in neuronal death after complete spinal cord injury. *Exp. Neurol.* **2014**, *261*, 65–75. [CrossRef]
22. Park, K.W.; Lin, C.Y.; Li, K.; Lee, Y.S. Effects of Reducing Suppressors of Cytokine Signaling-3 (SOCS3) Expression on Dendritic Outgrowth and Demyelination after Spinal Cord Injury. *PLoS ONE* **2015**, *10*, e0138301. [CrossRef] [PubMed]
23. Miao, T.; Wu, D.; Zhang, Y.; Bo, X.; Xiao, F.; Zhang, X.; Magoulas, C.; Subang, M.C.; Wang, P.; Richardson, P.M. SOCS3 suppresses AP-1 transcriptional activity in neuroblastoma cells through inhibition of c-Jun N-terminal kinase. *Mol. Cell. Neurosci.* **2008**, *37*, 367–375. [CrossRef] [PubMed]
24. Sun, F.; Park, K.K.; Belin, S.; Wang, D.; Lu, T.; Chen, G.; Zhang, K.; Yeung, C.; Feng, G.; Yankner, B.A.; et al. Sustained axon regeneration induced by co-deletion of PTEN and SOCS3. *Nature* **2011**, *480*, 372–375. [CrossRef] [PubMed]
25. Lin, C.; Chao, H.; Li, Z.; Xu, X.; Liu, Y.; Hou, L.; Liu, N.; Ji, J. Melatonin attenuates traumatic brain injury-induced inflammation: A possible role for mitophagy. *J. Pineal Res.* **2016**, *61*, 177–186. [CrossRef] [PubMed]
26. McGarry, T.; Orr, C.; Wade, S.; Biniecka, M.; Wade, S.; Gallagher, L.; Low, C.; Veale, D.J.; Fearon, U. JAK-STAT blockade alters synovial bioenergetics, mitochondrial function and pro-inflammatory mediators in Rheumatoid arthritis. *Arthritis Rheumatol.* **2018**, *70*, 1959–1970. [CrossRef] [PubMed]
27. Heiman-Patterson, T.D.; Deitch, J.S.; Blankenhorn, E.P.; Erwin, K.L.; Perreault, M.J.; Alexander, B.K.; Byers, N.; Toman, I.; Alexander, G.M. Background and gender effects on survival in the TgN(SOD1-G93A)1Gur mouse model of ALS. *J. Neurol. Sci.* **2005**, *236*, 1–7. [CrossRef] [PubMed]
28. Xie, Y.; Zhou, B.; Lin, M.Y.; Sheng, Z.H. Progressive endolysosomal deficits impair autophagic clearance beginning at early asymptomatic stages in fALS mice. *Autophagy* **2015**, *11*, 1934–1936. [CrossRef] [PubMed]
29. Xie, Y.; Zhou, B.; Lin, M.Y.; Wang, S.; Foust, K.D.; Sheng, Z.H. Endolysosomal Deficits Augment Mitochondria Pathology in Spinal Motor Neurons of Asymptomatic fALS Mice. *Neuron* **2015**, *87*, 355–370. [CrossRef]
30. Choi, C.I.; Lee, Y.D.; Gwag, B.J.; Cho, S.I.; Kim, S.S.; Suh-Kim, H. Effects of estrogen on lifespan and motor functions in female hSOD1 G93A transgenic mice. *J. Neurol. Sci.* **2008**, *268*, 40–47. [CrossRef]
31. Wooley, C.M.; Sher, R.B.; Kale, A.; Frankel, W.N.; Cox, G.A.; Seburn, K.L. Gait analysis detects early changes in transgenic SOD1(G93A) mice. *Muscle Nerve* **2005**, *32*, 43–50. [CrossRef] [PubMed]
32. Dobrowolny, G.; Giacinti, C.; Pelosi, L.; Nicoletti, C.; Winn, N.; Barberi, L.; Molinaro, M.; Rosenthal, N.; Musaro, A. Muscle expression of a local Igf-1 isoform protects motor neurons in an ALS mouse model. *J. Cell Biol.* **2005**, *168*, 193–199. [CrossRef] [PubMed]
33. Hayworth, C.R.; Gonzalez-Lima, F. Pre-symptomatic detection of chronic motor deficits and genotype prediction in congenic B6.SOD1(G93A) ALS mouse model. *Neuroscience* **2009**, *164*, 975–985. [CrossRef] [PubMed]
34. Banerjee, R.; Mosley, R.L.; Reynolds, A.D.; Dhar, A.; Jackson-Lewis, V.; Gordon, P.H.; Przedborski, S.; Gendelman, H.E. Adaptive immune neuroprotection in G93A-SOD1 amyotrophic lateral sclerosis mice. *PLoS ONE* **2008**, *3*, e2740. [CrossRef] [PubMed]
35. Boillee, S.; Yamanaka, K.; Lobsiger, C.S.; Copeland, N.G.; Jenkins, N.A.; Kassiotis, G.; Kollias, G.; Cleveland, D.W. Onset and progression in inherited ALS determined by motor neurons and microglia. *Science* **2006**, *312*, 1389–1392. [CrossRef] [PubMed]
36. Howell, B.N.; Newman, D.S. Dysfunction of central control of breathing in amyotrophic lateral sclerosis. *Muscle Nerve* **2017**, *56*, 197–201. [CrossRef] [PubMed]
37. Sales de Campos, P.; Olsen, W.L.; Wymer, J.P.; Smith, B.K. Respiratory therapies for Amyotrophic Lateral Sclerosis: A state of the art review. *Chron. Respir. Dis.* **2023**, *20*, 14799731231175915. [CrossRef]
38. Ikeda, K.; Kawakami, K.; Onimaru, H.; Okada, Y.; Yokota, S.; Koshiya, N.; Oku, Y.; Iizuka, M.; Koizumi, H. The respiratory control mechanisms in the brainstem and spinal cord: Integrative views of the neuroanatomy and neurophysiology. *J. Physiol. Sci.* **2017**, *67*, 45–62. [CrossRef]
39. Menuet, C.; Connelly, A.A.; Bassi, J.K.; Melo, M.R.; Le, S.; Kamar, J.; Kumar, N.N.; McDougall, S.J.; McMullan, S.; Allen, A.M. PreBotzinger complex neurons drive respiratory modulation of blood pressure and heart rate. *Elife* **2020**, *9*, e57288. [CrossRef]
40. Zhang, X.; Chen, S.; Li, L.; Wang, Q.; Le, W. Decreased level of 5-methyltetrahydrofolate: A potential biomarker for pre-symptomatic amyotrophic lateral sclerosis. *J. Neurol. Sci.* **2010**, *293*, 102–105. [CrossRef]
41. Hall, E.D.; Oostveen, J.A.; Gurney, M.E. Relationship of microglial and astrocytic activation to disease onset and progression in a transgenic model of familial ALS. *Glia* **1998**, *23*, 249–256. [CrossRef]

42. Diaz-Amarilla, P.; Olivera-Bravo, S.; Trias, E.; Cragnolini, A.; Martinez-Palma, L.; Cassina, P.; Beckman, J.; Barbeito, L. Phenotypically aberrant astrocytes that promote motoneuron damage in a model of inherited amyotrophic lateral sclerosis. *Proc. Natl. Acad. Sci. USA* **2011**, *108*, 18126–18131. [CrossRef]
43. Yamanaka, K.; Boillee, S.; Roberts, E.A.; Garcia, M.L.; McAlonis-Downes, M.; Mikse, O.R.; Cleveland, D.W.; Goldstein, L.S. Mutant SOD1 in cell types other than motor neurons and oligodendrocytes accelerates onset of disease in ALS mice. *Proc. Natl. Acad. Sci. USA* **2008**, *105*, 7594–7599. [CrossRef]
44. Sanagi, T.; Yuasa, S.; Nakamura, Y.; Suzuki, E.; Aoki, M.; Warita, H.; Itoyama, Y.; Uchino, S.; Kohsaka, S.; Ohsawa, K. Appearance of phagocytic microglia adjacent to motoneurons in spinal cord tissue from a presymptomatic transgenic rat model of amyotrophic lateral sclerosis. *J. Neurosci. Res.* **2010**, *88*, 2736–2746. [CrossRef] [PubMed]
45. Ohsawa, K.; Imai, Y.; Sasaki, Y.; Kohsaka, S. Microglia/macrophage-specific protein Iba1 binds to fimbrin and enhances its actin-bundling activity. *J. Neurochem.* **2004**, *88*, 844–856. [CrossRef]
46. Vrijsen, B.; Testelmans, D.; Belge, C.; Robberecht, W.; Van Damme, P.; Buyse, B. Non-invasive ventilation in amyotrophic lateral sclerosis. *Amyotroph. Lateral. Scler. Frontotemporal. Degener.* **2013**, *14*, 85–95. [CrossRef]
47. Zhao, W.; Beers, D.R.; Appel, S.H. Immune-mediated mechanisms in the pathoprogression of amyotrophic lateral sclerosis. *J. Neuroimmune Pharmacol.* **2013**, *8*, 888–899. [CrossRef] [PubMed]
48. McCombe, P.A.; Henderson, R.D. The Role of immune and inflammatory mechanisms in ALS. *Curr. Mol. Med.* **2011**, *11*, 246–254. [CrossRef]
49. Zhao, W.; Beers, D.R.; Hooten, K.G.; Sieglaff, D.H.; Zhang, A.; Kalyana-Sundaram, S.; Traini, C.M.; Halsey, W.S.; Hughes, A.M.; Sathe, G.M.; et al. Characterization of Gene Expression Phenotype in Amyotrophic Lateral Sclerosis Monocytes. *JAMA Neurol.* **2017**, *74*, 677–685. [CrossRef]
50. Liu, Y.; Stewart, K.N.; Bishop, E.; Marek, C.J.; Kluth, D.C.; Rees, A.J.; Wilson, H.M. Unique expression of suppressor of cytokine signaling 3 is essential for classical macrophage activation in rodents in vitro and in vivo. *J. Immunol.* **2008**, *180*, 6270–6278. [CrossRef]
51. Wilson, H.M. SOCS Proteins in Macrophage Polarization and Function. *Front. Immunol.* **2014**, *5*, 357. [CrossRef] [PubMed]
52. Okada, S.; Nakamura, M.; Katoh, H.; Miyao, T.; Shimazaki, T.; Ishii, K.; Yamane, J.; Yoshimura, A.; Iwamoto, Y.; Toyama, Y.; et al. Conditional ablation of Stat3 or Socs3 discloses a dual role for reactive astrocytes after spinal cord injury. *Nat. Med.* **2006**, *12*, 829–834. [CrossRef] [PubMed]
53. Boillee, S.; Vande Velde, C.; Cleveland, D.W. ALS: A disease of motor neurons and their nonneuronal neighbors. *Neuron* **2006**, *52*, 39–59. [CrossRef]
54. Bennett, M.L.; Viaene, A.N. What are activated and reactive glia and what is their role in neurodegeneration? *Neurobiol. Dis.* **2021**, *148*, 105172. [CrossRef] [PubMed]

Disclaimer/Publisher's Note: The statements, opinions and data contained in all publications are solely those of the individual author(s) and contributor(s) and not of MDPI and/or the editor(s). MDPI and/or the editor(s) disclaim responsibility for any injury to people or property resulting from any ideas, methods, instructions or products referred to in the content.

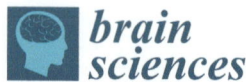

Article

Ventriculoperitoneal Shunt Treatment Increases 7 Alpha Hy-Droxy-3-Oxo-4-Cholestenoic Acid and 24-Hydroxycholesterol Concentrations in Idiopathic Normal Pressure Hydrocephalus

Emanuele Porru [1,†], Erik Edström [2,†], Lisa Arvidsson [2,†], Adrian Elmi-Terander [3,*], Alexander Fletcher-Sandersjöö [2], Anita Lövgren Sandblom [1], Magnus Hansson [1], Frida Duell [1] and Ingemar Björkhem [1]

[1] Division of Clinical Chemistry, Department of Laboratory Medicine, Karolinska University Hospital, 141 57 Huddinge, Sweden
[2] Department of Neurosurgery, Karolinska University Hospital, Department of Clinical Neuroscience, Karolinska Institutet, 171 77 Solna, Sweden
[3] Stockholm Spine Centre, Department of Clinical Neuroscience, Karolinska Institutet, 171 77 Solna, Sweden
* Correspondence: adrian.elmi.terander@ki.se
† These authors contributed equally to this work.

Abstract: Idiopathic normal pressure hydrocephalus (iNPH) is the most common form of hydrocephalus in the adult population, and is often treated with cerebrospinal fluid (CSF) drainage using a ventriculoperitoneal (VP) shunt. Symptoms of iNPH include gait impairment, cognitive decline, and urinary incontinence. The pathophysiology behind the symptoms of iNPH is still unknown, and no reliable biomarkers have been established to date. The aim of this study was to investigate the possible use of the oxysterols as biomarkers in this disease. CSF levels of the oxysterols 24S- and 27-hydroxycholesterol, as well as the major metabolite of 27-hydroxycholesterol, 7 alpha hydroxy-3-oxo-4-cholestenoic acid (7HOCA), were measured in iNPH-patients before and after treatment with a VP-shunt. Corresponding measurements were also performed in healthy controls. VP-shunt treatment significantly increased the levels of 7HOCA and 24S-hydroxycholesterol in CSF ($p = 0.014$ and $p = 0.037$, respectively). The results are discussed in relation to the beneficial effects of VP-shunt treatment. Furthermore, the possibility that CSF drainage may reduce an inhibitory effect of transiently increased pressure on the metabolic capacity of neuronal cells in the brain is discussed. This capacity includes the elimination of cholesterol by the 24S-hydroxylase mechanisms.

Keywords: oxysterols; 27-hydroxycholesterol; 7 alpha hydroxy-3-oxo-4-cholestenoic acid; 24S-hydroxycholesterol; CSF-drainage; idiopathic normal pressure hydrocephalus; ventriculoperitoneal shunt; shunt-treatment; biomarker; cerebrospinal fluid

1. Introduction

Idiopathic normal pressure hydrocephalus (iNPH) is a treatable neurological disorder affecting the elderly. The condition is characterized by gait and balance impairments, urinary incontinence and cognitive decline. Diagnostic imaging shows signs of disturbed cerebrospinal fluid (CSF) dynamics, including ventricular enlargement and widened sulci. These findings and the clinical symptoms are thought to reflect impaired CSF outflow and increased intracerebral pressure pulsatility [1,2]. The mechanisms involved in the transport of interstitial fluid and CSF across the blood–brain barrier have not been defined with certainty.

Similarly, the pathophysiology resulting in the triad of iNPH symptoms is also not clearly understood. However, clinical features of the disease include psychomotor slowing, executive dysfunction, impaired attention, decreased verbal fluency and worsened working memory, all of which correlate with the typical patterns of frontal lobe dysfunction [3–5].

Radiology studies have demonstrated that patients with iNPH mainly present with a hypoperfusion in the frontal lobe and reduced blood flow in the periventricular area [6–8]. Compared to those with Alzheimer's disease, who also have frontal lobe deficits, iNPH patients generally have milder symptoms.

The symptoms of this disease are potentially reversible if recognized early and treated with a ventriculoperitoneal (VP)-shunt. However, it is notable that the positive effects of the drainage of CSF are not accompanied by a reduction in ventricular size [9].

To evaluate the effect of drainage before VP-shunt surgery, CSF drainage through a lumbar puncture is routinely performed as a diagnostic tool. The patients are evaluated for relevant symptoms including gait, balance, cognition and incontinence before and after the lumbar puncture. The purpose is to identify those that are improved by CSF drainage and consequently have a greater chance of benefitting from VP-shunt treatment. A VP-shunt is a silicone tube with one end placed through the brain into the enlarged ventricles and the other end in the abdominal cavity. The rest of the tube is placed subcutaneously, and a valve defines the flow and pressure gradients needed for drainage.

iNPH is regarded as one of the most misdiagnosed diseases worldwide and may occur with varying combinations or degrees of other neurological conditions, including Alzheimer's disease, Parkinson's disease and vascular dementia [2]. Diagnosis is based on symptoms, clinical findings and radiological imaging. However, not all patients respond to CSF drainage and there is a need for improved diagnostic tools and markers to predict treatment outcomes. No distinct laboratory biomarker has been defined to date. However, levels of CSF cortisol, cortisone dehydroepiandrosterone (DHEA), 7 alpha hydroxy dehydroepiandrosterone (7DHEA), 7β-OH-DHEA, 7-oxo-DHEA, 16α-OH-DHEA and aldosterone have been shown to differ between iNPH patients and controls [10]. In the brain 27-OH is metabolized into 7HOCA [11]. 7HOCA may also be produced in extracerebral tissue from 7α-hydroxy-4-cholestene-3-one and naturally occurs in human blood [11,12]. An uptake of 7HOCA from the circulation occurs in the liver, where it is transformed into bile acid [13,14].

The most common oxysterols in CSF include 24S-hydroxycholesterol (24-OH), 27-hydroxycholesterol (27-OH) and the major oxysterol metabolite 7 alpha hydroxy-3-oxo-4-cholestenoic acid (7HOCA) [15,16]. The origin and metabolism of these three sterols are different, and their concentration in CSF is dependent on their sites of primary production, flux across the blood–brain barrier, rate of metabolism in, and elimination from the brain to the CSF [17] (Figure 1).

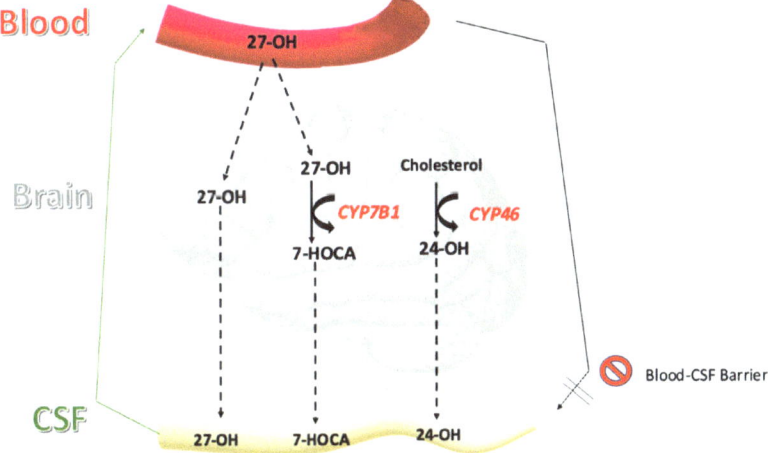

Figure 1. Flux of oxysterols into the cerebrospinal fluid.

In humans, 24-OH is almost exclusively formed in the brain and there is a continuous flux of 24-OH from the brain into the circulation. There is also a modest flux of this oxysterol from the brain into the CSF. The 24-OH present in CSF has a mixed origin: part of it originates directly from the brain and part of it originates from the circulation. This means that the integrity of the blood–brain barrier is important for the levels of 24-OH in CSF [18].

There is very little formation of 27-OH in the brain, and most of this oxysterol in the brain and CSF originates from the circulation. Despite the relatively high uptake of this oxysterol by the brain the levels in both brain and CSF are low, reflecting a very efficient metabolism. Given the negative effects of this oxysterol on various brain functions [19–28], this rapid metabolism can be regarded as a detoxification. The end metabolite of 27-OH in the brain is 7HOCA and there is a net flux of this steroid acid from the brain into the circulation. There is also a flux of this metabolite from the brain into CSF and the concentration in CSF is higher than that of any other oxysterol [15,16]. There is also an extracerebral formation of 7HOCA and there may be a small contribution from the circulation to the content in CSF. Most of the effect of blood–brain barrier defects on the concentration of 7HOCA in CSF is thought to be a consequence of the higher influx of the precursor 27-OH [16].

Previous studies have shown normal levels of 7HOCA in patients with Alzheimer's disease or vascular dementia [16]. In contrast, patients with subdural hematoma or subarachnoid hemorrhage demonstrate an increased level of 7HOCA [14,29,30]. In a review by Sodero, it is suggested that 24-OH has the potential to be used as a stable biomarker for various neurological diseases [31].

Based on the above findings, this study aims to investigate the possible use of the oxysterols 24-OH, 27-OH and 7HOCA as biomarkers in iNPH. In addition, the findings may further our mechanistic understanding of the effects of CSF drainage in iNPH.

2. Materials and Methods

2.1. Patient Selection and Study Setting

All adult patients (≥ 18 years) who were offered surgical treatment for iNPH between 2020 and 2022 were eligible for inclusion. The study hospital is a publicly funded and owned tertiary care center, serving a region of roughly 2.3 million inhabitants, and the only neurosurgical center in the region. As part of routine management, referrals to the study center for iNPH were evaluated at a multidisciplinary conference. Cases matching the clinical and radiological criteria for a diagnosis of iNPH were further evaluated in accordance with international guidelines [32], which include scores for gait, balance, incontinence and cognition. At the study hospital, the Hellstrom scale is used for the evaluation of these symptoms [33]. A lumbar tap test was performed to identify patients that improved after CSF-drainage. The tap test is the removal of 30ml of CSF through a lumbar puncture. In addition, a standardized grading of symptoms is performed before and after the removal of CSF. A positive response is defined as an improvement of 5 on a Hellstrom scale [33]. Medical records and imaging data from digital hospital charts were retrospectively reviewed using the health record software TakeCare (CompuGroup Medical Sweden AB, Farsta, Sweden). The study was approved by the National Ethical Review Board (Dnr 2019-04241).

Seventeen patients with iNPH (age 51–88, mean 74) accepted to participate in the study and signed informed consent after having received both written and oral information [32]. CSF samples were collected from 10 iNPH patients before and after treatment with an intraventricular VP-shunt. Seven patients provided CSF only before surgery. Postoperative samples were collected at a median of 4.5 months post-surgery. Twenty-eight patients of similar age, investigated with lumbar puncture for headaches and without pathological CSF findings, were used as controls.

2.2. Laboratory Analyses

Albumin was measured using Tina-quant Albumin Gen.2 kit (Roche, Basel, Switzerland). Analytical standards (pure > 98%) of each oxysterol were used for calibration and quantification. 7HOCA was measured by isotope dilution mass spectrometry as described previously [23,30]. The method for 7alpha-hydroxy dehydroepiandrosterone (7DHEA), along with 24-OH and 27OH, was developed and validated to obtain a new comprehensive analytical tool for endogenous oxysterols. The analyses were performed using deuterium labeled 27-OH and deuterium labeled 24- hydroxycholesterol as internal standard. Deuterium labeled 7DHEA was not available as internal standard. Instead, based on our results in terms of precision and accuracy, 27-OH-d5 was used as an internal standard for 7DHEA quantification. In brief, 500 mL of each sample was hydrolyzed by sodium hydroxide solution and heated at 60 °C for 1 h. Following two extractions with 3mL of chloroform, the samples were chemically derivatized by trimethylsylilation prior to analysis by ID-GCMS. Three μL of each sample were injected into a GC-MS system (Agilent GC4890, MS 5973, Santa Clara, CA, USA). The column used was a Agilent J&W HP-5ms 5%-phenyl)-methylpolysiloxane, (0.25 mm × 30 m, 0.25 μm), with the following analytical conditions: an injector temperature of 250 °C, splitless mode, gas flow rate 1 mL/min, oven temperature ramped from 180 °C to 250 in 3.5 min, and subsequently ramped to 300 °C in 12.5 min and held for 9 min, for a total run time of 25 min. The method was validated to satisfy analytical requirement in terms of accuracy (bias < 5%), reproducibility (CV < 5%) and recovery during the extraction step (>95%).

2.3. Statistical Analysis

The Shapiro–Wilk test was used to evaluate the normality of the data. As all continuous data significantly deviated from a normal distribution pattern (Shapiro–Wilk test p value < 0.05), it is presented as a median (range) and categorical data as numbers (proportion). The Mann–Whitney U test was used to compare pre- and postoperative metabolites in the treatment group to non-treated controls (non-matched continuous data), and the Wilcoxon signed-ranks test was used to compare metabolites in each treated patient before and after surgery (matched continuous data). All analyses were conducted using the statistical software program R. Statistical significance was set at $p < 0.05$.

2.4. Ethical Aspects

The study was approved by Swedish Ethical Authority and informed consent were obtained for each patient (Dnr 2019-04241). The CSF from anonymous control subjects was obtained from the clinical chemical routine lab. Only information about age and sex was given to the lab analyzing oxysterols.

3. Results

The oxysterols 7HOCA, 24-OH, and 27-OH as well as cholesterol, and albumin were measured in 17 iNPH patients and 28 controls. In 10 patients, a repeated analysis was performed at median 4.5 months after VP-shunt surgery.

The pre-operative concentrations of cholesterol, 24-OH and 27-OH were significantly lower in iNPH patients compared to controls, while no difference was seen for albumin or 7HOCA (Table 1, Figure 2). For the iNPH patients, surgery was then associated with a significant increase in 24-OH and 7HOCA, as well as a trend towards a significant increase for 27-OH (Table 2, Figure 2). As a result of this increase, post-operative analysis revealed that there was no longer any significant difference in 24-OH and 27-OH between iNPH patients and the control group (Table 3, Figure 2).

Table 1. Pre-operative metabolites in the treatment group vs. non-treated controls.

Oxysterol	Treatment ($n = 17$)	Control ($n = 28$)	p-Value
Albumin (mg/L)	243 (72–529)	205 (115–483), (5 missing)	0.547
Cholesterol (µg/mL)	2.3 (1.3–12), (1 missing)	3.9 (1.9–7.5)	**<0.001**
24-OH (ng/mL)	1.1 (0.5–4.0)	1.9 (0.8–5.4)	**0.006**
27-OH (ng/mL)	0.7 (0.3–1.7)	1.1 (0.4–2.5)	**0.001**
7HOCA (ng/mL)	14 (6.8–28)	17 (10–31), (2 missing)	0.186

Data is presented as median (range). Data compared using the Mann–Whitney U test (non-matched continuous data). Bold text in the p-value column indicates a statistically significant association ($p < 0.05$). Abbreviations: 24-OH = 24S-hydroxycholesterol; 27-OH = 27-hydroxycholesterol; 7HOCA = 7 alpha hydroxy-3-oxo-4-cholestenoic acid.

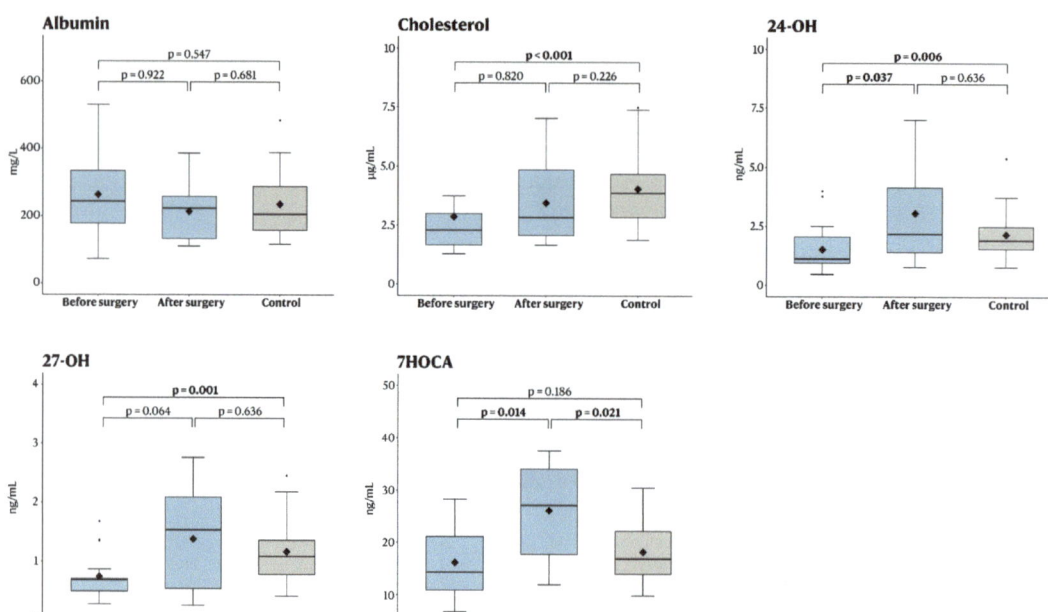

Figure 2. Boxplot showing concentrations before and after surgery, as well as compared to healthy controls. The Mann–Whitney U test was used to compare pre- and postoperative metabolites in the treatment group to non-treated controls (non-matched continuous data), and the Wilcoxon signed-ranks test was used to compare metabolites in each treated patient before and after surgery (matched continuous data).

Table 2. Matched comparisons between metabolites before and after surgery.

Oxysterol	Before Surgery ($n = 10$)	After Surgery ($n = 10$)	p-Value
Albumin (mg/L)	215 (72–518)	222 (110–386)	0.922
Cholesterol (µg/mL)	2.5 (1.3–12) (1 missing)	2.8 (1.7–7.0) (1 missing)	0.820
24-OH (ng/mL)	1.6 (0.6–4.0)	2.2 (0.8–7.0)	**0.037**
27-OH (ng/mL)	0.7 (0.4–1.7)	1.5 (0.2–2.8)	0.064
7HOCA (ng/mL)	17 (6.8–28)	27 (12–38)	**0.014**

Data is presented as median (range). Data compared using the Wilcoxon signed-ranks test (matched continuous data). Bold text in the p-value column indicates a statistically significant association ($p < 0.05$). Abbreviations: 24-OH = 24S-hydroxycholesterol; 27-OH = 27-hydroxycholesterol; 7HOCA = 7 alpha hydroxy-3-oxo-4-cholestenoic acid.

Table 3. Post-operative metabolites in the treatment group vs. non-treated controls.

Oxysterol	Treatment (n = 17)	Control (n = 28)	p-Value
Albumin (mg/L)	222 (110–386) (7 missing)	205 (115–483) (5 missing)	0.681
Cholesterol (µg/mL)	2.8 (1.7–7.0) (8 missing)	3.9 (1.9–7.5)	0.226
24-OH (ng/mL)	2.2 (0.8–7.0) (7 missing)	1.9 (0.8–5.4)	0.636
27-OH (ng/mL)	1.5 (0.2–2.8) (7 missing)	1.1 (0.4–2.5)	0.636
7HOCA (ng/mL)	27 (12–38) (7 missing)	17 (10–31) (2 missing)	**0.021**

Data is presented as median (range). Data compared using the Mann–Whitney U test (non-matched continuous data). Bold text in the p-value column indicates a statistically significant association ($p < 0.05$). Abbreviations: 24-OH = 24S-hydroxycholesterol; 27-OH = 27-hydroxycholesterol; 7HOCA = 7 alpha hydroxy-3-oxo-4-cholestenoic acid.

4. Discussion

In this study, we demonstrate that the CSF levels of 24-OH and 27-OH are lower in iNPH patients compared to controls, and that the levels of the metabolite 7-HOCA significantly increases in iNPH patients after VP-shunt treatment.

It should be emphasized that the major fluxes in oxysterols to and from the brain do not directly include the cerebrospinal fluid, but rather occur between the brain and the circulation. It is believed, however, that changes in these major fluxes as well as metabolic changes in the brain are reflected in the levels of oxysterols in the cerebrospinal fluid [34,35].

We hypothesized that measurements of oxysterols in CSF may give useful diagnostic information in iNPH, and that the beneficial effects of CSF drainage may be reflected in changes in the levels of specific oxysterols. Before treatment, the CSF levels of 24-OH and 27-OH were significantly higher in controls compared to iNPH patients (Table 1). VP-shunt treatment affected the fluxes by significantly increasing 7-HOCA. The similar effect of the drainage on all the different oxysterols studied suggests that it is a common factor affecting the fluxes of the different oxysterols. A possible factor is the metabolic capacity of the neuronal cells in the brain [36]. The metabolism of 24-OH by CYP46 and 7-HOCA by the CYP7B1 are dependent on neuronal cells. Since the shunt-treatment led to an increased level of 7HOCA, we would expect reduced metabolism levels of 27-OH. In this study, we did not see a reduction, but rather non-significant changes in the levels of 27-OH.

An increase in the levels of 7HOCA has previously been suggested as a marker for blood–brain barrier dysfunction [16]. In this study, the elevated postoperative 7HOCA levels might be due to the mechanical disruption of the parenchyma during surgery. Nagata et al. demonstrated an increased level of 7HOCA after craniotomy in a patient with subarachnoid hemorrhage [29]. The levels decreased during the first 24 hours post-surgery. However, a significant effect of the surgical procedure may not be so likely in our study, since the levels of 7HOCA were measured several months after surgery. Future studies may benefit from performing serial 7HOCA-sampling in these patients to further understand the mechanisms behind our results.

The levels of 27-OH in CSF are dependent upon the flux in this oxysterol from the circulation into the CSF. Since 27-OH is a precursor to 7HOCA, this is also the case for 7HOCA. The flux of 27-OH across the blood–brain barrier is, however, also combined with a corresponding flux in albumin across this barrier. Albumin is a strong binder of 7HOCA and thus a disrupted blood–brain barrier would be expected to result in increased levels of 7HOCA in the CSF by these two mechanisms [30].

Zhang et al studied the metabolism of oxysterols in cultured rat astrocytes, Schwann cells and neurons. They found that 27-OH, but not 24-OH, was metabolized into 7HOCA in all cell types. Adding 27-OH to the cell cultures resulted in elevated levels of 7-HOCA in astrocytes compered to neurons. Adding 24-OH to the cultures showed an increased metabolization to other cholesterols in astrocytes. This may be of relevance in the context of iNPH, since its pathophysiology may include disturbances in the glymphatic system that particularly affect astrocytes [37–39]. If this is the case, astrocytes may recover after CSF drainage and increase the levels of 7HOCA.

Liu et al demonstrated that hypercholesterolemia in the CNS is involved in inducing hydrocephalus [40]. Further research has to be done concerning this, but if the metabolization of 24-OH is affected by hydrocephalus, the increase in 24-OH may occur after VP-shunt treatment due to the increased level of cholesterol accumulated during the development of hydrocephalus.

The increased level of 7HOCA in CSF after VP- shunt treatment is noteworthy, and considering the neurotoxic effects of 27-OH on both neurons and astrocytes [19,28], it seems likely that this effect is beneficial. Further work is needed to evaluate the value of measuring 7HOCA in connection with iNPH treatment.

5. Limitations

The main limitation of this study is the limited sample size. Another limitation is the lack of simultaneous analysis of oxysterols in the blood, which could have provided valuable comparative data. This issue needs to be addressed in future studies. A strength of this study is the prospective patient inclusion, as well as the robust collection and analysis of the oxysterol concentrations.

6. Conclusions

Neither the etiology of iNPH nor the mechanisms explaining the beneficial effects of VP-shunt surgery are fully understood. This study analyzed CSF-levels of oxysterols before and after VP-shunt surgery, and showed that CSF from iNPH patients compared to controls had a significantly lower level of oxysterols before surgery and that there were significant increases in 24OH and 7HOCA after VP-shunt treatment. CSF drainage may reduce an inhibitory effect of transiently increased pressure on the metabolic capacity of neuronal cells in the brain. This capacity includes the elimination of cholesterol by the 24S-hydroxylase mechanisms. Thus, oxysterols may potentially be used as a biomarker in the diagnosis and management of iNPH.

Author Contributions: Conceptualization, E.E., L.A., A.E.-T. and I.B; methodology, I.B., E.P., A.L.S., M.H. and F.D.; validation, I.B.; formal analysis, A.F.-S.; investigation, E.P.; resources, I.B.; data curation, E.P. and A.F.-S.; writing—original draft preparation, E.P., E.E., L.A. and A.F.-S.; writing—review and editing, E.E., A.E.-T., L.A. and A.F.-S.; visualization, A.F.-S.; supervision, I.B., E.E., L.A. and A.E.-T.; project administration, I.B., L.A., E.E. and A.E.-T.; funding acquisition, I.B. All authors have read and agreed to the published version of the manuscript.

Funding: This work was supported by a grant from the Swedish Foundation "Gamla Tjänarinnor" and a grant from the Division of Clinical Chemistry ("Kliniknära Utvecklingsprojekt"). AET was supported by Region Stockholm (clinical research appointment). The funders had no role in the design, analysis or presentation of the manuscript.

Institutional Review Board Statement: The study was conducted in accordance with the Declaration of Helsinki, and approved by the Swedish National Ethical Review Board (Dnr 2019-04241).

Informed Consent Statement: Informed consent was obtained from all subjects involved in the study.

Data Availability Statement: Data is available from the corresponding author upon reasonable request.

Conflicts of Interest: The authors declare no conflict of interest.

Abbreviations

24-OH	24S-hydroxycholesterol
27-OH	27-hydroxycholesterol
7HOCA	7 alpha hydroxy-3-oxo-4-cholestenoic acid
DHEA	Cortisone dehydroepiandrosterone
7DHEA	7 alpha hydroxy dehydroepiandrosterone
CSF	Cerebrospinal fluid
CYP7B1	Cytochrome P450 family 7 subfamily B member 1
CYP46	Cytochrome P450 family 46
iNPH	Idiopathic normal pressure hydrocephalus
VP	ventriculoperitoneal

References

1. Adams, R.D.; Fisher, C.M.; Hakim, S.; Ojemann, R.G.; Sweet, W.H. Symptomatic Occult Hydrocephalus with Normal Cerebrospinal-Fluid Pressure. *N. Engl. J. Med.* **2010**, *97*, 693–695. [CrossRef] [PubMed]
2. Williams, M.A.; Malm, J. Diagnosis and Treatment of Idiopathic Normal Pressure Hydrocephalus. *Continuum* **2016**, *22*, 579–599. [CrossRef] [PubMed]
3. Picascia, M.; Zangaglia, R.; Bernini, S.; Minafra, B.; Sinforiani, E.; Pacchetti, C. A Review of Cognitive Impairment and Differential Diagnosis in Idiopathic Normal Pressure Hydrocephalus. *Funct. Neurol.* **2015**, *30*, 217–228. [CrossRef] [PubMed]
4. Tanaka, M.; Vécsei, L. Editorial of Special Issue "Dissecting Neurological and Neuropsychiatric Diseases: Neurodegeneration and Neuroprotection". *Int. J. Mol. Sci.* **2022**, *23*, 6991. [CrossRef]
5. Battaglia, S.; Harrison, B.J.; Fullana, M.A. Does the Human Ventromedial Prefrontal Cortex Support Fear Learning, Fear Extinction or Both? A Commentary on Subregional Contributions. *Mol. Psychiatry* **2021**, *27*, 784–786. [CrossRef]
6. Larsson, A.; Ärlig, A.; Bergh, A.C.; Bilting, M.; Jacobsson, L.; Stephensen, H.; Wikkelsö, C. Quantitative SPECT Cisternography in Normal Pressure Hydrocephalus. *Acta Neurol. Scand.* **1994**, *90*, 190–196. [CrossRef]
7. Kristensen, B.; Malm, J.; Fagerlund, M.; Hietala, S.O.; Johansson, B.; Ekstedt, J.; Karlsson, T. Regional Cerebral Blood Flow, White Matter Abnormalities, and Cerebrospinal Fluid Hydrodynamics in Patients with Idiopathic Adult Hydrocephalus Syndrome. *J. Neurol. Neurosurg. Psychiatry* **1996**, *60*, 282–288. [CrossRef]
8. Momjian, S.; Owler, B.K.; Czosnyka, Z.; Czosnyka, M.; Pena, A.; Pickard, J.D. Pattern of White Matter Regional Cerebral Blood Flow and Autoregulation in Normal Pressure Hydrocephalus. *Brain* **2004**, *127*, 965–972. [CrossRef]
9. Lenfeldt, N.; Hansson, W.; Larsson, A.; Birgander, R.; Eklund, A.; Malm, J. Three-Day CSF Drainage Barely Reduces Ventricular Size in Normal Pressure Hydrocephalus. *Neurology* **2012**, *79*, 237–242. [CrossRef]
10. Sosvorova, L.; Hill, M.; Mohapl, M.; Vitku, J.; Hampl, R. Steroid Hormones in Prediction of Normal Pressure Hydrocephalus. *J. Steroid Biochem. Mol. Biol.* **2015**, *152*, 124–132. [CrossRef]
11. Meaney, S.; Heverin, M.; Panzenboeck, U.; Ekström, L.; Axelsson, M.; Andersson, U.; Diczfalusy, U.; Pikuleva, I.; Wahren, J.; Sattler, W.; et al. Novel Route for Elimination of Brain Oxysterols across the Blood-Brain Barrier: Conversion into 7alpha-Hydroxy-3-Oxo-4-Cholestenoic Acid. *J. Lipid Res.* **2007**, *48*, 944–951. [CrossRef] [PubMed]
12. Axelson, M.; Mork, B.; Sjovallt, J. Occurrence of 3 Beta-Hydroxy-5-Cholestenoic Acid, 3 Beta,7 Alpha-Dihydroxy-5-Cholestenoic Acid, and 7 Alpha-Hydroxy-3-Oxo-4-Cholestenoic Acid as Normal Constituents in Human Blood. *J. Lipid Res.* **1988**, *29*, 629–641. [CrossRef]
13. Lund, E.; Andersson, O.; Zhang, J.; Babiker, A.; Ahlborg, G.; Diczfalusy, U.; Einarsson, K.; Sjövall, J.; Björkhem, I. Importance of a Novel Oxidative Mechanism for Elimination of Intracellular Cholesterol in Humans. *Arterioscler. Thromb. Vasc. Biol.* **1996**, *16*, 208–212. [CrossRef] [PubMed]
14. Nagata, K.; Axelson, M.; Bjorkhem, I.; Matsutani, M.; Takakura, K. Significance of Cholesterol Metabolites in Chronic Subdural Hematoma. *Recent Adv. Neurotraumatol.* **1993**, 49–52. [CrossRef]
15. Ogundare, M.; Theofilopoulos, S.; Lockhart, A.; Hall, L.J.; Arenas, E.; Sjövall, J.; Brenton, A.G.; Wang, Y.; Griffiths, W.J. Cerebrospinal Fluid Steroidomics: Are Bioactive Bile Acids Present in Brain? *J. Biol. Chem.* **2010**, *285*, 4666–4679. [CrossRef]
16. Saeed, A.; Floris, F.; Andersson, U.; Pikuleva, I.; Lövgren-Sandblom, A.; Bjerke, M.; Paucar, M.; Wallin, A.; Svenningsson, P.; BjÖrkhem, I. 7α-Hydroxy-3-Oxo-4-Cholestenoic Acid in Cerebrospinal Fluid Reflects the Integrity of the Blood-Brain Barrier. *J. Lipid Res.* **2014**, *55*, 313–318. [CrossRef]
17. Björkhem, I.; Leoni, V.; Svenningsson, P. On the Fluxes of Side-Chain Oxidized Oxysterols across Blood-Brain and Blood-CSF Barriers and Origin of These Steroids in CSF (Review). *J. Steroid Biochem. Mol. Biol.* **2019**, *188*, 86–89. [CrossRef]
18. Leoni, V.; Masterman, T.; Patel, P.; Meaney, S.; Diczfalusy, U.; Björkhem, I. Side Chain Oxidized Oxysterols in Cerebrospinal Fluid and the Integrity of Blood-Brain and Blood-Cerebrospinal Fluid Barriers. *J. Lipid Res.* **2003**, *44*, 793–799. [CrossRef]
19. Heverin, M.; Maioli, S.; Pham, T.; Mateos, L.; Camporesi, E.; Ali, Z.; Winblad, B.; Cedazo-Minguez, A.; Björkhem, I. 27-Hydroxycholesterol Mediates Negative Effects of Dietary Cholesterol on Cognition in Mice. *Behav. Brain Res.* **2015**, *278*, 356–359. [CrossRef]
20. Zhang, X.; Lv, C.; An, Y.; Liu, Q.; Rong, H.; Tao, L.; Wang, Y.; Wang, Y.; Xiao, R. Increased Levels of 27-Hydroxycholesterol Induced by Dietary Cholesterol in Brain Contribute to Learning and Memory Impairment in Rats. *Mol. Nutr. Food Res.* **2018**, *62*, 1–10. [CrossRef]
21. Ismail, M.A.M.; Mateos, L.; Maioli, S.; Merino-Serrais, P.; Ali, Z.; Lodeiro, M.; Westman, E.; Leitersdorf, E.; Gulyás, B.; Olof-Wahlund, L.; et al. 27-Hydroxycholesterol Impairs Neuronal Glucose Uptake through an IRAP/GLUT4 System Dysregulation. *J. Exp. Med.* **2017**, *214*, 699–717. [CrossRef] [PubMed]
22. Heverin, M.; Bogdanovic, N.; Lütjohann, D.; Bayer, T.; Pikuleva, I.; Bretillon, L.; Diczfalusy, U.; Winblad, B.; Björkhem, I. Changes in the Levels of Cerebral and Extracerebral Sterols in the Brain of Patients with Alzheimer's Disease. *J. Lipid Res.* **2004**, *45*, 186–193. [CrossRef] [PubMed]
23. Shafaati, M.; Marutle, A.; Pettersson, H.; Lövgren-Sandblom, A.; Olin, M.; Pikuleva, I.; Winblad, B.; Nordberg, A.; Björkhem, I. Marked Accumulation of 27-Hydroxycholesterol in the Brains of Alzheimer's Patients with the Swedish APP 670/671 Mutation. *J. Lipid Res.* **2011**, *52*, 1004–1010. [CrossRef] [PubMed]
24. Liu, Q.; An, Y.; Yu, H.; Lu, Y.; Feng, L.; Wang, C.; Xiao, R. Relationship between Oxysterols and Mild Cognitive Impairment in the Elderly: A Case-Control Study. *Lipids Health Dis.* **2016**, *15*, 1–6. [CrossRef] [PubMed]

25. Mateos, L.; Ismail, M.A.M.; Gil-Bea, F.J.; Schüle, R.; Schöls, L.; Heverin, M.; Folkesson, R.; Björkhem, I.; Cedazo-Mínguez, A. Side Chain-Oxidized Oxysterols Regulate the Brain Renin-Angiotensin System through a Liver X Receptor-Dependent Mechanism. *J. Biol. Chem.* **2011**, *286*, 25574–25585. [CrossRef] [PubMed]
26. Merino-Serrais, P.; Loera-Valencia, R.; Rodriguez-Rodriguez, P.; Parrado-Fernandez, C.; Ismail, M.A.; Maioli, S.; Matute, E.; Jimenez-Mateos, E.M.; Björkhem, I.; Defelipe, J.; et al. 27-Hydroxycholesterol Induces Aberrant Morphology and Synaptic Dysfunction in Hippocampal Neurons. *Cereb. Cortex* **2019**, *29*, 429–446. [CrossRef]
27. Sandebring-Matton, A.; Goikolea, J.; Björkhem, I.; Paternain, L. Reduction in Circulating 27-Hydroxycholesterol during Multidomaine Lifestyle/Vascular Intervention Is Associated with Improvement in Cognition. *Alzheimer Res. Ther.* **2021**, *13*, 56. [CrossRef]
28. Loera-Valencia, R.; Ismail, M.A.M.; Goikolea, J.; Lodeiro, M.; Mateos, L.; Björkhem, I.; Puerta, E.; Romão, M.A.; Gomes, C.M.; Merino-Serrais, P.; et al. Hypercholesterolemia and 27-Hydroxycholesterol Increase S100A8 and RAGE Expression in the Brain: A Link Between Cholesterol, Alarmins, and Neurodegeneration. *Mol. Neurobiol.* **2021**, *58*, 6063–6076. [CrossRef]
29. Nagata, K.; Seyama, Y.; Shimizu, T. Changes in the Level of 7 Alpha-Hydroxy-3-Oxo-4-Cholestenoic Acid in Cerebrospinal Fluid after Subarachnoid Hemorrhage. *Neurol. Med. Chir.* **1995**, *35*, 294–297. [CrossRef]
30. Saeed, A.A.; Edström, E.; Pikuleva, I.; Eggertsen, G.; Björkhem, I. On the Importance of Albumin Binding for the Flux of 7α-Hydroxy-3-Oxo-4-Cholestenoic Acid in the Brain. *J. Lipid Res.* **2017**, *58*, 455–459. [CrossRef]
31. Sodero, A.O. 24S-Hydroxycholesterol: Cellular Effects and Variations in Brain Diseases. *J. Neurochem.* **2021**, *157*, 899–918. [CrossRef] [PubMed]
32. Relkin, N.; Marmarou, A.; Klinge, P.; Bergsneider, M.; Black, P.M. Diagnosing Idiopathic Normal-Pressure Hydrocephalus. *Neurosurgery* **2005**, *57*, S24–S216. [CrossRef] [PubMed]
33. Hellström, P.; Klinge, P.; Tans, J.; Wikkelsø, C. A New Scale for Assessment of Severity and Outcome in INPH. *Acta Neurol. Scand.* **2012**, *126*, 229–237. [CrossRef] [PubMed]
34. Testa, G.; Staurenghi, E.; Zerbinati, C.; Gargiulo, S.; Iuliano, L.; Giaccone, G.; Fantò, F.; Poli, G.; Leonarduzzi, G.; Gamba, P. Changes in Brain Oxysterols at Different Stages of Alzheimer's Disease: Their Involvement in Neuroinflammation. *Redox Biol.* **2016**, *10*, 24–33. [CrossRef]
35. Björkhem, I. Crossing the Barrier: Oxysterols as Cholesterol Transporters and Metabolic Modulators in the Brain. *J. Intern. Med.* **2006**, *260*, 493–508. [CrossRef]
36. Lenfeldt, N.; Hauksson, J.; Birgander, R.; Eklund, A.; Malm, J. Improvement after Cerebrospinal Fluid Drainage Is Related to Levels of N-Acetyl-Aspartate in Idiopathic Normal Pressure Hydrocephalus. *Neurosurgery* **2008**, *62*, 135–141. [CrossRef]
37. Eide, P.K.; Hansson, H.A. Astrogliosis and Impaired Aquaporin-4 and Dystrophin Systems in Idiopathic Normal Pressure Hydrocephalus. *Neuropathol. Appl. Neurobiol.* **2018**, *44*, 474–490. [CrossRef]
38. Hasan-Olive, M.M.; Enger, R.; Hansson, H.A.; Nagelhus, E.A.; Eide, P.K. Loss of Perivascular Aquaporin-4 in Idiopathic Normal Pressure Hydrocephalus. *Glia* **2019**, *67*, 91–100. [CrossRef]
39. Trillo-Contreras, J.L.; Ramírez-Lorca, R.; Villadiego, J.; Echevarría, M. Cellular Distribution of Brain Aquaporins and Their Contribution to Cerebrospinal Fluid Homeostasis and Hydrocephalus. *Biomolecules* **2022**, *12*, 530. [CrossRef]
40. Liu, C.; Li, G.; Wang, P.; Wang, Y.; Pan, J. Characterization of Spontaneous Hydrocephalus Development in the Young Atherosclerosis-Prone Mice. *Neuroreport* **2017**, *28*, 1108–1114. [CrossRef]

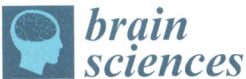

Review

Current Challenges in the Diagnosis of Progressive Neurocognitive Disorders: A Critical Review of the Literature and Recommendations for Primary and Secondary Care

Chiara Abbatantuono [1,†], Federica Alfeo [2,†], Livio Clemente [1], Giulio Lancioni [1,3], Maria Fara De Caro [1], Paolo Livrea [4] and Paolo Taurisano [1,*]

[1] Department of Translational Biomedicine and Neuroscience (DiBrain), University of Bari "Aldo Moro", 70121 Bari, Italy; chiara.abbatantuono@uniba.it (C.A.); livio.clemente@uniba.it (L.C.); giulio.lancioni@uniba.it (G.L.); maria.decaro@uniba.it (M.F.D.C.)
[2] Department of Education, Communication and Psychology (For.Psi.Com), University of Bari "Aldo Moro", 70121 Bari, Italy; federica.alfeo@uniba.it
[3] Lega F D'Oro Research Center, 60027 Osimo, Italy
[4] Villa Anita, SP22, 70038 Terlizzi, Italy; paololivrea@email.it
* Correspondence: paolo.taurisano@uniba.it; Tel.: +39-3491284088
† These authors contributed equally to this work.

Abstract: Screening for early symptoms of cognitive impairment enables timely interventions for patients and their families. Despite the advances in dementia diagnosis, the current nosography of neurocognitive disorders (NCDs) seems to overlook some clinical manifestations and predictors that could contribute to understanding the conversion from an asymptomatic stage to a very mild one, eventually leading to obvious disease. The present review examines different diagnostic approaches in view of neurophysiological and neuropsychological evidence of NCD progression, which may be subdivided into: (1) preclinical stage; (2) transitional stage; (3) prodromal or mild stage; (4) major NCD. The absence of univocal criteria and the adoption of ambiguous or narrow labels might complicate the diagnostic process. In particular, it should be noted that: (1) only neuropathological hallmarks characterize preclinical NCD; (2) transitional NCD must be assessed through proactive neuropsychological protocols; (3) prodromal/mild NCDs are based on cognitive functional indicators; (4) major NCD requires well-established tools to evaluate its severity stage; (5) insight should be accounted for by both patient and informants. Therefore, the examination of evolving epidemiological and clinical features occurring at each NCD stage may orient primary and secondary care, allowing for more targeted prevention, diagnosis, and/or treatment of both cognitive and functional impairment.

Keywords: neurocognitive disorders; cognitive impairment; stadial progression; diagnostic criteria

1. Introduction

Major neurocognitive disorder, previously referred to as dementia, is a clinical condition entailing a significant decline in patients' cognitive and daily living performances [1]. Screening for early symptoms of progressive, cognitive, and functional impairment would allow the use of early, more effective intervention to support patients and their caregivers [2]. Unfortunately, diagnostic criteria and tools currently available to detect subclinical, preclinical, and/or prodromal stages of neurocognitive disorders (NCDs) are not sufficiently developed and require further research work before one can rely on them as dependable means. The lack of harmonized neuropsychological assessment protocols [3] and the use of multiple measures for determining the onset/presence of impairment emphasize the need for more sensitive, specific, and culture-fair assessment tools and strategies [4]. In view of this challenging situation, healthcare professionals are charged with the daunting task of having to recognize the transitional stages between healthy and pathological aging to discriminate between individuals affected by dementing disorders and those who meet the diagnostic criteria for cognitive impairment no dementia (CIND) or mild cognitive impairment (MCI) [4].

Within any diagnostic approach, the professional will need to consider aging-related confounders and comorbidities, methodological deficiencies, and potential risks for clinical practice associated with "undetected" signs of dementia or cognitive impairment [5]. On the one hand, cognitive decline may advance over several years (or even decades) in the absence of overt clinical signs, making it difficult for the professional to recognize its development and the underlying pathophysiological processes [6]. On the other hand, assigning diagnostic labels to patients with subjective complaints or mild cognitive symptoms could prove to be a rushed and erroneous approach causing stress and anxiety for the patients and their caregivers [7] and leading to further/excessive testing and unnecessary interventions [8].

The present paper is an attempt to present and examine the stages that might define the time span leading from a condition of apparent wellbeing to an overt symptomatology of cognitive–functional impairment. Although the categorical diagnosis of NCDs represents the current diagnostic standard, it primarily relies on quantitative criteria addressing the severity of the neurocognitive impairment. Given NCD heterogeneity, this work focuses on delineating the progression of neurocognitive decline based on multiple models retrieved from the literature while also incorporating NCD manifestations that may arise at specific stages of decline. To this end, this review focuses on the stages of neurocognitive decline that can be identified as: (1) preclinical stage; (2) transitional stage; (3) prodromal or mild stage; (4) major NCD. As shown in Figures 1 and 2, the paper also addresses CIND as a separate nosographic entity encompassing clinically mild or moderate conditions that, however, do not reach the threshold for a major NCD diagnosis. The proposed stages, which have been conceptualized based on evidence and recommendations reported in the literature, require further research to be adopted as an operational framework for clinicians.

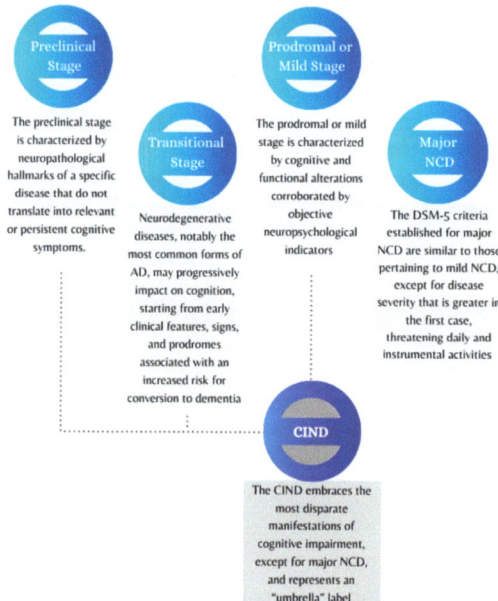

Figure 1. Graphical representation of four conventional stages of neurocognitive decline and cognitive impairment no dementia (CIND). The diagram shows the possible gradual progression of neurocognitive disorders from the preclinical stage to the onset of dementia. Abbreviations: AD = Alzheimer's disease; CIND = cognitive impairment no dementia; DSM-5 = Diagnostic and Statistical Manual of Mental Disorders, 5th edition; NCD = neurocognitive disorder.

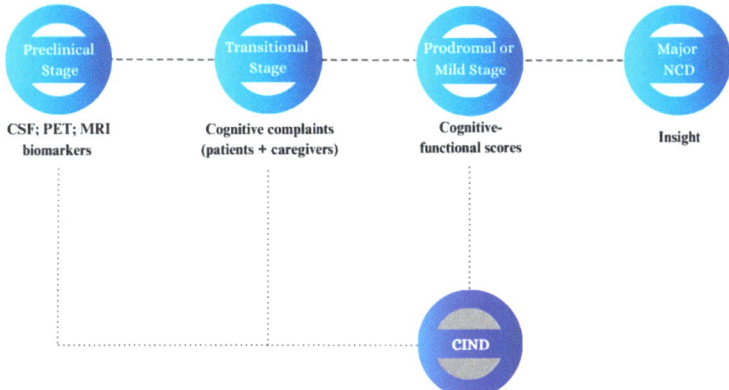

Figure 2. Graphical representation of the markers or indices covered by assessment procedures over the neurocognitive continuum. The figure summarizes selected measures and information that can be collected to support diagnosis and prognosis according to the most widely adopted classification models. Abbreviations: AD = Alzheimer's disease; CSF = cerebrospinal fluid; CIND = cognitive impairment no dementia; MRI = Magnetic Resonance Imaging; NCD = neurocognitive disorder; PET = positron emission tomography.

2. Methods

To yield a stadial progression of neurocognitive decline, a review of the most widely used criteria for NCDs [1,9] and MCI [10–12] was conducted. The search was also implemented using the online databases PubMed and Scopus to investigate the neurocognitive stages characterized by signs and clinical manifestations preceding the onset of mild and/or major NCDs. In addition to considering their epidemiological and clinical features, the diagnostic criteria and stadial models for NCDs are also critically discussed in relation to their applicability in primary and secondary care. All materials are available in the Open Science Framework (OSF) at https://osf.io/84wnp/ (accessed on 10 September 2023).

3. Results

3.1. Preclinical Stage (i.e., Stage 1)

The preclinical stage is characterized by neuropathological hallmarks of a specific disease (e.g., Alzheimer's disease, Parkinson's disease, frontotemporal degeneration, vascular injury or disease) that do not translate into relevant or persistent cognitive symptoms. Research has focused on this phase to highlight potential risk factors of cognitive decline and the need to prevent the onset of NCD manifestations through primary prevention measures [13]. Among these measures, early- and late-life engagement in cognitive, physical, and social activities is deemed to be associated with greater cognitive maintenance, and this could explain why most individuals who test positive for β-amyloid may not develop any NCDs [14].

Preclinical Alzheimer's disease (AD) consists of three distinct sub-stages that have been conceptualized based on in vivo studies [6]: (1) asymptomatic amyloidosis; (2) amyloidosis with "downstream" neurodegeneration; (3) amyloidosis with very mild cognitive and/or behavioral symptoms. Low cerebrospinal fluid β-amyloid protein 42 (CSF Aβ42) provides evidence of a neuropathological load that may be detected even before amyloidosis becomes visible on positron emission tomography (PET) imaging. Hence, isolated CSF Aβ positivity can be the first measurable sign of preclinical AD [15]. During that time, patients might start experiencing very mild neuropsychological alterations that require highly sensitive tools to be detected.

Overall, preclinical AD is prevalent in the elderly population. Considering a sample composed of 450 subjects aged more than 65 years and expected to be "cognitively normal", 43% showed no alterations (sub-stage 0), 16% fell into asymptomatic amyloidosis (sub-stage 1), 12% showed signs of neurodegeneration (sub-stage 2), 3% reported cognitive/behavioral alterations (sub-stage 3), 23% featured negative Aβ but positive neurodegeneration markers, and the remaining 3% were unclassified [16]. After one year, about 43% of sub-stage 3 developed MCI or dementia [17]. This indicates that early cognitive symptoms should be subject to clinical monitoring within the first few months following their onset.

Biomarkers emerging in preclinical AD can also contribute to differential diagnosis, as Aβ deposition detected by Aβ PET imaging and/or by low CSF Aβ1-42 levels represents a prerequisite (i.e., a risk factor) for clinical subjects to be included within the "Alzheimer continuum". However, the diagnosis of AD requires additional investigations through 18-F-fluorodeoxyglucose (FDG)-PET, structural MRI (sMRI), cortical Tau PET, and CSF biomarkers. Reduced glucose metabolism in specific brain regions (AD "signature"), temporal medial atrophy and regional cortical atrophy consistent with typical or atypical disease phenotypes, decreased Aβ1-42 combined with increased total Tau, and increased p-Tau in CSF all can support the diagnosis; the combination of different abnormalities depends on the spatiotemporal neuropathology trajectory over several years [18–20]. However, MRI findings show that neurodegeneration in atypical forms of AD may primarily cluster in brain areas other than medial temporal regions (e.g., posterior cortical or frontoparietal atrophy [21]).

Evidence of neurodegeneration markers (e.g., increased total CSF Tau; brain atrophy; glucose hypometabolism), in the absence of Aβ deposition demonstrated by Aβ cerebral PET and/or by low CSF Aβ1-42 levels, may instead characterize a wide range of clinical conditions called Suspected Non-Alzheimer Pathology (SNAP) [22]. It should be noted, however, that SNAP subjects may develop Aβ deposits over time [23], suggesting the possibility of becoming at risk or being affected by comorbid AD, the latter as indicated by the presence of increased Tau hyperphosphorylation. Different spatiotemporal trajectories of the p-Tau accumulation are known in AD and other tauopathies, the future availability of cerebral Tau PET being of great value for the differential diagnosis "in vivo" of these diseases [24].

3.2. Transitional Stage (i.e., Stage 2)

Neurodegenerative diseases, notably the most common forms of AD, may progressively impact on cognition, starting from early clinical features, signs, and prodromes associated with an increased risk for conversion to dementia [13]. During this stage, subjective experiences of cognitive impairment may occur and persist for at least six months, becoming a source of concern for patients and their caregivers. Subjective cognitive decline (SCD) may be perceived by the patient alone, without being noticed by further informants (e.g., caregivers, healthcare providers) through observable clinical signs [25]. Data from international cohort studies of aging indicate that almost a quarter of people aged over 60 years suffer from memory complaints, forgetfulness, and cognitive concerns [26] in the absence of informant-reported alterations in cognitive functioning and daily activities. Albeit self-experienced, SCD constitutes a risk factor for both MCI [26] and mild NCD [27], with a conversion rate of 6.67% cases per year [28]. Therefore, this condition arouses considerable clinical interest as it helps to clarify the gray zone between age-consistent changes and accelerated cognitive decline, allowing both patients and clinicians to intervene before NCD occurs [13].

Within the transitional stage, early yet persistent shifts in behavior may arise, which can be isolated or associated with slight cognitive issues (including SCD). Such symptoms do not meet the minimum criteria of severity and specificity to be included in a diagnostic cluster of psychiatric disorders; however, they may fall into the broad category of mild behavioral impairment (MBI) [29]. MBI affects 76.5% of people with SCD and 83.5% of people with mild cognitive impairment (MCI) [30]. From a longitudinal perspective, MBI can remain isolated, or can be followed by SCD or a mild NCD and subsequently evolve into a major NCD [31], thus representing a phenotype of transitional disease (stage 2). With specific reference to AD, isolated MBI may represent a phenotype of preclinical disease (stage 1) following asymptomatic amyloidosis [30].

3.3. Prodromal or Mild Stage (i.e., Stage 3)

The third stage (i.e., the prodromal or mild stage of NCD) is characterized by cognitive and functional alterations corroborated by objective neuropsychological indicators, such as cognitive test scores, which allow for the detection of mental state impairments and domain-specific deficits over the neurocognitive continuum. In contrast to major NCDs, such alterations do not interfere with daily routine. In order to classify an array of mild clinical conditions, the Diagnostic and Statistical Manual of Mental Disorders, Fifth Edition [1], has proposed the nosographic label of mild NCD in place of the MCI construct adopted for the previous two decades to discriminate between mild and severe patterns of cognitive decline [10]. The manual has set new diagnostic criteria that resemble those internationally proposed for MCI (i.e., acquired cognitive impairment with preserved independence in functional abilities [32]). The same core criteria have been maintained for the updated DSM-5-TR version [9]. Accordingly, clinicians are asked to assess cognitive functioning with specific reference to six cognitive domains: (1) complex attention; (2) executive function; (3) learning and memory; (4) language; (5) perceptual-motor function; and (6) social cognition. A selective, modest decline relating to one of these domains may be sufficient to allow diagnosis of mild NCD in self-reliant individuals [1].

In the case of minor cognitive symptoms, it is also advisable to consider the clinical presentation of MCI [33] as it encompasses diverse profiles of subthreshold alterations affecting dementia-free persons. Even if the "core" MCI criteria have remained unchanged, its clinical features have evolved and improved over fifteen years of research [11], reaching the current manifestations summarized in Table 1.

MCI sub-types have been operationalized based on the number and types of cognitive domains that may be found to be spared or impaired in MCI subjects. In particular, memory impairment can lead to two different MCI sub-types, consisting of amnesic single-domain MCI (a-MCI-sd) and amnesic multiple-domain MCI (a-MCI-md). If memory is spared, it is possible to discriminate between non-amnesic single-domain MCI (na-MCI-sd) and non-amnesic multiple-domain MCI (na-MCI-md) based on the same criterion. The highly variable MCI prevalence estimates mainly depend on the sample examined, according to the use of MCI macro-categories (i.e., a-MCI and na-MCI) or more specific diagnostic labels (e.g., a-MCI-sd). Indeed, the prevalence of MCI is still uncertain due to the heterogeneity of its diagnostic criteria and indices; however, there is agreement on its increased prevalence with advancing age, ranging from 2–5% (60 years of age) to 4–30% (over 90 years of age) [34]. The incidence of MCI is 6.37% cases per year in the age group between 70 and 89 years old and is higher in men (7.24%) than in women (5.73%) [35]. MCI progression has been extensively investigated through longitudinal studies, and its clinical patterns eventually fit a neuropsychological profile that largely overlaps with mild NCD, being prodromal to the onset of a major NCD. Indeed, about 5–10% of MCI subjects develop a major NCD [36], and conversion to dementia may also concern most people reverting from MCI to normal cognition [37].

The higher diagnostic specificity of mild NCD criteria (in terms of both number of impaired cognitive domains and etiologic hypotheses), compared to MCI criteria, results in different prevalence estimates regarding mild cognitive symptoms that may be smoothed through the harmonization of cognitive test scores for MCI [38]. According to both the aforementioned criteria, cognitive concerns can be reported by the patients themselves, or by reliable informants, and be supported by test results. With regard to this point, it is necessary to consider that patients' awareness about their slight cognitive deficits may involve anxiety-driven worsening in neuropsychological performances [7]. In a number of cases, self-awareness might be absent (anosognosia), entailing profound repercussions on diagnostic processes as well as prognostic trends as these patients may pay the cost of delayed diagnosis. Unawareness has not been included among mild NCD and MCI criteria that consider self- and informant-reported complaints as equally important for diagnostic purposes, yet anosognosia is associated with progressive neuropathological processes, representing a risk factor for MCI conversion to dementia [11,39].

One should note here that specific therapies for prodromal AD have provided disappointing or uncertain results that may also depend on misdiagnosis. Considering recent advances in the diagnosis of AD, such as the new discovery about Aβ plaques being a consequence (and not a cause) of cognitive impairment [40], the correction of cognitive risk factors still emerges as a key strategy to prevent the onset of major NCD [36,41].

Table 1. Sub-types of mild cognitive impairment (MCI) and related prevalence.

Memory		Impaired Amnestic MCI (a-MCI)		Spared Non-amnestic MCI (na-MCI)	
Other cognitive domains		Impaired Amnestic multiple-domain MCI (a-MCI-md)	Spared Amnestic single-domain MCI (a-MCI-sd)	Impaired Non-amnestic Multiple-domain MCI (na-MCI-md)	Spared Non-amnestic Single-domain MCI (na-MCI-sd)
Prevalence of each sub-type	[35] Roberts et al., 2012	~70%		~30%	
	[42] Rapp et al., 2010	42.8%	6.3%	26.7%	24.1%
	[43] Busse et al., 2006	26.2%	22.4%	9.3%	41.9%

Abbreviations: MCI = mild cognitive impairment; a-MCI = amnestic MCI; na-MCI = non-amnestic MCI; md = multiple-domain; sd = single-domain.

3.4. Major NCD (i.e., Stage 4)

The DSM-5 [1] has replaced the term dementia with the more comprehensive label of major NCD, redefining the number and type of impairments on which to base the diagnosis. Compared to the previous edition, the manual editions from 2013 onward no longer consider as mandatory the co-occurrence of memory decline and further acquired cognitive disturbances (e.g., executive and/or behavioral deficits) [1,9]. The most recent criteria established for major NCD are similar to those pertaining to mild NCD, except for disease severity that is greater in the first case, threatening daily and instrumental activities (as provided for in the DSM-IV). The presence of behavioral disturbances constitutes an additional specifier.

Given the lack of biomarkers for clinical differential diagnosis, the distinction between major and mild NCDs while patients are developing from early mild advanced disorder (late MCI) to initial major disorder is arbitrary. The differential process relies on the clinical and psychometric assessment of cognitive impairment and mostly depends on the tools and cut-off values adopted by clinicians. While test scores indicative of MCI generally fall within 1–1.5 standard deviation (SD), the cut-off proposed to discriminate between mild and major NCDs is conventionally set at 2 SDs below normative expectations [1,44]. The assessment of MCI severity can consist of annual cognitive screening that is, however, especially focused on memory impairment [45]. In view of the complexity of the neurocognitive decline, the Clinical Dementia Rating (CDR®) is one of the most used staging instruments to screen for patients' degree of impairment across cognitive and functional domains [46] with the following criteria: 0 = normal; 0.5 = very mild dementia (only partially overlapping with diagnostic criteria for MCI and mild NCD); 1 = mild dementia; 2 = moderate dementia; M dementia. Despite the wide use of the CDR in primary care, this tool provides a staging measure for senile dementia of Alzheimer's type [47]. In addition to the CDR, the use of comprehensive neuropsychological test batteries is recommended to account for the features that characterize the clinical progression of NCDs [3], also considering that the clinical picture may remain stable or evolve, entailing different healthcare outcomes. As primary neurodegenerative diseases progressively lead to disability and increasing needs for clinical care, it is necessary to monitor dementing conditions through quanti-/qualitative approaches to determine the different manifestations and degrees of NCDs.

The survival rate following the diagnosis of major NCD due to a primary neurodegenerative disease is significantly lower than that in the non-clinical population [48]. Reduced life expectancies may depend on several risk factors (e.g., age of the onset; male gender; disease severity and sub-type; comorbidities; socio-demographic variables) [48,49]. The mean survival time for patients diagnosed with AD is higher, up to 7–12 years depending on the disease onset, compared to individuals with mild-to-severe dementia stages assessed through the CDR® (approximately 3–3.5 years [50]). Patients suffering from vascular dementia (VaD) or Lewy body dementia (LBD) survive, in most cases, only up to 4 years after the diagnosis [48]. The reduced NCD mortality emerging from the last decade of research might be due to: (1) a greater control of risk factors, notably in high-income countries; (2) the overall effectiveness of secondary and tertiary prevention measures or therapies available for secondary neurodegenerative diseases. On the whole, reduced mortality and incidence may contribute to greater stability in NCD prevalence [51].

3.5. Cognitive Impairment No Dementia (CIND)

In addition to the aforementioned stages, it is also possible to contemplate further clinical entities (e.g., age-associated memory impairment (AAMI); age-associated cognitive decline (AACD); senescent forgetfulness; cognitive impairment no dementia (CIND)) [8,32] that still need to be operationalized through unambiguous indicators and markers. In particular, CIND has emerged as a widespread condition among subjects that do not reach the diagnostic threshold for major NCD [52]. Its prevalence estimates vary across studies and suggest that CIND may be unrelated to age, yet this broad clinical condition has been only partially considered in epidemiological research and is often confused with MCI and mild NCDs [34]. Given that CIND embraces the most disparate manifestations of cognitive impairment, except for major NCD, it is obvious that CIND represents an "umbrella" label expected to be more prevalent than MCI and major NCDs [53].

The phenomenology of CIND is so multifaceted that greater accuracy in defining the clinical characteristics and diagnostic criteria is required for this syndrome [52], considering patients' conversion rates from preclinical and/or subclinical conditions into NCDs. Previous studies indicate that about 10% of subjects affected by CIND may evolve into major NCD, 8.2% of whom may develop AD-type NCD and 5.7% cerebrovascular disease [52]. The combined effect of CIND and physical frailty is predictive of NCD, and people presenting simultaneously these two conditions have a fivefold risk of developing dementia [54]. These data endorse a broad conceptualization of CIND encompassing patients at higher risk for developing major NCD [53]. Accordingly, CIND is also associated with further conditions that may underlie cognitive decline, such as internal diseases (e.g., diabetes; heart failure) (24%); stroke (15%); cerebral vasculopathy (10%); depression and other psychiatric conditions (5%); neurological diseases (e.g., PD; traumatic brain injuries) (5%); past and recent alcohol abuse (2%); and neurodevelopmental disorders (1%) [52]. The early diagnosis and detection of CIND and its comorbid factors, therefore, pose a challenge to health professionals committed to chronic disease self-management [55].

To advance the diagnosis and treatments for such diverse etiologies of cognitive impairment, systematization of the diagnostic criteria of the CIND has been proposed in the last decade [56] based on previous conceptualizations [57]. These novel criteria have eventually placed the syndrome in an intermediate stage of impairment, which is included between MCI and major NCD and involves objective impairment in cognition that is more severe than MCI but not indicative of loss of functional abilities [56]. As a result, CIND appears to be similar to multiple-domain MCI or mild NCD (based on standardized testing); still, its clinical features have scarcely been investigated and seem too vague and unspecific [32] to allow for a clear placement of CIND within the stadial progression of NCDs.

4. Discussion

Although not exhaustive, this review intends to provide scholars as well as clinicians with a dimensional framework that stems from neurophysiological and neuropsychological approaches to the progression of neurocognitive decline. To this end, we focused on evolving epidemiologic and clinical features of cognitive impairment to orient primary care and secondary care in the early and differential diagnosis of NCDs through an integrated perspective. The detection, prevention, and/or treatment of such syndromes are indeed accompanied by new challenges and discoveries that may fit the above-described stages (i.e., preclinical stage; transitional stage; prodromal or mild stage; major NCD) and related neurocognitive profiles.

While there is agreement about the prevalence of cognitive decline among the elderly population, the current diagnostic gold standard for NCD [1] adopts categorical criteria that may result in a restricted view on unspecified, preclinical, and/or transitional syndromes. Moreover, the literature concerning preclinical NCDs is still lacking highly sensitive biological and cognitive indices, beyond AD hallmarks, that could contribute to understanding the subtle conversion from asymptomatic disease to early neuropsychological symptoms [6,17], including MBI [30]. Further issues requiring careful investigation concern hyperphosphorylation mechanisms underlying tauopathies, given the profound impact on cognitive functioning that may derive from comorbid SNAP and AD [24]. Overall, focusing on the preclinical stage is necessary to advance primary prevention measures against dementia, also considering that patients' $A\beta$ positivity may result from cognitive decline [40]. Nevertheless, empirical findings are still anchored on the so-called "Alzheimer continuum" as amyloidosis frequently occurs among individuals aged 65 years and over [14]. The asymptomatic disease may entail subjective experiences of cognitive decline (SCD) that persist over time and lead, in turn, to MCI or mild NCD [13,26,27]. During the transition from covert to overt disease, cognitive and behavioral symptoms gradually become a source of concern for patients and eventually result in prodromal patterns of cognitive decline based on domain-specific evaluation. In particular, it is advisable to use protocols for the early assessment of multiple cognitive–behavioral indices that may guide clinicians in the differential diagnosis (e.g., synucleinopathies [58]; neuropsychiatric syndromes; neuropsychiatric onset of NCDs). It follows that, over the preclinical–prodromal continuum, primary and specialized care should account for overdiagnosis and overtreatment risks, in addition to the opportunities offered by recommended screening procedures. Interpreting an array of reversible or benign conditions as NCDs is indeed a threat to public health, and the ethical implications of such overestimation should be detailed in guidelines and health programs [8]. Further challenges for clinical practices arise from the need to discriminate anosognosic from insightful individuals to recognize dementia predictors before the emergence of functional alterations. If cognitive and behavioral symptoms progress to daily living impairment, professionals are advised to monitor the severity of the NCD regularly through multi-level assessment procedures [3]. It should also be noted that a considerable proportion of MCI or CIND individuals never develop clinically overt dementia. Early/mild conditions could remain stable or even show spontaneous remission, emerging as risk factors or frailty manifestations rather than pathological entities.

The models of NCDs reported in the literature hold a dynamic view of such conditions that still reveals ambiguous and unclear aspects underlying the current nosography for cognitive impairment. These aspects might delay and complicate the diagnostic process as it relies on diverse theoretical and methodological frameworks. Novel imaging techniques and CSF biomarkers have shown great utility in the detection of early NCD manifestations, yet not all the aforementioned protocols have been adopted and validated across outpatient settings, resulting in poor clinical translatability. Further limitations apply to the DSM-5, as the NCD cluster does not cover specific criteria for progressive conditions (e.g., a diagnostic framework for subthreshold profiles of impairment, the clinical significance of brain areas and functions affected by neurodegeneration over time, and testing criteria). Hence, the widespread adoption of stadial criteria may represent an opportunity to set or advance screening and treatment standards. This scope could be afforded through the achievement of evidence-based protocols and reliable indicators of NCD progression that can be spent in a broader range of clinical and research contexts, granting early and appropriate care throughout the neurocognitive continuum.

Overall, the present stadial framework for NCDs may complement existing categorical diagnoses to offer practical benefits in the context of both primary and specialized care. This approach promotes early intervention through the identification of established hallmarks and symptoms that may convert to dementia, remain stable, or revert to a status of cognitive–functional wellbeing over time. Although no consensus on CIND makes it even harder to predict the prognosis of different "no dementia" syndromes, some proactive strategies can be adopted to counter mild-to-major conversion. Based on epidemiological data on the potential remissions of mild symptoms up to the prodromal stage, it becomes crucial to target the modifiable factors of dementia (e.g., cardiovascular health and lifestyle choices) aimed at fostering patients' functioning and quality of life. While medications and cognitive-enhancing drugs can be effective in managing specific symptoms [59,60], favorable outcomes in the early stages of the neurocognitive continuum may be partially ascribable to brain and cognitive reserves, which act as protective factors against both age- and disease-related decline [14,61–63]. To this end, the involvement of caregivers from the onset of very mild symptoms is key. Caregivers can indeed engage the patients in stimulating experiences as well as monitor the persistence and impact of symptoms that may become evident at neuropsychological follow ups. Their role in informal care, which is being increasingly recognized by institutional care teams, is equally important when patients' functioning and insight begin to decline [64].

By categorizing cognitive decline into stages, the healthcare system can also allocate resources efficiently, directing support to individuals at higher risk from the preclinical phase and evaluating cases where undergoing invasive exams can be avoided and integrated treatment strategies [60,65–68] can be advised. Moreover, this framework contributes to overtreatment and stigma reduction by acknowledging cognitive impairment as a continuum, encouraging individuals to seek medical help earlier and participate actively in their care decisions, and mitigating concerns that usually occur when undergoing screening [68].

5. Conclusions

The recognition and monitoring of individuals at the stages from preclinical to overt dementia are essential for optimizing clinical efforts against neurocognitive decline. These strategies may allow healthcare professionals to assess the progression of cognitive decline stepwise, orient care plans to evolving patient needs, and provide timely interventions to enhance their quality of life. In view of the validation of further assessment techniques and dementia biomarkers, the adoption of a perspective that accounts for clinical–temporal progression can enrich the diagnostic systems and supportive measures currently in use, ultimately advocating wellbeing and independence for individuals experiencing neurocognitive symptoms.

Author Contributions: C.A., F.A. and L.C. contributed to the study design and manuscript drafting; G.L., M.F.D.C., P.L. and P.T. contributed to the study conceptualization and design and revisions of contents. All authors have read and agreed to the published version of the manuscript.

Funding: This research received no external funding.

Institutional Review Board Statement: Not applicable.

Informed Consent Statement: Not applicable.

Data Availability Statement: All materials are available on the Open Science Framework (OSF): https://osf.io/84wnp/ (accessed on 10 September 2023).

Conflicts of Interest: The authors declare no conflict of interest.

References

1. American Psychiatric Association. *Diagnostic and Statistical Manual of Mental Disorders*, 5th ed.; DSM-5; American Psychiatric Association: Washington, DC, USA, 2013.
2. Robinson, L.; Tang, E.; Taylor, J.-P. Dementia: Timely diagnosis and early intervention. *BMJ* **2015**, *350*, h3029. [CrossRef] [PubMed]
3. Costa, A.; Bak, T.; Caffarra, P.; Caltagirone, C.; Ceccaldi, M.; Collette, F.; Crutch, S.; Della Sala, S.; Démonet, J.F.; Dubois, B.; et al. The need for harmonisation and innovation of neuropsychological assessment in neurodegenerative dementias in Europe: Consensus document of the Joint Program for Neurodegenerative Diseases Working Group. *Alzheimer's Res. Ther.* **2017**, *9*, 27. [CrossRef] [PubMed]
4. Huang, L.; Chen, K.; Liu, Z.; Guo, Q. A Conceptual Framework for Research on Cognitive Impairment with no Dementia in Memory Clinic. *Curr. Alzheimer Res.* **2020**, *17*, 517–525. [CrossRef] [PubMed]
5. Aldus, C.F.; Arthur, A.; Dennington-Price, A.; Millac, P.; Richmond, P.; Dening, T.; Fox, C.; Matthews, F.E.; Robinson, L.; Stephan, B.C.; et al. Undiagnosed dementia in primary care: A record linkage study. *Health Serv. Deliv. Res.* **2020**, *8*, 1–108. [CrossRef] [PubMed]
6. Sperling, R.A.; Aisen, P.S.; Beckett, L.A.; Bennett, D.A.; Craft, S.; Fagan, A.M.; Iwatsubo, T.; Jack, C.R.; Kaye, J.; Montine, T.J.; et al. Toward defining the preclinical stages of Alzheimer's disease: Recommendations from the National Institute on Aging-Alzheimer's Association workgroups on diagnostic guidelines for Alzheimer's disease. *Alzheimer's Dement.* **2011**, *7*, 280–292. [CrossRef]
7. Gruters, A.A.A.; Christie, H.L.; Ramakers, I.H.G.B.; Verhey, F.R.J.; Kessels, R.P.C.; de Vugt, M.E. Neuropsychological assessment and diagnostic disclosure at a memory clinic: A qualitative study of the experiences of patients and their family members. *Clin. Neuropsychol.* **2021**, *35*, 1398–1414. [CrossRef]
8. Vanacore, N.; Pucchio, A.D.; Lacorte, E.; Bacigalupo, I.; Mayer, F.; Grande, G.; Cesari, M.; Canevelli, M. Dal mild cognitive impairment alla demenza: Qual è il ruolo della sanità pubblica? *Recent. Progress. Med.* **2017**, *108*, 211–215. [CrossRef]
9. American Psychiatric Association. *Diagnostic and Statistical Manual of Mental Disorders*, 5th ed.; Text Revision; DSM-5-TR; American Psychiatric Association Publishing: Washington, DC, USA, 2022; ISBN 978-0-89042-575-6.
10. Petersen, R.C.; Smith, G.E.; Waring, S.C.; Ivnik, R.J.; Tangalos, E.G.; Kokmen, E. Mild Cognitive Impairment: Clinical Characterization and Outcome. *Arch. Neurol.* **1999**, *56*, 303. [CrossRef]
11. Petersen, R.C.; Caracciolo, B.; Brayne, C.; Gauthier, S.; Jelic, V.; Fratiglioni, L. Mild cognitive impairment: A concept in evolution. *J. Intern. Med.* **2014**, *275*, 214–228. [CrossRef]
12. Petersen, R.C. Mild cognitive impairment as a diagnostic entity. *J. Intern. Med.* **2004**, *256*, 183–194. [CrossRef]
13. Dubois, B.; Hampel, H.; Feldman, H.H.; Scheltens, P.; Aisen, P.; Andrieu, S.; Bakardjian, H.; Benali, H.; Bertram, L.; Blennow, K.; et al. Preclinical Alzheimer's disease: Definition, natural history, and diagnostic criteria. *Alzheimer's Dement.* **2016**, *12*, 292–323. [CrossRef] [PubMed]
14. Livingston, G.; Huntley, J.; Sommerlad, A.; Ames, D.; Ballard, C.; Banerjee, S.; Brayne, C.; Burns, A.; Cohen-Mansfield, J.; Cooper, C.; et al. Dementia prevention, intervention, and care: 2020 report of the Lancet Commission. *Lancet* **2020**, *396*, 413–446. [CrossRef] [PubMed]
15. Palmqvist, S.; Mattsson, N.; Hansson, O.; Alzheimer's Disease Neuroimaging Initiative. Cerebrospinal fluid analysis detects cerebral amyloid-β accumulation earlier than positron emission tomography. *Brain* **2016**, *139*, 1226–1236. [CrossRef] [PubMed]
16. Jack, C.R.; Knopman, D.S.; Weigand, S.D.; Wiste, H.J.; Vemuri, P.; Lowe, V.; Kantarci, K.; Gunter, J.L.; Senjem, M.L.; Ivnik, R.J.; et al. An operational approach to National Institute on Aging-Alzheimer's Association criteria for preclinical Alzheimer disease. *Ann. Neurol.* **2012**, *71*, 765–775. [CrossRef]
17. Knopman, D.S.; Jack, C.R.; Wiste, H.J.; Weigand, S.D.; Vemuri, P.; Lowe, V.; Kantarci, K.; Gunter, J.L.; Senjem, M.L.; Ivnik, R.J.; et al. Short-term clinical outcomes for stages of NIA-AA preclinical Alzheimer disease. *Neurology* **2012**, *78*, 1576–1582. [CrossRef]
18. Ebenau, J.L.; Timmers, T.; Wesselman, L.M.P.; Verberk, I.M.W.; Verfaillie, S.C.J.; Slot, R.E.R.; van Harten, A.C.; Teunissen, C.E.; Barkhof, F.; van den Bosch, K.A.; et al. ATN classification and clinical progression in subjective cognitive decline: The SCIENCe project. *Neurology* **2020**, *95*, e46–e58. [CrossRef]
19. Jack, C.R.; Bennett, D.A.; Blennow, K.; Carrillo, M.C.; Feldman, H.H.; Frisoni, G.B.; Hampel, H.; Jagust, W.J.; Johnson, K.A.; Knopman, D.S.; et al. A/T/N: An unbiased descriptive classification scheme for Alzheimer disease biomarkers. *Neurology* **2016**, *87*, 539–547. [CrossRef]
20. Jack, C.R.; Bennett, D.A.; Blennow, K.; Carrillo, M.C.; Dunn, B.; Haeberlein, S.B.; Holtzman, D.M.; Jagust, W.; Jessen, F.; Karlawish, J.; et al. NIA-AA Research Framework: Toward a biological definition of Alzheimer's disease. *Alzheimer's Dement.* **2018**, *14*, 535–562. [CrossRef]
21. Graff-Radford, J.; Yong, K.X.X.; Apostolova, L.G.; Bouwman, F.H.; Carrillo, M.; Dickerson, B.C.; Rabinovici, G.D.; Schott, J.M.; Jones, D.T.; Murray, M.E. New insights into atypical Alzheimer's disease in the era of biomarkers. *Lancet Neurol.* **2021**, *20*, 222–234. [CrossRef]
22. Wisse, L.E.M.; Das, S.R.; Davatzikos, C.; Dickerson, B.C.; Xie, S.X.; Yushkevich, P.A.; Wolk, D.A.; Alzheimer's Disease Neuroimaging Initiative. Defining SNAP by cross-sectional and longitudinal definitions of neurodegeneration. *Neuroimage Clin.* **2018**, *18*, 407–412. [CrossRef]
23. Young, A.L.; Oxtoby, N.P.; Daga, P.; Cash, D.M.; Fox, N.C.; Ourselin, S.; Schott, J.M.; Alexander, D.C. A data-driven model of biomarker changes in sporadic Alzheimer's disease. *Brain* **2014**, *137*, 2564–2577. [CrossRef] [PubMed]

24. Duquette, A.; Pernègre, C.; Veilleux Carpentier, A.; Leclerc, N. Similarities and Differences in the Pattern of Tau Hyperphosphorylation in Physiological and Pathological Conditions: Impacts on the Elaboration of Therapies to Prevent Tau Pathology. *Front. Neurol.* **2021**, *11*, 607680. [CrossRef] [PubMed]
25. Abdulrab, K.; Heun, R. Subjective Memory Impairment. A review of its definitions indicates the need for a comprehensive set of standardised and validated criteria. *Eur. Psychiatr.* **2008**, *23*, 321–330. [CrossRef] [PubMed]
26. Röhr, S.; Pabst, A.; Riedel-Heller, S.G.; Jessen, F.; Turana, Y.; Handajani, Y.S.; Brayne, C.; Matthews, F.E.; Stephan, B.C.M.; Mbelesso, P.; et al. Estimating prevalence of subjective cognitive decline in and across international cohort studies of aging: A COSMIC study. *Alzheimer's Res. Ther.* **2020**, *12*, 167. [CrossRef]
27. van Harten, A.C.; Mielke, M.M.; Swenson-Dravis, D.M.; Hagen, C.E.; Edwards, K.K.; Roberts, R.O.; Geda, Y.E.; Knopman, D.S.; Petersen, R.C. Subjective cognitive decline and risk of MCI: The Mayo Clinic Study of Aging. *Neurology* **2018**, *91*, e300–e312. [CrossRef]
28. Mitchell, A.J.; Beaumont, H.; Ferguson, D.; Yadegarfar, M.; Stubbs, B. Risk of dementia and mild cognitive impairment in older people with subjective memory complaints: Meta-analysis. *Acta Psychiatr. Scand.* **2014**, *130*, 439–451. [CrossRef]
29. Ismail, Z.; Agüera-Ortiz, L.; Brodaty, H.; Cieslak, A.; Cummings, J.; Fischer, C.E.; Gauthier, S.; Geda, Y.E.; Herrmann, N.; Kanji, J.; et al. The Mild Behavioral Impairment Checklist (MBI-C): A Rating Scale for Neuropsychiatric Symptoms in Pre-Dementia Populations. *J. Alzheimer's Dis.* **2017**, *56*, 929–938. [CrossRef]
30. Sheikh, F.; Ismail, Z.; Mortby, M.E.; Barber, P.; Cieslak, A.; Fischer, K.; Granger, R.; Hogan, D.B.; Mackie, A.; Maxwell, C.J.; et al. Prevalence of mild behavioral impairment in mild cognitive impairment and subjective cognitive decline, and its association with caregiver burden. *Int. Psychogeriatr.* **2018**, *30*, 233–244. [CrossRef]
31. Lussier, F.Z.; Pascoal, T.A.; Chamoun, M.; Therriault, J.; Tissot, C.; Savard, M.; Kang, M.S.; Mathotaarachchi, S.; Benedet, A.L.; Parsons, M.; et al. Mild behavioral impairment is associated with β-amyloid but not tau or neurodegeneration in cognitively intact elderly individuals. *Alzheimer's Dement.* **2020**, *16*, 192–199. [CrossRef]
32. Bermejo-Pareja, F.; Contador, I.; del Ser, T.; Olazarán, J.; Llamas-Velasco, S.; Vega, S.; Benito-León, J. Predementia constructs: Mild cognitive impairment or mild neurocognitive disorder? A narrative review. *Int. J. Geriatr. Psychiatry* **2021**, *36*, 743–755. [CrossRef]
33. Winblad, B.; Palmer, K.; Kivipelto, M.; Jelic, V.; Fratiglioni, L.; Wahlund, L.-O.; Nordberg, A.; Bäckman, L.; Albert, M.; Almkvist, O.; et al. Mild cognitive impairment--beyond controversies, towards a consensus: Report of the International Working Group on Mild Cognitive Impairment. *J. Intern. Med.* **2004**, *256*, 240–246. [CrossRef]
34. Alexander, M.; Perera, G.; Ford, L.; Arrighi, H.M.; Foskett, N.; Debove, C.; Novak, G.; Gordon, M.F. Age-Stratified Prevalence of Mild Cognitive Impairment and Dementia in European Populations: A Systematic Review. *J. Alzheimer's Dis.* **2015**, *48*, 355–359. [CrossRef] [PubMed]
35. Roberts, R.O.; Geda, Y.E.; Knopman, D.S.; Cha, R.H.; Pankratz, V.S.; Boeve, B.F.; Tangalos, E.G.; Ivnik, R.J.; Rocca, W.A.; Petersen, R.C. The incidence of MCI differs by subtype and is higher in men: The Mayo Clinic Study of Aging. *Neurology* **2012**, *78*, 342–351. [CrossRef] [PubMed]
36. Langa, K.M.; Levine, D.A. The diagnosis and management of mild cognitive impairment: A clinical review. *JAMA* **2014**, *312*, 2551–2561. [CrossRef] [PubMed]
37. Roberts, R.O.; Knopman, D.S.; Mielke, M.M.; Cha, R.H.; Pankratz, V.S.; Christianson, T.J.H.; Geda, Y.E.; Boeve, B.F.; Ivnik, R.J.; Tangalos, E.G.; et al. Higher risk of progression to dementia in mild cognitive impairment cases who revert to normal. *Neurology* **2014**, *82*, 317–325. [CrossRef]
38. Sachdev, P.S.; Lipnicki, D.M.; Kochan, N.A.; Crawford, J.D.; Thalamuthu, A.; Andrews, G.; Brayne, C.; Matthews, F.E.; Stephan, B.C.M.; Lipton, R.B.; et al. The Prevalence of Mild Cognitive Impairment in Diverse Geographical and Ethnocultural Regions: The COSMIC Collaboration. *PLoS ONE* **2015**, *10*, e0142388. [CrossRef]
39. Wilson, R.S.; Barnes, L.L.; Rajan, K.B.; Boyle, P.A.; Sytsma, J.; Weuve, J.; Evans, D.A. Antecedents and consequences of unawareness of memory impairment in dementia. *Neuropsychology* **2018**, *32*, 931–940. [CrossRef]
40. Sturchio, A.; Dwivedi, A.K.; Young, C.B.; Malm, T.; Marsili, L.; Sharma, J.S.; Mahajan, A.; Hill, E.J.; Andaloussi, S.E.; Poston, K.L.; et al. High cerebrospinal amyloid-β 42 is associated with normal cognition in individuals with brain amyloidosis. *EClinicalMedicine* **2021**, *38*, 100988. [CrossRef]
41. Hsu, D.; Marshall, G.A. Primary and Secondary Prevention Trials in Alzheimer Disease: Looking Back, Moving Forward. *Curr. Alzheimer Res.* **2017**, *14*, 426–440. [CrossRef]
42. Rapp, S.R.; Legault, C.; Henderson, V.W.; Brunner, R.L.; Masaki, K.; Jones, B.; Absher, J.; Thal, L. Subtypes of Mild Cognitive Impairment in Older Postmenopausal Women: The Women's Health Initiative Memory Study. *Alzheimer Dis. Assoc. Disord.* **2010**, *24*, 248–255. [CrossRef]
43. Busse, A.; Hensel, A.; Guhne, U.; Angermeyer, M.C.; Riedel-Heller, S.G. Mild cognitive impairment: Long-term course of four clinical subtypes. *Neurology* **2006**, *67*, 2176–2185. [CrossRef] [PubMed]
44. Tractenberg, R.E.; Schafer, K.; Morris, J.C. Interobserver disagreements on clinical dementia rating assessment: Interpretation and implications for training. *Alzheimer Dis. Assoc. Disord.* **2001**, *15*, 155–161. [CrossRef] [PubMed]
45. Lin, S.-Y.; Lin, P.-C.; Lin, Y.-C.; Lee, Y.-J.; Wang, C.-Y.; Peng, S.-W.; Wang, P.-N. The Clinical Course of Early and Late Mild Cognitive Impairment. *Front. Neurol.* **2022**, *13*, 685636. [CrossRef]
46. Lowe, D.A.; Balsis, S.; Miller, T.M.; Benge, J.F.; Doody, R.S. Greater Precision when Measuring Dementia Severity: Establishing Item Parameters for the Clinical Dementia Rating Scale. *Dement. Geriatr. Cogn. Disord.* **2012**, *34*, 128–134. [CrossRef] [PubMed]

47. Morris, J.C. Clinical Dementia Rating: A Reliable and Valid Diagnostic and Staging Measure for Dementia of the Alzheimer Type. *Int. Psychogeriatr.* **1997**, *9*, 173–176. [CrossRef] [PubMed]
48. Strand, B.H.; Knapskog, A.-B.; Persson, K.; Edwin, T.H.; Amland, R.; Mjørud, M.; Bjertness, E.; Engedal, K.; Selbæk, G. Survival and years of life lost in various aetiologies of dementia, mild cognitive impairment (MCI) and subjective cognitive decline (SCD) in Norway. *PLoS ONE* **2018**, *13*, e0204436. [CrossRef] [PubMed]
49. Garre-Olmo, J.; Ponjoan, A.; Inoriza, J.M.; Blanch, J.; Sánchez-Pérez, I.; Cubí, R.; de Eugenio, R.; Turró-Garriga, O.; Vilalta-Franch, J. Survival, effect measures, and impact numbers after dementia diagnosis: A matched cohort study. *Clin. Epidemiol.* **2019**, *11*, 525–542. [CrossRef]
50. Brodaty, H.; Seeher, K.; Gibson, L. Dementia time to death: A systematic literature review on survival time and years of life lost in people with dementia. *Int. Psychogeriatr.* **2012**, *24*, 1034–1045. [CrossRef]
51. Prince, M.; Ali, G.-C.; Guerchet, M.; Prina, A.M.; Albanese, E.; Wu, Y.-T. Recent global trends in the prevalence and incidence of dementia, and survival with dementia. *Alzheimer's Res. Ther.* **2016**, *8*, 23. [CrossRef]
52. Plassman, B.L.; Langa, K.M.; Fisher, G.G.; Heeringa, S.G.; Weir, D.R.; Ofstedal, M.B.; Burke, J.R.; Hurd, M.D.; Potter, G.G.; Rodgers, W.L.; et al. Prevalence of cognitive impairment without dementia in the United States. *Ann. Intern. Med.* **2008**, *148*, 427–434. [CrossRef]
53. Ritchie, L.J.; Tuokko, H. Clinical Decision Trees for Predicting Conversion from Cognitive Impairment No Dementia (CIND) to Dementia in a Longitudinal Population-Based Study. *Arch. Clin. Neuropsychol.* **2011**, *26*, 16–25. [CrossRef] [PubMed]
54. Grande, G.; Haaksma, M.L.; Rizzuto, D.; Melis, R.J.F.; Marengoni, A.; Onder, G.; Welmer, A.-K.; Fratiglioni, L.; Vetrano, D.L. Co-occurrence of cognitive impairment and physical frailty, and incidence of dementia: Systematic review and meta-analysis. *Neurosci. Biobehav. Rev.* **2019**, *107*, 96–103. [CrossRef] [PubMed]
55. Lovett, R.M.; Curtis, L.M.; Persell, S.D.; Griffith, J.W.; Cobia, D.; Federman, A.; Wolf, M.S. Cognitive impairment no dementia and associations with health literacy, self-management skills, and functional health status. *Patient Educ. Couns.* **2020**, *103*, 1805–1811. [CrossRef] [PubMed]
56. Roberts, R.; Knopman, D.S. Classification and Epidemiology of MCI. *Clin. Geriatr. Med.* **2013**, *29*, 753–772. [CrossRef]
57. Canadian Medical Association study of health and aging: Study methods and prevalence of dementia. *Can. Med. Assoc. J.* **1994**, *150*, 899–913.
58. McKeith, I.G.; Ferman, T.J.; Thomas, A.J.; Blanc, F.; Boeve, B.F.; Fujishiro, H.; Kantarci, K.; Muscio, C.; O'Brien, J.T.; Postuma, R.B.; et al. Research criteria for the diagnosis of prodromal dementia with Lewy bodies. *Neurology* **2020**, *94*, 743–755. [CrossRef]
59. Frederiksen, K.S.; Cooper, C.; Frisoni, G.B.; Frölich, L.; Georges, J.; Kramberger, M.G.; Nilsson, C.; Passmore, P.; Mantoan Ritter, L.; Religa, D.; et al. A European Academy of Neurology guideline on medical management issues in dementia. *Eur. J. Neurol.* **2020**, *27*, 1805–1820. [CrossRef]
60. Pizzi, S.D.; Granzotto, A.; Bomba, M.; Frazzini, V.; Onofrj, M.; Sensi, S.L. Acting Before; A Combined Strategy to Counteract the Onset and Progression of Dementia. *Curr. Alzheimer Res.* **2020**, *17*, 790–804. [CrossRef]
61. Song, S.; Stern, Y.; Gu, Y. Modifiable lifestyle factors and cognitive reserve: A systematic review of current evidence. *Ageing Res. Rev.* **2022**, *74*, 101551. [CrossRef]
62. Stern, Y.; Arenaza-Urquijo, E.M.; Bartrés-Faz, D.; Belleville, S.; Cantilon, M.; Chetelat, G.; Ewers, M.; Franzmeier, N.; Kempermann, G.; Kremen, W.S.; et al. Whitepaper: Defining and investigating cognitive reserve, brain reserve, and brain maintenance. *Alzheimer's Dement.* **2020**, *16*, 1305–1311. [CrossRef]
63. Stern, Y. How Can Cognitive Reserve Promote Cognitive and Neurobehavioral Health? *Arch. Clin. Neuropsychol.* **2021**, *36*, 1291–1295. [CrossRef] [PubMed]
64. Reckrey, J.M.; Boerner, K.; Franzosa, E.; Bollens-Lund, E.; Ornstein, K.A. Paid Caregivers in the Community-based Dementia Care Team: Do Family Caregivers Benefit? *Clin. Ther.* **2021**, *43*, 930–941. [CrossRef] [PubMed]
65. Chowdhary, N.; Barbui, C.; Anstey, K.J.; Kivipelto, M.; Barbera, M.; Peters, R.; Zheng, L.; Kulmala, J.; Stephen, R.; Ferri, C.P.; et al. Reducing the Risk of Cognitive Decline and Dementia: WHO Recommendations. *Front. Neurol.* **2022**, *12*, 765584. [CrossRef]
66. De Caro, M.F.; Taurisano, P.; Calia, C.; Abbatantuono, C. *Modelli e Profili Neuropsicologici Delle Patologie Neurodegenerative*; Franco Angeli: Milano, Italy, 2022. Available online: https://www.francoangeli.it/Libro/Modelli-e-profili-neuropsicologici-delle-patologie-neurodegenerative?Id=27924 (accessed on 25 September 2023).
67. Huang, X.; Zhao, X.; Li, B.; Cai, Y.; Zhang, S.; Yu, F.; Wan, Q. Biomarkers for evaluating the effects of exercise interventions in patients with MCI or dementia: A systematic review and meta-analysis. *Exp. Gerontol.* **2021**, *151*, 111424. [CrossRef]
68. Pini, L.; Manenti, R.; Cotelli, M.; Pizzini, F.B.; Frisoni, G.B.; Pievani, M. Non-Invasive Brain Stimulation in Dementia: A Complex Network Story. *Neurodegener. Dis.* **2018**, *18*, 281–301. [CrossRef] [PubMed]

Disclaimer/Publisher's Note: The statements, opinions and data contained in all publications are solely those of the individual author(s) and contributor(s) and not of MDPI and/or the editor(s). MDPI and/or the editor(s) disclaim responsibility for any injury to people or property resulting from any ideas, methods, instructions or products referred to in the content.

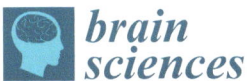

Article

CSF, Blood, and MRI Biomarkers in Skogholt's Disease—A Rare Neurodegenerative Disease in a Norwegian Kindred

Klaus Thanke Aspli [1,2], Jan O. Aaseth [3], Trygve Holmøy [2,4], Kaj Blennow [5,6,7,8], Henrik Zetterberg [5,6,9,10,11,12], Bjørn-Eivind Kirsebom [2,13,14], Tormod Fladby [2,4] and Per Selnes [2,15,*]

1. Department of Neurology, Innlandet Hospital Trust, 2381 Lillehammer, Norway; klaus.aspli@sykehuset-innlandet.no
2. Institute of Clinical Medicine, University of Oslo, 0316 Oslo, Norway; trygve.holmoy@medisin.uio.no (T.H.); bjorn-eivind.kirsebom@unn.no (B.-E.K.); tormod.fladby@medisin.uio.no (T.F.)
3. Research Department, Innlandet Hospital Trust, 2381 Brumunddal, Norway; jan.aaseth@inn.no
4. Department of Neurology, Akershus University Hospital, 1478 Nordbyhagen, Norway
5. Institute of Neuroscience and Physiology, Department of Psychiatry and Neurochemistry, The Sahlgrenska Academy at the University of Gothenburg, 43153 Mölndal, Sweden; kaj.blennow@neuro.gu.se (K.B.); henrik.zetterberg@clinchem.gu.se (H.Z.)
6. Clinical Neurochemistry Laboratory, Sahlgrenska University Hospital, 43153 Mölndal, Sweden
7. Institut du Cerveau et de la Moelle Épinière (ICM), Pitié-Salpêtrière Hospital, Sorbonne Université, 75651 Paris, France
8. First Affiliated Hospital of USTC, University of Science and Technology of China, Hefei 230001, China
9. Department of Neurodegenerative Disease, UCL Institute of Neurology, Queen Square, London WC1N 3BG, UK
10. UK Dementia Research Institute, University College London, London WC1N 3AR, UK
11. Hong Kong Center for Neurodegenerative Diseases, Hong Kong, China
12. Wisconsin Alzheimer's Disease Research Center, University of Wisconsin School of Medicine and Public Health, University of Wisconsin-Madison, Madison, WI 53706, USA
13. Department of Neurology, University Hospital of North Norway, 9019 Tromsø, Norway
14. Department of Psychology, Faculty of Health Sciences, UiT, the Arctic University of Norway, 9019 Tromsø, Norway
15. Department of Research, Akershus University Hospital, 1478 Nordbyhagen, Norway
* Correspondence: per.selnes@medisin.uio.no

Abstract: Skogholt's disease is a rare neurological disorder that is only observed in a small Norwegian kindred. It typically manifests in adulthood with uncharacteristic neurological symptoms from both the peripheral and central nervous systems. The etiology of the observed cerebral white matter lesions and peripheral myelin pathology is unclear. Increased cerebrospinal fluid (CSF) concentrations of protein have been confirmed, and recently, very high concentrations of CSF total and phosphorylated tau have been detected in Skogholt patients. The symptoms and observed biomarker changes in Skogholt's disease are largely nonspecific, and further studies are necessary to elucidate the disease mechanisms. Here, we report the results of neurochemical analyses of plasma and CSF, as well as results from the morphometric segmentation of cerebral magnetic resonance imaging. We analyzed the biomarkers $A\beta_{1-42}$, $A\beta_{1-40}$, $A\beta_{x-38}$, $A\beta_{x-40}$, $A\beta_{x-42}$, total and phosphorylated tau, glial fibrillary acidic protein, neurofilament light chain, platelet-derived growth factor receptor beta, and beta-trace protein. All analyzed CSF biomarkers, except neurofilament light chain and $A\beta_{1/x-42}$, were increased several-fold. In blood, none of these biomarkers were significantly different between the Skogholt and control groups. MRI volumetric segmentation revealed decreases in the ventricular, white matter, and choroid plexus volumes in the Skogholt group, with an accompanying increase in white matter lesions. The cortical thickness and subcortical gray matter volumes were increased in the Skogholt group. Pathophysiological changes resulting from choroidal dysfunction and/or abnormal CSF turnover, which may cause the increases in CSF protein and brain biomarker levels, are discussed.

Keywords: tau protein; amyloid beta; PDGFRβ; β-trace protein; NFL; GFAP; blood–brain barrier; Skogholt's disease; MRI

1. Introduction

Skogholt's disease is a rare, slowly progressing, central and peripheral neurodegenerative disorder only observed with maternal inheritance in a small Norwegian family line. So far, it has been diagnosed in four generations in a community in the southeastern part of Norway, and it was named after the local community physician who first described it [1,2]. Minor symptoms may develop before the age of 30, but clinical symptoms typically present between the ages of 30 and 70 in affected family members and include cognitive decline, progressive muscle weakness, unsteady gait, and dysarthria [2]. The disorder was first described in 1998 by Hagen and co-workers [2], who reported the clinical characteristics and the results of laboratory, imaging, and nerve conduction studies, as well as histopathological results and a preliminary genetic workup.

They found greatly elevated cerebrospinal fluid (CSF) concentrations of total protein and extensive cerebral white matter lesions, together with signs of peripheral nervous system involvement, originally interpreted as a combined central and peripheral demyelinating disorder [2]. In three of four selected cases examined using electroencephalography (EEG), there were signs of general slowing. In three sural nerve biopsies from selected cases, they found demyelination with teased fibers, great variation in myelin thickness, paranodal globules, onion-bulb formations, and Pi granules but no axonal degeneration. Neurography showed reduced motor conduction velocities and prolonged distal latencies in the peroneal or tibial nerves in three cases. The needle electromyography of two cases showed signs of peripheral neurogenic lesions predominantly in the lower extremities. Agarose gel electrophoresis of CSF showed what were described as transudative patterns (increased protein concentrations) but few or no traces of intrathecal IgG synthesis [2].

Later findings included greatly increased concentrations in the CSF of copper (Cu), iron (Fe), total tau (t-tau), and phosphorylated tau (p-tau), combined with normal to low levels of amyloid beta 42 protein ($A\beta_{42}$) [3,4], but normal CSF cell counts and no signs of intrathecal synthesis of immunoglobulins [3].

Subjectively experienced cognitive difficulties are common, and a cognitive screening battery disclosed a significantly prolonged Trail-Making-Test-B time, suggesting some difficulty in executive functioning [3].

The cause of the strikingly unusual combination of clinical and paraclinical findings in Skogholt's disease is unknown but likely represents a genetically linked neurodegenerative condition not described outside the affected family line [1–4].

In the present study, our objective was to further study the pathophysiology of Skogholt's disease, as well as to disclose the characteristics of this disease. We applied a comprehensive battery of markers in CSF and blood, including the core markers of Alzheimer's disease (AD), specifically the amyloid-β species $A\beta_{x-42}$, $A\beta_{x-40}$, and $A\beta_{x-38}$; phosphorylated tau (p-tau); and total tau (t-tau), as well as the astroglia-associated glial fibrillary acidic protein (GFAP), the axonal biomarker neurofilament light chain (NfL), the microvascular marker platelet-derived growth factor receptor beta (PDGFRβ), and beta-trace protein (βTP). In addition, we obtained segmental data of the cortical thicknesses and volumes of brain substructures using algorithmic processing of brain MRI data.

2. Materials and Methods

2.1. Subjects

We included three separate groups: Skogholt cases, lab controls, and MRI controls. Table 1 shows the demographic data of each group.

2.2. Diagnostic Criteria

Belonging to the affected family line was a prerequisite to consider a diagnosis of Skogholt's disease. An additional increase in CSF total protein above 1 g/L (normal range: 0.15–0.45 g/L) was considered sufficient for the diagnosis. Increased CSF total protein in the range between 0.45 and 1.0 g/L was also considered sufficient for a definite diagnosis if accompanied by clinical symptoms or MRI findings consistent with Skogholt's disease.

Table 1. Demographics of study groups.

Characteristic	Skogholt (n = 11)	Lab Control (n = 14)	MRI Control (n = 60)
Sex: Female	6 (55%)	11 (79%)	29 (48%)
Male	5 (45%)	3 (21%)	31 (52%)
Age (Yrs)	57 (45, 67)	64 (56, 70)	64 (58, 68)
Coffee (Cups/d)	3.0 (2.2, 4.2)	2.5 (<1, 4.0)	-
Smoking (pkgYrs) [a]	9 (4, 29)	1 (<1, 22)	-
Alcohol (U/m) [b]	9 (3, 14)	3 (1, 6)	-
Exercise (H/w) [c]	≥3 (1–2, ≥3)	1–2 (1–2, ≥3)	-
Education (Yrs)	9 (8, 11)	12 (12, 16)	14 (12, 16)

Summary statistics presented for sex are given by numbers, with groupwise percentages in parentheses; otherwise, data are given as the medians along with the 1st and 3rd quartiles. [a] A pack year (pkgYrs) equals smoking 20 cigarettes daily for one year. [b] Alcohol consumption in Norwegian alcohol units per month. [c] Hours per week.

2.3. Skogholt Group

Eleven Skogholt patients that were capable of informed consent and physically fit enough to attend were included in the study. All cases belonged to one kindred from a community in the southeastern inland part of Norway. Three additional cases were unable to participate due to age-related frailty or concurrent morbidity at the time of inclusion.

2.4. Laboratory Controls

The lab control group consisted of 14 individuals recruited from the Department of Neurology at the Innlandet Hospital Trust in Lillehammer. Patients not expected to receive an inflammatory or neurodegenerative diagnosis were targeted for inclusion, while patients with certain multiple sclerosis or known dementia were not considered eligible. The lab control group was thus heterogeneous, as previously described [3]. Samples of blood and CSF were obtained from the lab controls and compared with the Skogholt group.

2.5. Cerebral MRI Controls

For the comparison of cortical and parenchymal segmentation data, we included 60 MRI controls from the Dementia Disease Initiation (DDI) project, which has more than 500 participants [5]. We only included healthy controls, i.e., individuals without biomarker evidence of cerebral amyloidosis (based either on a negative flutemetamol-PET scan or a CSF A$\beta_{42/40}$ ratio ≤ 0.077), with normal results on a cognitive screening battery, and without subjective cognitive complaints. Two eligible controls were excluded due to failed algorithmic parcellation of MRI data.

2.6. Ethics

The study protocol was approved by the Regional Committee for Medical and Health Research Ethics, South-East Region, Norway, Ref. No. 556-04224 and No. 2013/1017. The study was conducted in accordance with the Declaration of Helsinki. Written informed consent was obtained from all patients before enrollment.

2.7. Lab Pre-Analytics

Samples of plasma and CSF were obtained and prepared as described previously [3]. Before collection, CSF opening pressure was measured. Skogholt patients were sampled in the morning while fasting. A fasting regimen was not feasible for the controls, who were sampled as soon as possible upon inclusion.

2.8. Lab Analytics

From CSF and EDTA-plasma samples obtained previously [3], we analyzed an expanded set of brain biomarkers at the Clinical Neurochemistry Lab in Mölndal. CSF total and phosphorylated tau (T-tau and P-tau) as well as Aβ_{1-42} and Aβ_{1-40} concentrations were measured using a fully automated Lumipulse instrument (Fujirebio, Ghent, Belgium) as described previously [6]. The Aβ species $Aβ_{x-38}$, $Aβ_{x-40}$, and $Aβ_{x-42}$ were measured using a MesoScale Discovery triplex assay. CSF NfL and GFAP concentrations were measured using in-house ELISAs as previously described [7–9]. Soluble PDGF-receptor β (PDGFRβ) was measured using a PDGFR beta Human ELISA Kit (Thermo Scientific, Frederick, MD, USA).

The beta-trace protein (prostaglandin D synthase) concentration was measured via nephelometry on an Atellica NEPH 630 System (Siemens Healthineers, Erlangen, Germany).

The measurements were performed by board-certified laboratory technicians who were blinded to the clinical data.

2.9. MRI Systems, Sequence Parameters, and Software for Postprocessing Statistics

Cerebral MRI of Skogholt patients was obtained on a Philips Achieva MRI system with a magnetic field strength of 1.5 Tesla. The MRI protocol included 3D FLAIR, axial T2, diffusion, inflow angio, and SWI as well as 3DT1 scanning before and after contrast enhancement with a macrocyclic gadolinium contrast agent (gadoteric acid).

MRI from the DDI controls used in the current study were obtained on eight scanners distributed in six centers. The scanner systems, sequence parameters, and number of subjects are detailed in Table S1.

Cortical reconstruction and volumetric segmentation were performed with FastSurfer [10,11]. This included the segmentation of the subcortical white matter (WM) and deep gray matter structures and the parcellation of the cortical surface [12,13] according to a previously published parcellation scheme [14]. This labeled the cortical sulci and gyri, and mean thickness values were calculated in the regions of interest (ROIs). All segmentations were visually inspected.

White matter hyperintensities [15] (WMHs) were segmented from 3D FLAIR MRI using an in-house deep learning algorithm [16].

2.10. Statistics

All statistical computing and data visualizations were performed in RStudio using R version 4.1.3 (and 4.2.2 for the final graphs) [17] with extension packages [18–22].

Due to the small numbers of cases and controls, judgements regarding the distribution of data were unreliable. Therefore, we used both Student's two-tailed two-sample t-test and the Wilcoxon rank-sum test, i.e., the Mann–Whitney U-test, with α pragmatically set to 0.01 when judging group differences and correspondingly provide the raw data of descriptive statistics for each group using the mean and median with the standard deviation (SD) and interquartile, i.e., 1st to 3rd quartile, range (IQR). Group differences in standardized measurements or standardized ratios (measurements with ICV for MRI volume markers) are explored in graphs showing the standardized linear regression coefficients (with 95% confidence intervals) of group status for each marker.

The adjustment of coefficients was carried out by including appropriate covariates in the regression models. Continuous variables such as age and ICV were standardized, while dichotomous variables, e.g., sex or MRI magnetic field strength (1.5 or 3T), were kept unchanged as binary variables.

To verify the confidence intervals, they are also shown as the 2.5th to 97.5th percentile ranges of the bootstrap distributions of the estimates/coefficients based on 20,000 resampled datapoints in the dataset stratified by group and gender.

3. Results

3.1. Demographics

The Demographics of the Skogholt cases and the two control groups are given in Table 1.

3.2. CSF Biomarkers

The opening pressure upon lumbar puncture was normal in all Skogholt patients, ranging from 10.5 to 19.5 cm water, with a mean of 14.4 cm, which was not significantly different from the controls.

The measured CSF biomarkers were significantly increased in the Skogholt group (*t*-test and Mann–Whitney U-test), except for $A\beta_{1-42}$, $A\beta_{x-42}$, and NfL, as shown in Table 2 and Figure S1. ($A\beta_{1-42}$, $A\beta_{x-42}$, and NfL were borderline significantly increased according to the U-test but not the *t*-test).

Table 2. CSF biomarkers.

Analyte	Mean (SD)		Median (IQR)		*p*-Values		Ratio of	
	Skogholt (n = 7)	Control (n = 11)	Skogholt (n = 7)	Control (n = 11)	t [a]	U [b]	Means [c]	Medians [d]
$A\beta_{1-42}$	1687 (1214)	922 (341)	1464 (950–1718)	921 (721–1068)	0.15	0.079	1.83	1.59
$A\beta_{1-40}$	35,385 (7596)	10,868 (2936)	38,528 (29,796–40,531)	10,614 (8788–12,940)	<0.001	<0.001	3.26	3.63
p-Tau	424 (87.1)	44.2 (29.3)	464 (346–476)	36.5 (27.2–49.5)	<0.001	<0.001	9.61	12.7
t-Tau	3147 (467)	400 (250)	3160 (2814–3562)	342 (236–397)	<0.001	<0.001	7.87	9.23
$A\beta_{1-42/1-40}$	0.050 (0.0277)	0.0842 (0.0194)	0.042 (0.034–0.0485)	0.091 (0.0885–0.0963)	0.017	0.022	0.60	0.46
GFAP	51,497 (10,622)	16,677 (7867)	52,373 (45,109–56,718)	16,974 (9830–22,089)	<0.001	<0.001	3.09	3.09
NfL	9138 (11,486)	4738 (9626)	4210 (2851–8818)	1200 (881–4027)	0.403	0.046	1.93	3.51
PDGFRβ	1915 (283)	422 (118)	1936 (1752–2051)	410 (316–523)	<0.001	<0.001	4.53	4.72
βTP	112 (9.41)	16.6 (3.69)	108 (107–120)	16 (15–18.8)	<0.001	<0.001	6.75	6.75
$A\beta_{x-38}$	5497 (504)	1812 (631)	5359 (5211–5829)	1628 (1370–2302)	<0.001	<0.001	3.03	3.29
$A\beta_{x-40}$	12,319 (2361)	4428 (1097)	13,106 (10,829–14,016)	4326 (3820–4901)	<0.001	<0.001	2.78	3.03
$A\beta_{x-42}$	619 (407)	331 (142)	558 (340–663)	307 (266–361)	0.113	0.031	1.87	1.82

Clinical neurochemistry results from analysis of various species of amyloid beta (Aβ) and results from analysis of total tau protein (t-Tau), phosphorylated tau protein (p-Tau), glial fibrillary acidic protein (GFAP), neurofilament light chain (NfL), platelet-derived growth factor receptor beta (PDGFRβ), and beta-trace protein (βTP). All measurements are in pg/mL except for βTP (mg/mL). [a] *p*-values from Student's *t*-test, not adjusted for multiple testing. [b] *p*-values from Mann–Whitney U-tests with continuity correction, not adjusted for multiple testing. [c] Ratio of means between Skogholt and control patients. [d] Ratio of medians between Skogholt and control patients.

All directly measured CSF markers except NfL were significantly increased in proportion to the CSF total protein content. The $A\beta_{1-42/1-40}$ ratio was decreased with borderline significance.

3.3. Plasma Biomarkers

Only plasma GFAP was decreased with borderline significance in the Skogholt group, while all other examined plasma biomarkers were not significantly different between the groups (plasma NFL was decreased with borderline significance according to the U-test but not the *t*-test) (Table 3).

Table 3. Plasma biomarkers.

Analyte	Mean (SD)		Median (IQR)		p-Values		Ratio of	
	Skogholt ($n = 11$)	Control ($n = 14$)	Skogholt ($n = 11$)	Control ($n = 14$)	t [a]	U [b]	Means [c]	Medians [d]
tTau	38.8 (24.6)	49 (40.8)	33.2 (28.7–39.2)	39.3 (24.6–47.7)	0.447	0.536	0.791	0.844
GFAP	58.8 (27.8)	128 (107)	56.8 (35–81.2)	82 (68.6–153)	0.034	0.033	0.459	0.693
NfL	22.5 (33.7)	83.3 (186)	9.49 (8.46–15.7)	30.1 (14.3–61.2)	0.251	0.025	0.270	0.316
$A\beta_{40}$	97.6 (20.1)	108 (28.1)	92 (89–101)	94.6 (89.2–123)	0.306	0.647	0.906	0.973
$A\beta_{42}$	6.66 (0.9)	6.95 (1.28)	6.47 (6.18–7.03)	6.97 (6.3–7.3)	0.514	0.501	0.958	0.928
pTau181	7.74 (3.24)	8.23 (4.71)	7.33 (5.92–9.34)	5.85 (5.45–10.8)	0.760	0.687	0.940	1.250
$A\beta_{42}/A\beta_{40}$	0.0693 (0.00801)	0.0668 (0.0132)	0.0705 (0.063–0.0761)	0.069 (0.0626–0.0766)	0.566	0.851	1.040	1.020

Clinical neurochemistry results: amyloid beta (Aβ), total tau protein (tTau), phosphorylated tau protein 181 (pTau181), glial fibrillary acidic protein (GFAP), and neurofilament light chain (NfL). All measurements are in pg/mL. [a] p-values from Students t-test, not adjusted for multiple testing. [b] p-values from Mann–Whitney U-tests with continuity correction, not adjusted for multiple testing. [c] Ratio of means between Skogholt and control patients. [d] Ratio of medians between Skogholt and control patients.

3.4. MRI Findings

The majority of the examined Skogholt cases had grade-three Fazekas, i.e., confluent deep white matter T2 hyperintensities on cerebral MRI (Table 4 and Figure 1), while most controls had minimal to no observable deep white matter lesions [23]. The observed white matter lesions were not like the typical lesions observed in multiple sclerosis and were considered nonspecific regarding etiology.

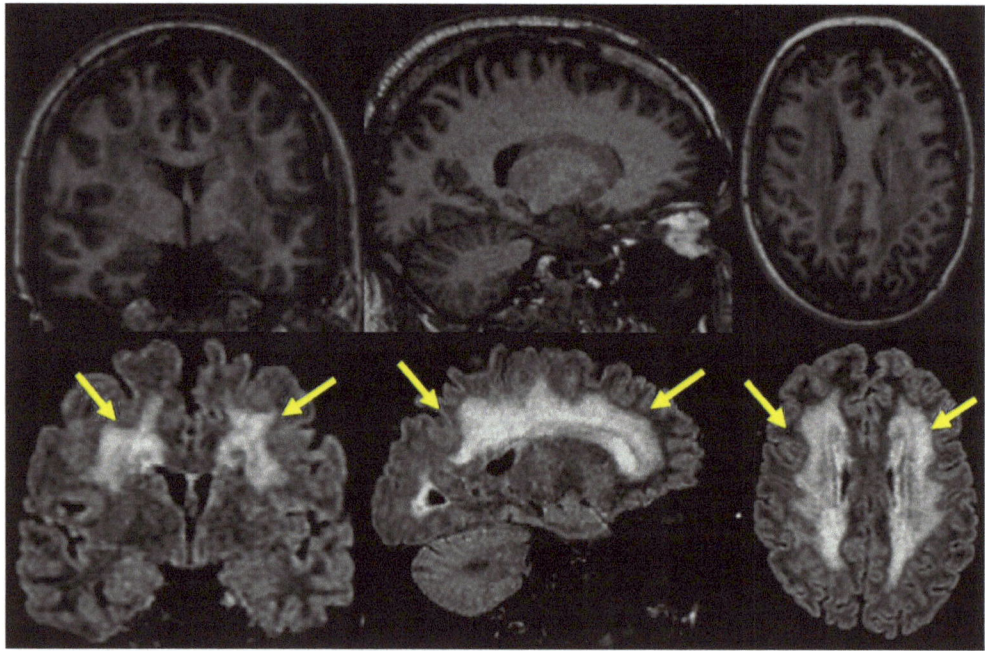

Figure 1. Representative cerebral MRI-T1 (top) and MRI-FLAIR (below) images from a 50-year-old Skogholt patient. Note the extensive white matter hyperintensities (WMHs) typical of the disease (see arrows).

Table 4. Fazekas scores of white matter lesions.

Fazekas Score	Skogholt Group $n = 11$	MRI Control Group $n = 60$
0	2 (18%)	13 (23%)
1	1 (9.1%)	36 (64%)
2	2 (18%)	7 (12%)
3	6 (55%)	0 (0%)
missing	0	4

Semiquantitative scores of white matter hyperintensities on cerebral MRI T2 sequences. Statistics presented as n (%). Fisher's exact test gives a p-value < 0.001.

The intracranial volume (ICV) was significantly smaller in the Skogholt group, even when adjusting for age, sex, and magnetic field strength (Figure 2). Only a few Skogholt patients had more than minimal cerebral cortical atrophy (Table 5). Two cases had minor microhemorrhages on their SWI sequences, and one additional case had changes in their SWI and diffusion sequences, interpreted as a subacute stroke.

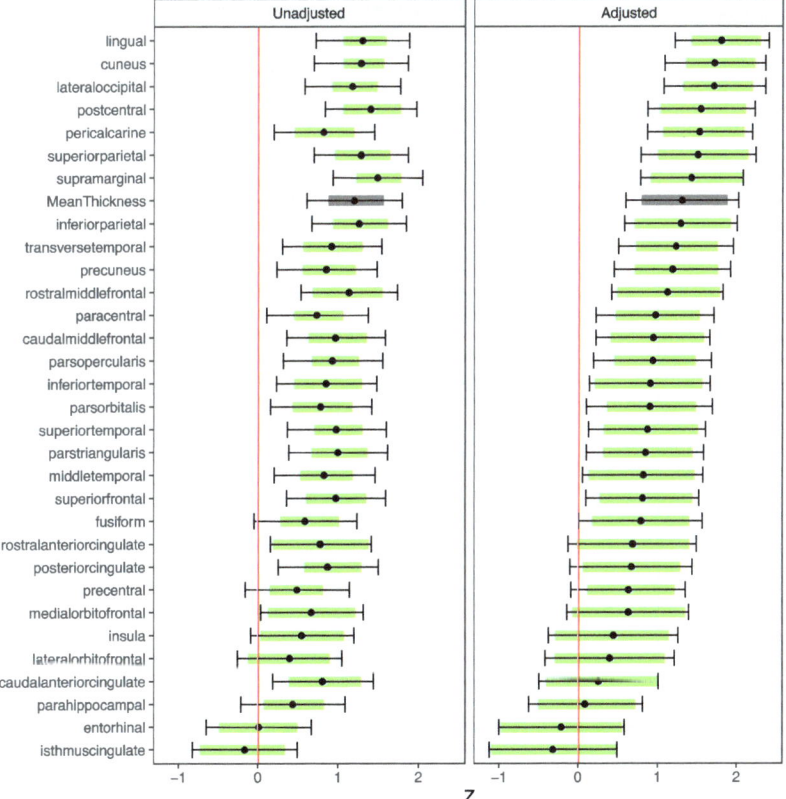

Figure 2. Differences in regional cortical thickness between the Skogholt subjects and controls. Group differences in unadjusted standard scores (left pane) and standard scores adjusted for covariates (right pane) of thicknesses of cortical segments on MRI. Dots show estimated differences in standard scores between Skogholt patients and MRI controls. Error bars indicate the 95% CIs, and shaded areas represent the 2.5–97.5 percentile ranges of the bootstrap distributions of the estimated differences from 20,000 resampled datapoints. The standard scores were adjusted for intracranial volume, age, sex, and MRI magnetic field strength using linear regression. Green indicates a particular cortical area, while gray indicates the cortex in general.

Table 5. MRI cerebral atrophy scores.

Score	GCA	MTA	Koedam
0	6 (55%)	6 (55%)	5 (45%)
1	3 (27%)	5 (45%)	5 (45%)
2	2 (18%)	0 (0%)	1 (9.1%)

Atrophy scores from cerebral MRI of eleven cases with Skogholt's disease. Statistics presented as n (%). GCA = Global Cortical Atrophy, MTA = Medial Temporal lobe Atrophy, Koedam = Posterior atrophy.

An algorithmic evaluation of the MRI scans showed generally increased cortical thickness in the Skogholt group, even when adjusting for age, gender, magnetic field strength, and ICV (Figure 3). The cortical thickening was most prominent in the lingual, cuneus, and lateral occipital regions.

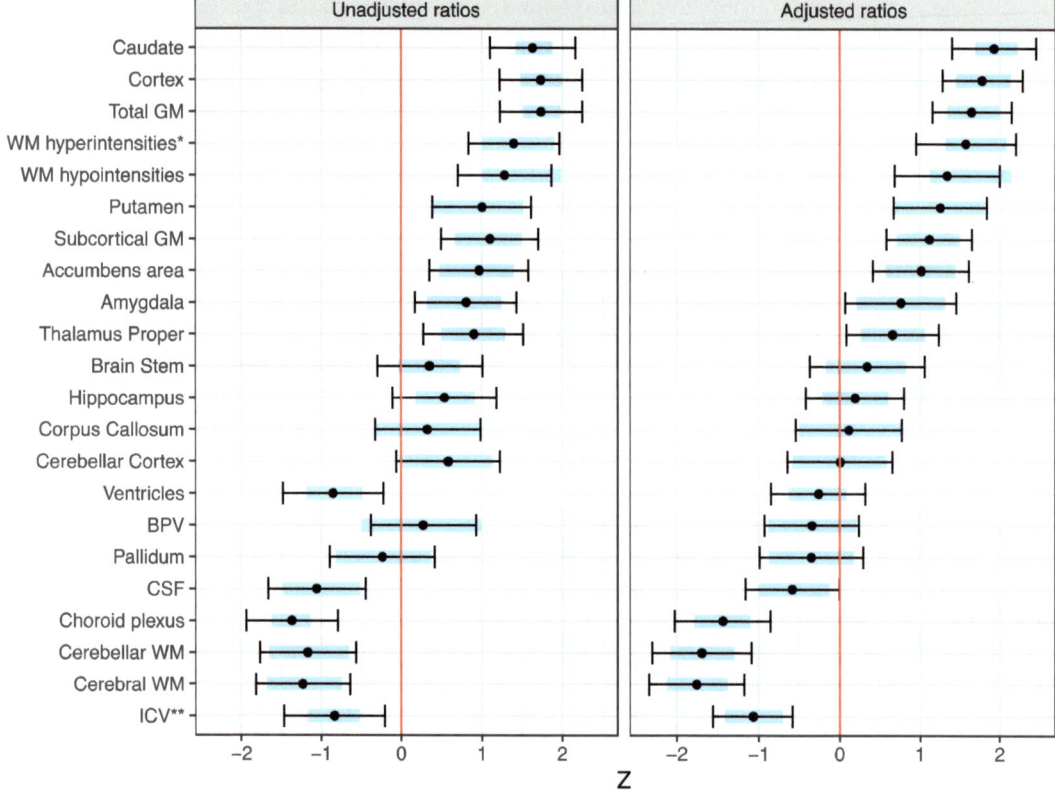

Figure 3. Differences in brain structure volumes between the Skogholt subjects and controls. Group differences in unadjusted standardized ratios (left pane) and standardized ratios adjusted for covariates (right pane) of brain segments to intracranial volume (ICV), based on MRI segmentation data from 3D T1 sequences. GM = gray matter, WM = white matter, WMH* = WM hyperintensities on 3D FLAIR sequence. Dots show standard scores for the differences between Skogholt patients and MRI controls. Error bars indicate the 95% CIs, and shaded areas represent the 2.5th to 97.5th percentile ranges of the bootstrap distributions of the estimated differences from 20,000 resampled datapoints. The differences in standardized ratios were adjusted for age, sex, and MRI magnetic field strength using a linear regression with standardization of continuous variables. ICV** = ICV with linear model using standardized ICV value rather than standardized ICV/ICV ratio.

Relative to the ICV (and adjusted for age, gender, and magnetic field strength) and compared to healthy controls from the DDI project, the Skogholt cases had reduced total white matter, CSF, and choroid plexus volumes and increased white matter changes (Figure 3). The volumes of cortical and subcortical gray matter were modestly increased in the Skogholt group.

Summary statistics of the raw data from MRI parcellation are provided in Supplementary Tables S2 and S3.

4. Discussion

Increased CSF total protein concentrations, extensive white matter hyperintensities, and pathological CSF biomarkers of neurodegeneration are established characteristics of Skogholt's disease [2–4].

The present work adds to the literature on Skogholt's disease with an expanded set of CSF and plasma biomarkers and with MRI morphometry. MRI data revealed strikingly decreased white matter volumes, decreased choroid plexus volumes, increased gray matter volumes, and increased cortical thickness compared to the control group. The extended biomarker panel confirmed previous findings of increased CSF T-tau and P-tau [3] and revealed increased CSF levels of several other biomarkers. In contrast, we did not find increased levels of the same markers in plasma. Such exceptionally high levels of CSF biomarkers cannot be explained by any differences in lifestyle risk factors (Table 1).

Although the previously reported low levels of CSF $A\beta_{42}$ in Skogholt's disease [3] appear to be inconsistent with the higher levels found in the current analysis, this discrepancy may be explained by the even higher levels of $A\beta_{x-40}$ and $A\beta_{x-38}$ found in Skogholt CSF in this study. The ELISA technique (Innotest kit) previously used to measure the $A\beta_{42}$ concentration [3] is susceptible to interference from $A\beta_{40}$ or $A\beta_{38}$ [24]. The current analysis included two different assays for the quantification of Aβ species: a Lumipulse instrument for $A\beta_{1-40}$ and $A\beta_{1-42}$ and a triplex method for $A\beta_{x-38}$, $A\beta_{x-40}$, and $A\beta_{x-42}$.

The CSF beta-trace protein (βTP) was increased almost seven-fold, substantially more than what can be accounted for by the, on average, 3.5-fold increase in CSF total protein previously reported [3]. Increased βTP concentrations stand in contrast to the low mean choroid plexus volume, as the "brain" isoform of βTP mostly originates in choroid epithelial cells [25]. However, the possibly deficient CSF production seems to primarily affect the watery phase of the liquor. Nevertheless, the speciation of the βTP isoforms in CSF and plasma in comparison to other groups may be of interest in future studies. It is notable that other CSF markers were also increased (Table 2 and Figure S1).

High CSF protein concentrations have previously been reported in conditions with slow CSF turnover [26,27]. It is possible that many of the observed protein changes in Skogholt CSF may be explained by perturbed CSF dynamics, reflecting impaired CSF production. An impaired blood–cerebrospinal fluid barrier with a failing dilution of CSF constituents would also increase the concentration of CNS-derived proteins. An intriguing observation was that the CSF levels of the brain biomarkers were markedly increased, from 2–3-fold (for $A\beta_{38}$, $A\beta_{40}$, NfL, and GFAP) up to 8–10-fold (for t-tau and p-tau). The lack of brain atrophy on MRI indicates that these increases are not related to neurodegeneration. A possible explanation is deranged CSF production affecting the dilution and turnover of constituents, which would allow for a higher CSF concentration of brain proteins. Future research should specifically determine the CSF production and clearance rates in Skogholt's disease. With MRI, we find that the choroid plexus is smaller in Skogholt's disease compared to controls, a possible clue to the primary pathology of the condition. CSF protein concentrations are traditionally used as a surrogate marker for the blood–brain barrier (BBB) as well as blood–nerve barrier (BNB) integrity. In chronic inflammatory polyneuropathy, which appears to exist in some patients with Skogholt's disease [2], a disruption of these barriers is thought to cause the clinical symptoms, resulting in an elevation of the CSF protein level. Damage to the blood–CSF barrier causes altered CSF flow rates, modulating the CSF protein content [28]. BNB damage causes an influx of serum proteins into the CSF [29]. Based on present and previous observations, it is tempting to suggest that Skogholt's disease is precipitated by primary defects in the BBB and BNB. However, normal levels of tau species in plasma argue against the degeneration of the BBB with leakage (as seen in, e.g., cerebral small vessel disease), and alternative explanations related to the hampered production or release of CSF cannot be excluded.

The MRI findings in the Skogholt cases were unexpected. Compared to the controls, we report decreased white matter and increased gray matter volumes. Additionally, we report decreased choroid plexus and ventricle volumes. The decreased white matter volume may be explained by demyelination or degeneration secondary to the pathological composition of the CSF [30]. Previous studies have found that BBB disruption is linked with white matter degeneration [31,32], again strengthening the hypothesis that BBB dysfunction is a primary or central feature of Skogholt's disease.

Increased gray matter volumes may be explained by swelling or alternatively by compensatory mechanisms, e.g., an increased number of local interneuronal connections and dysmyelination. Dysmyelination and BBB integrity in Skogholt's disease are topics for future studies.

The scope of the current study is limited by its small numbers of cases and controls available for fluid marker comparison. The lab control group was diverse and was not sampled as early in the morning as was possible for the Skogholt group. The MRI control group was sufficiently large, but lab results were not available for comparison. Furthermore, the cases and the MRI controls were not examined using the same MRI scanner, introducing the possibility for biased scanner results. However, the morphometric differences were consistent for the different MRI systems, and we corrected for field strength. Additionally, if there were differences due to scanner effects, we would not expect to see the present pattern of group differences. Morphometry on 3T systems is known to report increased cortical thickness compared to 1.5 T systems [33], the opposite of what we found in the present publication.

5. Conclusions

The extraordinarily high CSF biomarker levels in Skogholt's disease are remarkable but must be considered together with the overall increase in CSF proteins, which are altogether more compatible with disturbed CSF dynamics than neurodegeneration. MRI findings of confluent white matter lesions are typical but not necessary to establish a diagnosis of Skogholt's disease. Our algorithmic processing of MRI data showed decreases in white matter and choroid plexus volumes accompanied by increases in cortical thickness and volume, as well as an increased volume of subcortical gray matter.

Future studies on Skogholt's disease will benefit from including more cases and avoiding systematic biases when the laboratory analysis and neuroimaging are not distributed over several locations.

Supplementary Materials: The following supporting information can be downloaded at https://www.mdpi.com/article/10.3390/brainsci13111511/s1, Table S1: MRI scanner system parameters and number of scans; Table S2: Cortical thickness; Table S3: Region of interest volumes; Figure S1: Violin plots with individual CSF biomarker datapoints.

Author Contributions: Conceptualization, K.T.A., T.H., K.B., H.Z., J.O.A. and P.S.; methodology, K.T.A. and P.S.; validation, K.T.A., J.O.A., B.-E.K. and P.S.; formal analysis, K.T.A.; investigation, K.T.A.; resources, K.T.A., K.B., H.Z., P.S. and T.F.; data curation, K.T.A.; writing—original draft preparation, K.T.A.; writing—review and editing, K.T.A., T.H., K.B., H.Z., J.O.A., T.F. and P.S.; visualization, K.T.A.; supervision, P.S. and J.O.A.; project administration, J.O.A.; funding acquisition, J.O.A. and T.F. All authors have read and agreed to the published version of the manuscript.

Funding: This research was funded by the Innlandet Hospital Trust, Norway. HZ is a Wallenberg Scholar supported by grants from the Swedish Research Council (#2022-01018); the European Union's Horizon Europe research and innovation programme under grant agreement No. 101053962; Swedish State Support for Clinical Research (#ALFGBG-71320), the Alzheimer Drug Discovery Foundation (ADDF), USA (#201809-2016862); the AD Strategic Fund and the Alzheimer's Association (#ADSF-

21-831376-C, #ADSF-21-831381-C, and #ADSF-21-831377-C); the Bluefield Project; the Olav Thon Foundation; the Erling-Persson Family Foundation; Stiftelsen för Gamla Tjänarinnor, Hjärnfonden, Sweden (#FO2022-0270); the European Union's Horizon 2020 research and innovation programme under Marie Skłodowska-Curie grant agreement No. 860197 (MIRIADE); the European Union Joint Programme—Neurodegenerative Disease Research (JPND2021-00694), and the UK Dementia Research Institute at UCL (UKDRI-1003). The sponsors had no role in the design of the study; in the collection, analyses, or interpretation of the data; in the writing of the manuscript; or in the decision to publish the results. BEK was supported by a grant from Helse-Nord (HNF1540-20). The DDI project was funded by the Norwegian Research Council and JPND/PMI-AD (NRC 311993).

Institutional Review Board Statement: The study protocol was approved by the Regional Committee for Medical and Health Research Ethics, South-East Region, Norway, Ref. No. 556-04224 and No. 2013/1017. The study was conducted in accordance with the Declaration of Helsinki.

Informed Consent Statement: Written informed consent was obtained from all patients before enrollment.

Data Availability Statement: The data presented in this study are available on request from the corresponding author. The data are not publicly available due to restrictions in consent.

Acknowledgments: We thank bioengineer Vigdis Kalkvik in the Department of Medical Biochemistry, Innlandet Hospital Trust, Lillehammer, for technical assistance. We thank radiologists Torunn Gabrielsen and Eivind Alhaug in the Department of Diagnostic Imaging, Innlandet Hospital Trust, Lillehammer, for setting up the project's MRI protocol and scoring the MRI findings. We thank occupational therapist Ole Fredrik Korsnes for contributing to the cognitive screening protocol.

Conflicts of Interest: Trygve Holmøy has received speaker's honoraria from Roche, Novartis, Biogen, Merck, and Sanofi. Kaj Blennow has served as a consultant or on advisory boards for Abcam, Axon, BioArctic, Biogen, JOMDD/Shimadzu, Julius Clinical, Lilly, MagQu, Novartis, Ono Pharma, Pharmatrophix, Prothena, Roche Diagnostics, and Siemens Healthineers. Henrik Zetterberg has served on scientific advisory boards and/or as a consultant for Abbvie, Acumen, Alector, Alzinova, ALZPath, Annexon, Apellis, Artery Therapeutics, AZTherapies, CogRx, Denali, Eisai, Nervgen, Novo Nordisk, Optoceutics, Passage Bio, Pinteon Therapeutics, Prothena, Red Abbey Labs, reMYND, Roche, Samumed, Siemens Healthineers, Triplet Therapeutics, and Wave and has given lectures at symposia sponsored by Cellectricon, Fujirebio, Alzecure, Biogen, and Roche. Kaj Blennow and Henrik Zetterberg are co-founders of Brain Biomarker Solutions in Gothenburg AB (BBS), which is a part of the GU Ventures Incubator Program (outside the submitted work). Bjørn-Eivind Kirsebom has served as a consultant for Biogen. Per Selnes has served as a consultant for Roche. Tormod Fladby reports receiving consulting fees from Biogen and Novo Nordisk; having several planned, issued, and pending patents regarding innate immune amyloid beta clearance and the regulation of inflammation; and participating on the Data Safety Monitoring Board or Advisory Board of Biogen, Novo, and Nordisk and is the leader of the board of Nansen Neuroscience (unpaid).

References

1. Aspli, K.T.; Flaten, T.P.; Roos, P.M.; Holmøy, T.; Skogholt, J.H.; Aaseth, J. Iron and copper in progressive demyelination—New lessons from Skogholt's disease. *J. Trace Elem. Med. Biol.* **2015**, *31*, 183–187. [CrossRef] [PubMed]
2. Hagen, K.; Boman, H.; Mellgren, S.I.; Lindal, S.; Bovim, G. Progressive central and peripheral demyelinating disease of adult onset in a Norwegian family. *Arch. Neurol.* **1998**, *55*, 1467–1472. [CrossRef] [PubMed]
3. Aspli, K.T.; Holmøy, T.; Flaten, T.P.; Whist, J.E.; Aaseth, J.O. Skogholt's disease—A tauopathy precipitated by iron and copper? *J. Trace Elem. Med. Biol.* **2022**, *70*, 126915. [CrossRef] [PubMed]
4. Gellein, K.; Skogholt, J.H.; Aaseth, J.; Thoresen, G.B.; Lierhagen, S.; Steinnes, E.; Syversen, T.; Flaten, T.P. Trace elements in cerebrospinal fluid and blood from patients with a rare progressive central and peripheral demyelinating disease. *J. Neurol. Sci.* **2008**, *266*, 70–78. [CrossRef]
5. Fladby, T.; Pålhaugen, L.; Selnes, P.; Waterloo, K.; Bråthen, G.; Hessen, E.; Almdahl, I.S.; Arntzen, K.A.; Auning, E.; Eliassen, C.F.; et al. Detecting At-Risk Alzheimer's Disease Cases. *J. Alzheimers Dis.* **2017**, *60*, 97–105. [CrossRef]
6. Gobom, J.; Parnetti, L.; Rosa-Neto, P.; Vyhnalek, M.; Gauthier, S.; Cataldi, S.; Lerch, O.; Laczo, J.; Cechova, K.; Clarin, M.; et al. Validation of the LUMIPULSE automated immunoassay for the measurement of core AD biomarkers in cerebrospinal fluid. *Clin. Chem. Lab. Med.* **2022**, *60*, 207–219. [CrossRef]
7. Gaetani, L.; Höglund, K.; Parnetti, L.; Pujol-Calderon, F.; Becker, B.; Eusebi, P.; Sarchielli, P.; Calabresi, P.; Di Filippo, M.; Zetterberg, H.; et al. A new enzyme-linked immunosorbent assay for neurofilament light in cerebrospinal fluid: Analytical validation and clinical evaluation. *Alzheimer's Res. Ther.* **2018**, *10*, 8. [CrossRef]

8. Rosengren, L.E.; Ahlsén, G.; Belfrage, M.; Gillberg, C.; Haglid, K.G.; Hamberger, A. A sensitive ELISA for glial fibrillary acidic protein: Application in CSF of children. *J. Neurosci. Methods* **1992**, *44*, 113–119. [CrossRef]
9. Zetterberg, H. Glial fibrillary acidic protein: A blood biomarker to differentiate neurodegenerative from psychiatric diseases. *J. Neurol. Neurosurg. Psychiatry* **2021**, *92*, 1253. [CrossRef]
10. Henschel, L.; Conjeti, S.; Estrada, S.; Diers, K.; Fischl, B.; Reuter, M. FastSurfer—A fast and accurate deep learning based neuroimaging pipeline. *Neuroimage* **2020**, *219*, 117012. [CrossRef]
11. Henschel, L.; Kügler, D.; Reuter, M. FastSurferVINN: Building resolution-independence into deep learning segmentation methods—A solution for HighRes brain MRI. *Neuroimage* **2022**, *251*, 118933. [CrossRef] [PubMed]
12. Fischl, B.; van der Kouwe, A.; Destrieux, C.; Halgren, E.; Ségonne, F.; Salat, D.H.; Busa, E.; Seidman, L.J.; Goldstein, J.; Kennedy, D.; et al. Automatically parcellating the human cerebral cortex. *Cereb. Cortex* **2004**, *14*, 11–22. [CrossRef] [PubMed]
13. Fischl, B.; Dale, A.M. Measuring the thickness of the human cerebral cortex from magnetic resonance images. *Proc. Natl. Acad. Sci. USA* **2000**, *97*, 11050–11055. [CrossRef] [PubMed]
14. Desikan, R.S.; Ségonne, F.; Fischl, B.; Quinn, B.T.; Dickerson, B.C.; Blacker, D.; Buckner, R.L.; Dale, A.M.; Maguire, R.P.; Hyman, B.T.; et al. An automated labeling system for subdividing the human cerebral cortex on MRI scans into gyral based regions of interest. *Neuroimage* **2006**, *31*, 968–980. [CrossRef]
15. Wardlaw, J.M.; Smith, E.E.; Biessels, G.J.; Cordonnier, C.; Fazekas, F.; Frayne, R.; Lindley, R.I.; O'Brien, J.T.; Barkhof, F.; Benavente, O.R.; et al. Neuroimaging standards for research into small vessel disease and its contribution to ageing and neurodegeneration. *Lancet Neurol.* **2013**, *12*, 822–838. [CrossRef]
16. Røvang, M.S.; Selnes, P.; MacIntosh, B.J.; Rasmus Groote, I.; Pålhaugen, L.; Sudre, C.; Fladby, T.; Bjørnerud, A. Segmenting white matter hyperintensities on isotropic three-dimensional Fluid Attenuated Inversion Recovery magnetic resonance images: Assessing deep learning tools on a Norwegian imaging database. *PLoS ONE* **2023**, *18*, e0285683. [CrossRef]
17. R Core Team. *R: A Language and Environment for Statistical Computing*; R Foundation for Statistical Computing: Vienna, Austria, 2022.
18. Gohel, D.; Panagiotis, S. *ggiraph: Make 'ggplot2' Graphics Interactive, R Package Version 0.8.7*; R Foundation for Statistical Computing: Vienna, Austria, 2023.
19. Wickham, H.; François, R.; Henry, L.; Müller, K.; Vaughan, D. *dplyr: A Grammar of Data Manipulation, R Package Version 1.0.7*; R Foundation for Statistical Computing: Vienna, Austria, 2021.
20. Sjoberg, D.D.; Whiting, K.; Curry, M.; Lavery, J.A.; Larmarange, J. Reproducible Summary Tables with the gtsummary Package. *R J.* **2021**, *13*, 570–580. [CrossRef]
21. Wickham, H. *ggplot2: Elegant Graphics for Data Analysis*; Springer: New York, NY, USA, 2016.
22. Wickham, H.; Averick, M.; Bryan, J.; Chang, W.; McGowan, L.D.A.; François, R.; Grolemund, G.; Hayes, A.; Henry, L.; Hester, J. Welcome to the Tidyverse. *J. Open Source Softw.* **2019**, *4*, 1686. [CrossRef]
23. Fazekas, F.; Chawluk, J.B.; Alavi, A.; Hurtig, H.I.; Zimmerman, R.A. MR signal abnormalities at 1.5 T in Alzheimer's dementia and normal aging. *AJR Am. J. Roentgenol.* **1987**, *149*, 351–356. [CrossRef]
24. Keshavan, A.; Wellington, H.; Chen, Z.; Khatun, A.; Chapman, M.; Hart, M.; Cash, D.M.; Coath, W.; Parker, T.D.; Buchanan, S.M.; et al. Concordance of CSF measures of Alzheimer's pathology with amyloid PET status in a preclinical cohort: A comparison of Lumipulse and established immunoassays. *Alzheimers Dement.* **2021**, *13*, e12131. [CrossRef]
25. Lafer, I.; Michaelis, S.; Schneider, C.; Baranyi, A.; Schnedl, W.J.; Holasek, S.; Zelzer, S.; Niedrist, T.; Meinitzer, A.; Enko, D. Beta-trace protein concentrations at the blood-cerebrospinal fluid barrier—Acute phase affects protein status. *Excli. J.* **2021**, *20*, 1446–1452. [CrossRef] [PubMed]
26. Reiber, H. Blood-cerebrospinal fluid (CSF) barrier dysfunction means reduced CSF flow not barrier leakage—Conclusions from CSF protein data. *Arq. Neuropsiquiatr.* **2021**, *79*, 56–67. [CrossRef] [PubMed]
27. Schaefer, J.H.; Yalachkov, Y.; Friedauer, L.; Kirchmayr, K.; Miesbach, W.; Wenger, K.J.; Foerch, C.; Schaller-Paule, M.A. Measurement of prothrombin fragment 1 + 2 in cerebrospinal fluid to identify thrombin generation in inflammatory central nervous system diseases. *Mult. Scler. Relat. Disord.* **2022**, *60*, 103720. [CrossRef]
28. Reiber, H. Dynamics of brain-derived proteins in cerebrospinal fluid. *Clin. Chim. Acta* **2001**, *310*, 173–186. [CrossRef] [PubMed]
29. Brettschneider, J.; Petzold, A.; Süssmuth, S.; Tumani, H. Cerebrospinal fluid biomarkers in Guillain-Barré syndrome—Where do we stand? *J. Neurol.* **2009**, *256*, 3–12. [CrossRef]
30. Jhelum, P.; David, S. Ferroptosis: Copper-iron connection in cuprizone-induced demyelination. *Neural. Regen. Res.* **2022**, *17*, 89–90. [CrossRef]
31. Kerkhofs, D.; Wong, S.M.; Zhang, E.; Staals, J.; Jansen, J.F.A.; van Oostenbrugge, R.J.; Backes, W.H. Baseline Blood-Brain Barrier Leakage and Longitudinal Microstructural Tissue Damage in the Periphery of White Matter Hyperintensities. *Neurology* **2021**, *96*, e2192–e2200. [CrossRef]

32. Zhang, C.E.; Wong, S.M.; Uiterwijk, R.; Backes, W.H.; Jansen, J.F.A.; Jeukens, C.; van Oostenbrugge, R.J.; Staals, J. Blood-brain barrier leakage in relation to white matter hyperintensity volume and cognition in small vessel disease and normal aging. *Brain Imaging Behav.* **2019**, *13*, 389–395. [CrossRef]
33. Buchanan, C.R.; Muñoz Maniega, S.; Valdés Hernández, M.C.; Ballerini, L.; Barclay, G.; Taylor, A.M.; Russ, T.C.; Tucker-Drob, E.M.; Wardlaw, J.M.; Deary, I.J.; et al. Comparison of structural MRI brain measures between 1.5 and 3 T: Data from the Lothian Birth Cohort 1936. *Hum. Brain Mapp.* **2021**, *42*, 3905–3921. [CrossRef]

Disclaimer/Publisher's Note: The statements, opinions and data contained in all publications are solely those of the individual author(s) and contributor(s) and not of MDPI and/or the editor(s). MDPI and/or the editor(s) disclaim responsibility for any injury to people or property resulting from any ideas, methods, instructions or products referred to in the content.